W9-ARD-529

NEUROLOGY
SECRETS

NEUROLOGY SECRETS

Loren A. Rolak, M.D.
Associate Professor of Clinical Neurology
Department of Neurology
Baylor College of Medicine
Assistant Chief of Neurology
Houston Veterans Affairs Medical Center
Houston, Texas

HANLEY & BELFUS, INC./ Philadelphia

Publisher: HANLEY & BELFUS, INC.
                210 S. 13th Street
                Philadelphia, PA 19107
                (215) 546-7293
                FAX (215) 790-9330

NEUROLOGY SECRETS   ISBN 1-56053-056-1

© 1993 by Hanley & Belfus, Inc. All rights reserved. No part of this book may be reproduced, reused, republished, or transmitted in any form or by any means without written permission of the publisher.

Library of Congress catalog card number   93-77759

Last digit is the print number: 9 8 7 6 5 4

DEDICATION

For Roxann, Kelley, and Stacey

CONTENTS

CONTRIBUTORS

Richard M. Armstrong, M.D., FRCP(C)
Associate Professor, Department of Neurology, Baylor College of Medicine, Houston, Texas

Tetsuo Ashizawa, M.D.
Associate Professor, Department of Neurology, Baylor College of Medicine, Houston, Texas

Sudhir S. Athni, M.D.
Resident, Department of Neurology, Baylor College of Medicine, Houston, Texas

Francisco Cardoso, M.D.
Assistant Professor, Departments of Morphology and Neurology, Federal University of Minas Gerais, Belo Horizonte, Minas Gerais, Brazil

Igor Cherches, M.D.
Resident, Department of Neurology, Baylor College of Medicine, Houston, Texas

Howard S. Derman, M.D.
Assistant Professor, Department of Neurology, Baylor College of Medicine, Houston, Texas

Rachelle S. Doody, M.D., Ph.D.
Assistant Professor, Department of Neurology, Baylor College of Medicine, Houston, Texas

Everton A. Edmondson, M.D.
Private practitioner, Houston, Texas

James D. Frost, Jr., M.D.
Professor, Department of Neurology, Baylor College of Medicine, Houston, Texas

E. Patricia Gill, M.D.
Fellow in Infectious Diseases, Department of Internal Medicine, Baylor College of Medicine, Houston, Texas

Yadollah Harati, M.D., FACP
Associate Professor, Department of Neurology, Baylor College of Medicine, Houston; Director, Muscle and Nerve Pathology Laboratory, and Chief, Neurology Service, Houston Veterans Affairs Medical Center, Houston, Texas

Richard L. Harris, M.D.
Associate Professor of Clinical Medicine, Department of Internal Medicine, Section of Infectious Diseases, Baylor College of Medicine, Houston, Texas

Richard A. Hrachovy, M.D.
Associate Professor, Department of Neurology, Baylor College of Medicine, Houston, Texas

Steven B. Inbody, M.D.
Assistant Professor, Department of Neurology, Baylor College of Medicine, Houston, Texas

Joseph Jankovic, M.D.
Professor, Department of Neurology, and Director, Parkinson's Disease Center and
Movement Disorders Clinic, Baylor College of Medicine, Houston, Texas

James M. Killian, M.D.
Professor and Vice Chairman, Department of Neurology, Baylor College of Medicine,
Houston, Texas

Eugene C. Lai, M.D., Ph.D.
Assistant Professor, Department of Neurology, Baylor College of Medicine, Houston,
Texas

Brian Loftus, M.D.
Resident, Department of Neurology, Baylor College of Medicine, Houston, Texas

Loren A. Rolak, M.D.
Associate Professor of Clinical Neurology, Department of Neurology, Baylor College of
Medicine, Houston Veterans Affairs Medical Center, Houston, Texas

Davis B. Rosenfield, M.D.
Professor, Department of Neurology, Baylor College of Medicine, Houston, Texas

Paul A. Rutecki, M.D.
Associate Professor, Department of Neurology, and Director, Francis Forster Epilepsy
Center, University of Wisconsin Medical School, Madison, Wisconsin

R. Glenn Smith, M.D., Ph.D.
Assistant Professor, Department of Neurology, Baylor College of Medicine, Houston,
Texas

Angus A. Wilfong, M.D.
Assistant Professor, Department of Pediatrics, University of Saskatchewan College of
Medicine, Saskatoon, Saskatchewan, Canada

John P. Winikates, M.D.
Instructor, Department of Neurology, Baylor College of Medicine, Houston, Texas

FOREWORD

The excitement of Neurology is related not only to new information developing from the tremendous advances in basic neurosciences, but also to the elegance of the nervous system itself and to the increasingly sophisticated methods that we use to learn how it functions and how it can be disturbed in disease. There are a large number of textbooks in the field, as well as a large number of computerized learning systems in medicine. But none of them has yet replaced the effectiveness of the Socratic approach to education, both in an academic and in a clinical setting. In Neurology, as well as in other areas of medicine, one of the most difficult tasks is knowing how to ask the right questions. For the medical student just starting out, pertinent questions relate to where the lesion may be and to the tempo of the process, which may suggest the etiology. For the house officer, the questions may relate more to the patterns of symptoms and signs characteristic of certain diseases, whereas for the practitioner the prognosis of untreated disease and the efficacy of various therapies may be the focus of inquiry. For all individuals concerned with problem solving in neurologic disease, asking the right question the right way is of greatest importance.

In the present volume, Dr. Loren Rolak and other members of the Department of Neurology at Baylor College of Medicine have employed the question and answer approach, which is the hallmark of The Secrets Series®. The book is intended to cover the kinds of questions commonly encountered in an academic institution on teaching rounds for medical students and residents, and also in clinical problem solving in the office. *Neurology Secrets* is not intended to be an in-depth approach to disease etiology and pathogenesis. Instead, it is intended to phrase questions in a way that provides "the big picture." From that point on, the student—and all of us continue to be students for our entire careers—must use original source material as well as the patients themselves to continue the educational process.

The authors have been extremely successful in accomplishing their goals, and all of us will benefit. No field will change more than the field of Neurology in the future, and *Neurology Secrets* lets you in on the ground floor of what promises to be one of the most exciting voyages ever taken by man—one that results in an understanding of our humanity through an understanding of the brain.

Stanley H. Appel, M.D.
Professor and Chairman
Department of Neurology
Baylor College of Medicine
Houston, Texas

1. CLINICAL NEUROANATOMY

Sudhir S. Athni, M.D., Igor Cherches, M.D., and Brian Loftus, M.D.

EMBRYOLOGY

1. How is the neural tube formed?

Beginning around the 18th gestational day, a midline notochordal thickening anterior to the blastopore forms the neural plate. A midsagittal groove appears in the plate—the neural groove—and the sides elevate to form the neural folds. As the folds fuse, the neural tube is formed. Some cells at the edges of the fold do not fuse into the tube, and become neural crest cells.

2. What types of cells are derived from the neural crest cells?

Neural crest cells give rise to (1) unipolar sensory cells, (2) postganglionic cells of sympathetic and parasympathetic ganglia, (3) chromaffin cells of the adrenal medulla, (4) some microglial cells, (5) pia mater, (6) some arachnoid cells, (7) melanocytes, and (8) Schwann cells.

3. What are the alar plate and the basal plate?

As the neural tube is formed, a longitudinal groove appears on each side and divides the neural tube into a dorsal half, or alar plate, and a ventral half, or basal plate. The **alar plate** gives rise to the prosencephalon, the sensory and coordinating nuclei of the thalamus, the sensory neurons of the cranial nerves, the coordinating nuclei including cerebellum, inferior olives, red nucleus, and quadrigeminal plate, and the posterior horn area (sensory) of the spinal cord. The **basal plate** stops at the level of the diencephalon and gives rise to the motor neurons of the cranial nerves and anterior horn (motor) area of the spinal cord.

4. What is the process of formation of the ventricles, prosencephalon, mesencephalon, and rhombencephalon?

Around the end of the first gestational month, a series of bulges anterior to the first cervical somites appears. The first bulge is the prosencephalon, or forebrain. The cavity of this bulge will form the lateral ventricles and third ventricle. Secondary outpouchings from the forebrain are called optic vesicles, and these eventually form the retina, pigment epithelium, and optic nerve. The second bulge is the mesencephalon, or midbrain. The cavity of this bulge will form the cerebral aqueduct. The third bulge is the rhombencephalon, or hindbrain. This cavity gives rise to the fourth ventricle.

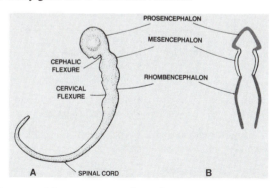

Development of the nervous system in the fourth week (A and B) of gestation.

1

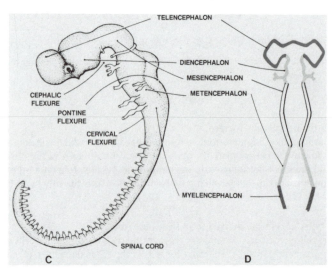

Development of the nervous system in the sixth week (C and D) of gestation. (Reprinted with permission from Gilman S, Newman SW: Manter and Gatz's Essentials of Clinical Neuroanatomy and Neurophysiology, 8th ed. Philadelphia, F.A. Davis, 1992.)

5. Which structures arise from the prosencephalon?

The prosencephalon develops into the telencephalon, which includes the cerebral cortex and basal ganglia, and the diencephalon, which includes the thalamus and the hypothalamus.

6. Which structures arise from the mesencephalon?

The mesencephalon gives rise to the midbrain.

7. Which structures arise from the rhombencephalon?

The rhombencephalon gives rise to the metencephalon (pons + cerebellum) and myelencephalon (medulla).

Embryonic Divisions of the Central Nevous System

EMBRYONIC DIVISIONS		ADULT DERIVATIVES	VENTRICULAR CAVITIES
Forebrain (prosencephalon)	Telencephalon	Cerebral cortex Basal ganglia	Lateral ventricles
	Diencephalon	Thalamus Hypothalamus Subthalamus Epithalamus	Third ventricle
Midbrain (mesencephalon)	—	Tectum Cerebral peduncles	Aqueduct
Hindbrain (rhombencephalon)	Metencephalon	Cerebellum Pons	Fourth ventricle
	Myelencephalon	Medulla	
Spinal cord	—	Spinal cord	No cavity

MUSCLE

8. What is the histologic organization of skeletal muscle?
Skeletal muscle is composed of long, thin, cylindrical, multinucleated cells called muscle fibers (or myofibrils). Each fiber has a motor endplate at its neuromuscular junction. Each fiber is surrounded by connective tissue called endomysium. Groups of fibers, or a fascicle, are surrounded by a connective tissue layer called the perimysium. Fascicles are grouped together and surrounded by epimysium.

9. What is found at the A band, H band, I band, and Z line?
The **A band** contains the thin filaments (actin) and the thick filaments (myosin). The **H band** is the portion of the A band that contains only myosin, and the **I band** is the portion that contains only actin. The **Z line** is where the actin is anchored.

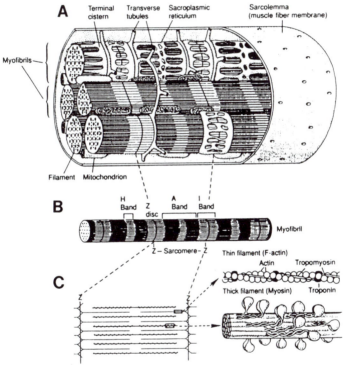

The histologic anatomy of the human skeletal muscle. (Reprinted with permission from Kandel E, Schwartz JH, Jessell TM (eds): Principles of Neuroscience, 3rd ed. New York, Elsevier, 1991, p 549.)

10. How does the muscle contract?
When the sarcoplasmic reticulum is depolarized, calcium ions enter the cell and bind to troponin. This causes a conformational change that allows the actin binding site to be exposed to myosin. The myosin attaches to the actin binding site and flexes, causing the actin filament to slide by the myosin filament. Adenosine triphosphate (ATP) is required to allow the myosin-actin crossbridge to release and the muscle to relax.

11. What is meant by the term "motor unit"?
The motor unit is one motor nerve (lower motor neuron) and all muscle fibers that it innervates.

The Muscle Stretch Reflex

12. What type of nerve fiber innervates the muscle?
An anterior horn motor neuron, called an alpha motor neuron, innervates the muscle. It is the final common pathway for muscle contraction.

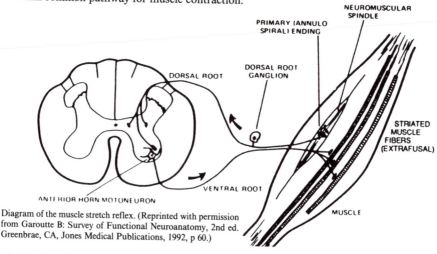

Diagram of the muscle stretch reflex. (Reprinted with permission from Garoutte B: Survey of Functional Neuroanatomy, 2nd ed. Greenbrae, CA, Jones Medical Publications, 1992, p 60.)

13. What are Renshaw cells?
Renshaw cells are interneurons that are stimulated by the alpha motor neuron and then, by feedback to inhibit the alpha motor neuron, cause autoinhibition.

14. In the spinal cord, which nerve fibers synapse on the alpha motor neuron?
Both the corticospinal tract and afferent Ia sensory nerves regulate the alpha motor neuron by synapsing on it in the anterior horn of the spinal cord.

15. What is the function of the Ia nerve fiber?
When the muscle spindle is stretched, the Ia sensory nerve, via the dorsal root, monosynaptically stimulates the alpha motor neuron, which fires and contracts (shortens) the muscle. In this way, the muscle stretch reflex maintains the tone and tension in the muscle.

16. Is the Ia reflex monosynaptic or polysynaptic?
It is monosynaptic but does initiate polysynaptic inhibition of the antagonist muscle group.

17. What is the role of the gamma efferent nerve?
The gamma efferent nerve fibers keep the muscle spindles "tight" by innervating and contracting the intrafusal fibers in the muscle spindle. This ensures that the spindle remains sensitive to any stretch.

18. Where does the Ib fiber originate?
The Ib originates from the Golgi tendon organ, another structure that monitors muscle stretch and acts to inhibit muscle contraction.

19. Where does the Ib neuron synapse?
At the spinal cord level, the Ib sensory nerve polysynaptically inhibits the alpha motor neuron to prevent muscle contraction and stimulates the gamma efferent fiber to reset the muscle tone.

20. Is the Ib reflex monosynaptic or polysynaptic?
The Ib reflex is polysynaptic.

LUMBOSACRAL PLEXUS AND LEG INNERVATION

21. Which roots make up the lumbar plexus?
Roots of L1,2,3,4 and sometimes T12 make up the lumbar plexus.

22. What are the two largest branches of the lumbar plexus?
    1. **Obturator nerve (L2,3,4).** It leaves the pelvis through the obturator foramen and supplies the adductors of the thigh.
    2. **Femoral nerve (L2,3,4).** It exits the pelvis with the femoral artery and supplies the hip flexors and knee extensors. Distally it continues as the saphenous nerve to supply the medial anterior knee and medial distal leg, including the medial malleolus.

23. What are the other branches of the lumbar plexus?
    1. **Iliohypogastric nerve (L1)**—to skin over hypogastric and gluteal areas; to abdominal muscles
    2. **Ilioinguinal nerve (L1)**—to skin over groin and scrotum (labia)
    3. **Genitofemoral nerve (L1,2)**—enters the internal inguinal ring and runs in the inguinal canal
    4. **Lateral femoral cutaneous nerve (L2,3)**—to skin over anterior and lateral parts of the thigh

24. Which nerve is at risk during appendectomy (McBurney's incision)?
The iliohypogastric nerve may be cut as it passes between the external and internal oblique muscles. This results in weakness in the area of inguinal canal, putting the patient at risk for direct inguinal hernia.

25. What is meralgia paraesthetica?
Meralgia paraesthetica is numbness and tingling in the lateral thigh secondary to compression of the lateral femoral cutaneous nerve as it runs over the inguinal ligament. It commonly occurs in obese persons.

26. Which nerve supplies the gluteus maximus?
The inferior gluteal nerve (L5, S1,2) supplies the gluteus maximus muscle.

27. What is the largest nerve in the body?
The sciatic nerve (L4,5, S1,2,3), the largest in the body, is composed of the common peroneal nerve (L4,5, S1,2) in its dorsal division, and the tibial nerve (L4,5 S1,2,3) in its ventral division.

28. What is the only nerve in the sacral plexus that emerges through the greater sciatic foramen, superior to the piriformis muscle?
The superior gluteal nerve (L4,5 and S1) supplies the gluteus medius and minimus and tensor fascia lata (abduction and medial rotation of the thigh).

29. Which nerve supplies the inferior buttock and posterior thigh?
The posterior femoral cutaneous nerve (S1,2,3), which runs with the inferior gluteal nerve, supplies the inferior buttock and posterior thigh.

30. Which nerve supplies the structures in the perineum?
The pudendal nerve (S2,3,4) supplies the perineum.

31. What is the only muscle supplied by the sciatic nerve that receives innervation exclusively from the ventral division?
The biceps femoris has only ventral innervation. This is important clinically when trying to differentiate lesions caused by damage to the common peroneal nerve vs. the sciatic nerve itself.

32. Which muscles are supplied by the tibial nerve?
The tibial nerve supplies plantar flexors and invertors of the foot.

33. What are the two divisions of the common peroneal nerve?
   1. **Deep peroneal nerve**—dorsiflexion of the foot and toes, and sensation to a small area of skin between the first and second toes.
   2. **Superficial peroneal nerve**—evertors of the foot and sensation to the skin of the dorsal and lateral foot.

BRACHIAL PLEXUS AND ARM INNERVATION

34. The brachial plexus comprises which roots?
The brachial plexus comprises the ventral rami of C5,6,7,8 and T1.

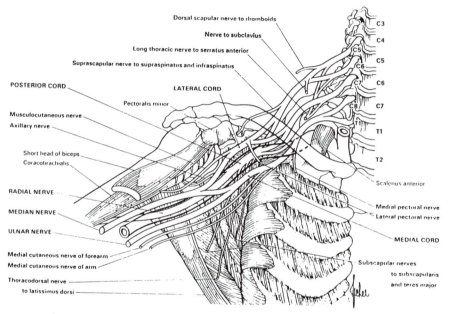

The brachial plexus. (Reprinted with permission from Tindall B: Aids to the Examination of the Peripheral Nervous System. London, W.B. Saunders, 1990.)

35. Which nerves arise from the ventral rami of the roots prior to the formation of the brachial plexus?
   1. **Dorsal scapular nerve**, from C5—to rhomboid and levator scapula muscles; responsible for elevation and stabilization of the scapula.
   2. **Long thoracic nerve**, from C5,6,7—to serratus anterior responsible for abduction of the scapula.
   Testing these nerves is very useful when trying to differentiate between root and plexus lesions. If there is a deficit in one of these nerves (clinically or electrically), then the lesion is proximal to the plexus.

36. Which roots form the three trunks of the brachial plexus?
(1) Superior trunk, formed by C5 and C6; (2) middle trunk, formed by C7; and (3) lower trunk, formed by C8 and T1.

37. What is the only branch from the trunks of the brachial plexus?
The suprascapular nerve (C5) comes off the upper trunk and supplies the supraspinatus (abduction) and infraspinatus (external rotation) of the shoulder.

38. Which vascular structure is associated with the three cords of the brachial plexus?
The lateral cord (C5,6,7), medial cord (C8, T1), and posterior cord (C5,6,7,8) are named in relationship to the axillary artery.

39. What are the branches of the cords of the brachial plexus?
Lateral cord
1. Lateral pectoral nerve (C5,6,7)—to pectoralis minor
2. Musculocutaneous nerve (C5,6)—to brachialis and coracobrachialis (elbow flexion)
Medial cord
3. Medial pectoral nerve (C8, T1)—to pectoralis major (shoulder adduction)
4. Ulnar nerve (C8, T1)—ulnar wrist and long finger flexors
5. Medial root of median nerve (C8, T1)—long finger flexors and small hand muscles
6. Medial brachial cutaneous nerve—skin over medial surface of arm and proximal forearm
7. Medial antebrachial cutaneous nerve—skin over medial surface of forearm
Posterior cord
8. Upper subscapular nerve (C5,6)—to subscapularis (medial rotation of the humerus)
9. Thoracodorsal nerve (C6,7,8)—to latissimus dorsi (shoulder adduction)
10. Lower subscapular nerve (C5,6)—to teres major (adducts the humerus)
11. Axillary nerve (C5, C6)—to deltoid (abduction of the humerus) and teres minor (lateral rotation of humerus)
12. Radial nerve (C5,6,7,8 and T1)—to extensor muscles of upper limb.

40. What is Erb's palsy?
Erb's palsy is an injury to the upper brachial plexus (C5 and C6) resulting from excessive separation or stretch of the neck and shoulder (such as from a sliding injury or from pulling on an infant's neck during delivery). The result is decreased sensation in the C5 and C6 dermatomes and paralysis of scapular muscles. The arm may be held in adduction, with the fingers pointing backward, so-called waiter's tip position. Distal strength in the upper extremity remains intact.

41. What is Klumpke's palsy?
Klumpke's palsy results from maximum abduction of the shoulder, causing injury to the lower brachial plexus (C8 and T1) and leading to weakness and anesthesia in a primarily ulnar distribution.

42. What is Parsonage-Turner syndrome?
Parsonage-Turner syndrome is an acute brachial plexus neuritis, commonly also affecting the long thoracic, musculocutaneous, and axillary nerves. It causes patchy upper extremity weakness and numbness, usually accompanied by pain. Symptoms are bilateral in 20% of patients. This condition is associated with diabetes, systemic lupus erythematosus, and polyarteritis nodosa, and may follow immunizations or viral infections. One-third of patients will recover within 1 year and 90% within 3 years.

43. Poorly fitting crutches results in what deficit?
Pressure from crutches results in a lesion of the posterior cord or the radial nerve, leading to weakness of the elbow, wrist, and digits.

44. Which nerve is commonly affected in shoulder dislocation or fracture of the humerus?
The axillary nerve is affected, resulting in a lesion that causes decreased abduction of the shoulder and anesthesia over the lateral part of the proximal arm.

45. What is thoracic outlet syndrome (TOS)?
Classically, TOS consists of decreased upper-extremity pulses with tingling and numbness in the medial aspect of the arm secondary to compression of the medial cord of the brachial plexus and the axillary artery by a cervical rib or other structures.

ROOTS AND DERMATOMES

46. What is found in the ventral nerve root?
The ventral nerve root contains principally motor axons.

47. What is found in the dorsal nerve root?
The dorsal nerve root contains principally sensory axons.

48. What synapse is found in the dorsal root ganglia?
There is no synapse in the dorsal root ganglia. The dorsal root ganglia is made up of unipolar cell bodies for the sensory system.

49. What are the dermatomes of the following landmarks: thumb, middle finger, little finger, breast nipple, umbilicus, medial knee, big toe, and little toe?

Thumb	C6	Little finger	C8	Umbilicus	T10	Big toe	L4
Middle finger	C7	Breast nipple	T4	Medial knee	L3	Little toe	S1

The dermatomes corresponding to each spinal root. (Reprinted, with modifications, with permission from Garoutte B: Survey of Functional Neuroanatomy, 2nd ed. Greenbrae, CA, Jones Medical Publications, 1992, p 76.)

50. What are the common signs and symptoms of lumbar radiculopathies?

Lumbar radiculopathies cause back pain with radiation below the knee. The pain increases with a Valsalva maneuver or leg stretch (such as the straight leg raising test). Weakness or numbness may develop in the distribution of the involved root. An S1 radiculopathy diminishes ankle reflexes, whereas an L4 radiculopathy decreases knee reflexes. Statistically, an L5 radiculopathy is more common than S1, followed by L4. This is because the intervertebral discs at these levels are under greatest pressure from the curvature of normal lumbar lordosis, and thus are most vulnerable to herniation and compression of the spinal roots.

51. What are the common signs and symptoms of cervical radiculopathies?

Cervical radiculopathies usually involve the lower cervical roots (C6, C7, and C8). Patients typically complain of pain in the back of the neck, frequently with radiation to the arm in a dermatomal distribution. Paresthesias are often present in one or two digits. Absent brachioradialis, biceps, or triceps reflexes suggest lesions of C5, C6, and C7, respectively, and these muscles may also lose strength.

SPINAL CORD: Gross Anatomy

52. How is the spinal cord organized?

Sections of the spinal cord cut perpendicular to the length of the cord reveal a butterfly-shaped area of gray matter with surrounding white matter. The white matter consists mainly of longitudinal nerve fibers, carrying the ascending and descending tracts up and down the cord. Midline grooves are present on the dorsal and ventral surfaces (the dorsal median sulcus and ventral median fissure). The gray matter of the cord contains dorsal and ventral enlargements known as dorsal horns and ventral horns.

53. In a given transverse section of the spinal cord, how is the gray matter subdivided?

The gray matter can be subdivided into groups of nuclei. When the spinal cord is cut along its length, these nuclei appear to be arranged in cell columns or "laminae." Rexed divided the cord into 10 laminae. Each lamina extends the length of the cord, with lamina I at the most dorsal aspect of the dorsal horn, lamina IX at the most ventral aspect of the ventral horn, and lamina X surrounding the central canal. Lamina II is also called the substantia gelatinosa and is the area of synapse for the spinothalamic tract. Lamina IX is the site of the cell bodies for the anterior horn motor cells.

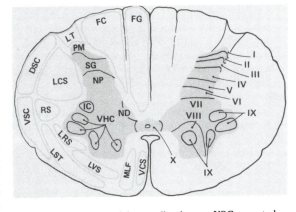

Diagram of the cross-section of the spinal cord in the lower cervical region, showing the major ascending and descending tracts, spinal nuclei, and Rexed's laminae. DSC = dorsal spinocerebellar tract; FC = fasciculus cuneatus; FG = fasciculus gracilis; IC = intermedial lateral cell column; LCS = lateral cortical spinal tract; LRS = lateral reticular spinal tract; LST = lateral spinothalamic tract; LT = Lissauer's tract; LVS = lateral vestibular spinal tract; MLF = medial longitudinal fasciculus; ND = nucleus dorsalis; NP = nucleus proprius; PM = posteromarginal nucleus; RS = rubrospinal tract; SG = substantia gelatinosa; VCS = ventral cortical spinal tract; VHC = ventral horn cell columns; VSC = ventral spinocerebellar tract. (Reprinted with permission from Gilman S, Newman SW: Manter and Gatz's Essentials of Clinical Neuroanatomy and Neurophysiology, 8th ed. Philadelphia, F.A. Davis, 1992.)

54. What are the major ascending tracts in the spinal cord?
The major ascending tracts are (1) dorsal columns, (2) spinothalamic tract, (3) dorsal spinocerebellar tract, and (4) ventral spinocerebellar tract.

55. What are the major descending tracts in the spinal cord?
The major descending tracts are (1) intermediolateral columns, (2) lateral corticospinal tract, (3) lateral reticulospinal tract, (4) lateral vestibulospinal tract, (5) medial longitudinal fasciculus, and (6) ventral corticospinal tract.

56. Going from rostral to caudal, what are the five divisions of the spinal cord?
The five divisions of the spinal cord are cervical, thoracic, lumbar, sacral, and coccygeal.

57. At what vertebral level does the spinal cord end?
The spinal cord ends at vertebral level L1–L2.

58. How many spinal nerves exit from each region of the spinal cord?
Spinal nerves exit the spinal cord in pairs: 8 cervical, 12 thoracic, 5 lumbar, 5 sacral, and 1 coccygeal. Each spinal nerve is composed of the union of the dorsal sensory root and the ventral motor root.

59. What is the filum terminale?
Although the spinal cord ends at the lower border of vertebral level L1, the pia mater continues caudally as a connective tissue filament, the filum terminale, which passes through the subarachnoid space to the end of the dural sac, where it receives a covering of dura and continues to its attachment to the coccyx.

60. What is the cauda equina?
The lumbar and sacral spinal nerves have very long roots, descending from their respective points in the spinal cord to their exit points in the intervertebral foramina. These roots descend in a bundle from the conus, termed the cauda equina for its resemblance to a horse's tail.

61. What is the blood supply of the spinal cord?
The one anterior spinal artery and the two posterior spinal arteries travel along the length of the cord to supply blood to the cord. These arteries originate from the vertebral arteries. Other arteries that replenish the anterior and posterior spinal arteries and enter the spinal canal through the intervertebral foramina in association with the spinal nerves. They are called radicular arteries if they supply only the nerve roots, and radiculospinal arteries if they supply blood to both the roots and the cord. Each radiculospinal artery supplies blood to approximately six spinal cord segments, with the exception of the great radicular artery of Adamkiewicz, which usually enters with the left second lumbar ventral root (range T10–L4) and supplies most of the caudal third of the cord.

62. How much of the spinal cord is supplied by the anterior spinal artery?
The anterior spinal artery furnishes blood to the anterior two-thirds of the spinal cord.

63. How much of the spinal cord is supplied by the posterior spinal arteries?
The two posterior spinal arteries furnish blood to the posterior one-third of the spinal cord.

Sensory: Dorsal Columns and Proprioception

64. What type of information is carried in the dorsal columns?
The dorsal columns convey tactile discrimination, vibration, and joint position sense.

65. What type of receptors are stimulated to sense this information?
Muscle spindles and Golgi tendon organs perceive position sense, pacinian corpuscles perceive vibration, and Meissner corpuscles perceive superficial touch sensation needed for tactile discrimination. The latter two are examples of mechanoreceptors.

66. What type of peripheral nerve fiber is involved with transmission of "dorsal column" information?
Large, myelinated, fast-conducting nerve fibers carry "dorsal-column-type" information.

67. What is the pathway by which this information reaches the cerebral cortex?
Sensation on skin → afferent sensory nerve → dorsal column on ipsilateral side (fasciculus gracilis and cuneatus) → lower medulla → synapse in nucleus gracilis and cuneatus → arcuate fibers → cross to the contralateral side into the medial lemniscus → ascend to the ventralis posterolateralis (VPL) nucleus of the thalamus → synapse → through the posterior limb of the internal capsule → postcentral gyrus of the cortex.

68. Where do dorsal column fibers decussate? At what locations do they synapse?
The dorsal columns decussate in the lower medulla, after synapsing in the nucleus gracilis and cuneatus. They also synapse in the VPL of the thalamus before going to the cortex.

Sensory: Spinothalamic

69. What type of information is carried in the spinothalamic tract?
The spinothalamic tract conveys pain, temperature, and crude touch.

70. What type of peripheral nerve fiber is involved with transmission of "spinothalamic" information?
Small, myelinated, and unmyelinated fibers carry "spinothalamic-type" information.

71. What is the pathway by which this information reaches the cerebral cortex?
Sensation on skin → afferent sensory nerve → substantia gelatinosa of the ipsilateral dorsal horn → synapse → cross via the anterior white commissure → contralateral spinothalamic tract → ascend to the VPL nucleus of the thalamus → synapse → through the posterior limb of the internal capsule → postcentral gyrus of the cortex.

72. Where do the spinothalamic fibers decussate? At what locations do they synapse?
These fibers decussate at the level they enter the spinal cord, after synapsing in Rexed's lamina II (substantia gelatinosa). They also synapse in the VPL of the thalamus before going to the cortex.

73. What type of receptors are stimulated to sense this information?
Pain and temperature are perceived by naked terminals of A-delta and C fibers and by many specialized chemoreceptors that are excited by tissue substances released in response to noxious and inflammatory stimuli. Substance P is thought to be the neurotransmitter released by A-delta and C fibers at their connections with the interneurons in the spinal cord.

74. Where in the internal capsule do the afferents travel from the VPL thalamic nucleus?
The sensory tracts from the VPL travel in the posterior aspect of the posterior limb of the internal capsule.

75. To which anatomic locations do these afferents from the VPL project?
They project to the postcentral gyrus (Brodmann's area 3,1,2; also called somatosensory I), and to somatosensory II (the posterior aspect of the superior lip of the lateral fissure).

Sensory: Spinocerebellar

76. Which pathway carries proprioception from the lower limbs to the cerebellum?
Proprioception travels from the legs to the cerebellum in the dorsal columns.

77. Where does cerebellar proprioception for the lower limb synapse?
These fibers synapse in the mid-thoracic level of the spinal cord in the nucleus dorsalis of Clark.

78. Where is the spinocerebellar tract located?
The spinocerebellar tract lies lateral to corticospinal in the cord.

Motor: Corticospinal

79. Where do the motor fibers originate?
The motor fibers originate from the precentral gyrus (Brodmann's area 4). Initiation of movement arises from the premotor cortex (Brodmann's area 6), which lies anterior to the precentral gyrus.

80. Where do the motor fibers travel in the internal capsule?
The corticospinal fibers travel in the anterior portion of the posterior limb of the internal capsule. The motor fibers to the face (corticobulbar fibers) travel in the genu of the internal capsule.

81. Where do the motor fibers travel in the midbrain?
In the midbrain, the corticospinal fibers travel in the central part of the crus (the crus is the most ventral part of the midbrain).

82. Which cranial nerve exits the midbrain in close proximity to the corticospinal fibers?
Cranial nerve III exits the midbrain in close proximity to the corticospinal fibers, which explains the symptomatology of a common vascular syndrome: in Weber's syndrome, a stroke here causes an ipsilateral third nerve palsy with contralateral hemiparesis.

83. Where do the motor fibers decussate?
The corticospinal tract decussates in the lower ventral medulla, and most fibers continue in the cord as the lateral corticospinal tract, with a small percentage descending in the ventral corticospinal tract.

84. On what type of neurons in the spinal cord do the corticospinal fibers synapse?
In the spinal cord, the corticospinal fibers synapse on the alpha and gamma motor neurons in Rexed's lamina IX.

Motor: Other Tracts

85. What is the reticulospinal tract?
The reticulospinal tract also originates in the precentral gyrus, but instead of descending uninterrupted to the spinal cord, these fibers synapse in the reticular formation of the brainstem as they descend to the spinal cord. These fibers mainly have an inhibitory effect on the alpha and gamma motor neurons.

86. What is the vestibulospinal tract?
The vestibulospinal tract is the efferent from the lateral vestibular nucleus. This tract descends the spinal cord, residing lateral to the spinothalamic tract, and coordinates motor and vertibular performance.

87. What is the medial longitudinal fasciculus (MLF)?
The medial longitudinal fasciculus is also an efferent of the lateral vestibular nucleus. This tract ascends to the sixth and third cranial nuclei, as well as descends the spinal cord. Its main function is to coordinate head and truncal posture with eye movements.

BRAINSTEM

Cranial Nerves

88. What are the three parts of the brainstem?
The brainstem consists of the midbrain, pons, and medulla.

89. What is the reticular formation?
The reticular formation is a loosely organized longitudinal collection of interneurons that fill the central core of the brainstem, concerned with modulating awareness and behavioral performance.

90. Name the 12 cranial nerves.

I Olfactory	IV Trochlear	VII Facial	X Vagus
II Optic	V Trigeminal	VIII Auditory	XI Spinal accessory
III Oculomotor	VI Abducens	IX Glossopharyngeal	XII Hypoglossal

91. What are general somatic afferent nerves? Which cranial nerves carry them?
General somatic afferent fibers carry extroceptive (pain, temperature, touch) and proprioceptive impulses. Cranial nerves (for proprioception): III, IV, V, VI, XII, and (for pain, temperature, touch) V, VII, IX, X.

92. What are general visceral afferent nerves? Which cranial nerves carry them?
General visceral afferent fibers carry impulses from the visceral structures, and cranial nerves IX and X contain these fibers.

93. What are special somatic afferent nerves? Which cranial nerves carry them?
Special somatic afferent fibers carry sensory impulses from the special senses (vision, hearing, equilibrium), and cranial nerves II and VIII contain these fibers.

94. What are special visceral afferent nerves? Which cranial nerves carry them?
Special visceral afferent fibers carry impulses from the olfactory and gustatory senses, and cranial nerve I (olfactory) and VII, IX, and X (gustatory) contain these fibers.

95. What are general somatic efferent nerves? Which cranial nerves carry them?
General somatic efferent fibers carry motor impulses to somatic skeletal muscles. In the head, the tongue and extraocular muscles are of this type. Cranial nerves III, IV, VI, and XII carry these fibers.

96. What are general visceral efferent nerves? Which cranial nerves carry them?
General visceral efferent fibers carry parasympathetic autonomic axons. The cranial nerves that carry general visceral efferent fibers are:

    1. **Cranial nerve III** (Edinger-Westphal nucleus): the preganglionic fibers from the Edinger-Westphal nucleus terminates in the ciliary ganglion, and the postganglionic fibers innervate the pupil.

    2. **Cranial nerve VII** (superior salivatory nucleus): the preganglionic fibers from the superior salivatory nucleus terminate in the pterygopalatine and submandibular ganglion.

The postganglionic fibers innervate the lacrimal gland (from the pterygopalatine ganglion) and the submandibular and sublingual gland (from the submandibular ganglion).

3. **Cranial nerve IX** (inferior salivatory nucleus): the preganglionic fibers from the inferior salivatory nucleus terminate in the otic ganglion, and the postganglionic fibers innervate the parotid gland.

4. **Cranial nerve X** (dorsal motor nucleus): the dorsal motor nucleus innervates the abdominal viscera.

97. What are special visceral efferent nerves? Which cranial nerves carry them?
Special visceral efferent fibers innervate skeletal muscle derived from the branchial arches. Cranial nerves V (muscles of mastication, first branchial arch), VII (muscles of facial expression, second branchial arch), IX (stylopharyngeus muscle, third branchial arch), X (muscles of the soft palate and pharynx, fourth branchial arch), and XI (muscles of the larynx/sternocleidomastoid/trapezius, sixth branchial arch) carry them.

Midbrain

98. What are the three anatomic subdivisions of the midbrain?
The midbrain can be divided into the tectum, tegmentum, and cerebral crus.

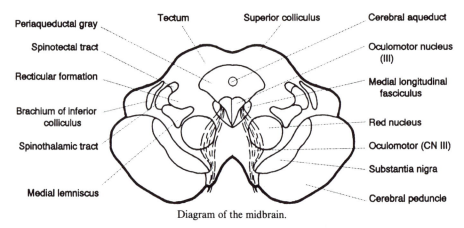

Periaqueductal gray
Spinotectal tract
Recticular formation
Brachium of inferior colliculus
Spinothalamic tract
Medial lemniscus

Tectum   Superior colliculus

Cerebral aqueduct
Oculomotor nucleus (III)
Medial longitudinal fasciculus
Red nucleus
Oculomotor (CN III)
Substantia nigra
Cerebral peduncle

Diagram of the midbrain.

99. What is the quadrigeminal plate?
The quadrigeminal plate is formed by the tectum and the superior and inferior colliculi.

100. What is the substantia nigra?
The substantia nigra, a motor nucleus in the basal ganglia system, lies anterior to the tegmentum but posterior to the crus (pyramidal tract) in the midbrain.

101. Which disease affects the substantia nigra? What is the pathology?
The primary efferent neurotransmitter from the substantia nigra is dopamine. Parkinson's disease damages the substantia nigra. Pathologically, the neurons lose their melanin so the nucleus becomes depigmented. Many neurons also contain inclusion bodies called Lewy bodies.

102. What is the red nucleus?
The red nucleus is a globular mass located in the ventral portion of the tegmentum of the midbrain. It is a relay center for many of the efferent cerebellar tracts. The crossed fibers of the superior cerebellar peduncle pass through and around its edges.

103. What is the Edinger-Westphal nucleus?
The Edinger-Westphal nucleus, in the posterior midbrain, supplies parasympathetic fibers that terminate in the ciliary ganglion via cranial nerve III. It is mainly involved in pupillary constriction and the light accommodation reflex.

104. What is the function of cranial nerve III?
Cranial nerve III innervates all the extraocular muscles except for the lateral rectus and superior oblique. It innervates the medial rectus, superior rectus, inferior rectus, and inferior oblique muscles.

105. Where does cranial nerve III originate and exit the brainstem?
Cranial nerve III, the oculomotor nerve, exits the brainstem medially from the midbrain, between the posterior cerebral artery and the superior cerebellar artery.

106. What is the function of cranial nerve IV?
Cranial nerve IV, the trochlear nerve, innervates the superior oblique muscle.

107. What is the route of cranial nerve IV?
Cranial nerve IV travels posteriorly and medially, crosses the midline, wraps around the midbrain, and exits the brainstem laterally between the posterior cerebral artery and superior cerebellar artery. It has the longest intracranial route (approximately 7.5 cm) of any cranial nerve. It then travels through the cavernous sinus and enters the orbit through the superior orbital fissure. Because it crosses the midline, the right trochlear nerve innervates the left superior oblique muscle.

108. In a superior oblique palsy, which way would the patient tilt his or her head?
If the left superior oblique muscle is weak, then tilting the head to the right would reduce the diplopia, and tilting the head to the left would worsen the diplopia. So, patients tilt their head away from the affected eye.

Pons

109. Which cranial nerves exit at the pontomedullary junction?
Cranial nerve VI exits medially and cranial nerves VII and VIII exit laterally.

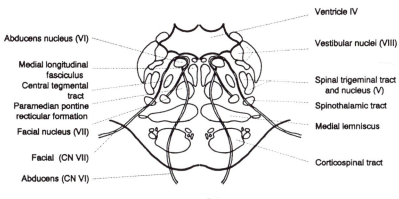

Anatomy of the pons.

110. Where does cranial nerve V exit the brainstem?
Cranial nerve V, the trigeminal nerve, exits the brainstem laterally at the mid-pons level. It divides into three main branches: V1 = ophthalmic; V2 = maxillary; and V3 = mandibular.

111. What are the four subdivisions of the trigeminal nucleus?
(1) Mesencephalic nucleus (which is a nucleus of unipolar cell bodies similar to the dorsal root ganglion, with no synapse), (2) the chief sensory nucleus, (3) the descending spinal nucleus, and (4) the motor nucleus.

112. What type of information does cranial nerve V carry?
The trigeminal nerve carries sensation (general somatic afferent) from the anterior two-thirds of the face, and motor innervation (special visceral efferent) to the muscles of mastication (medial/lateral pterygoid, masseter, temporalis), the mylohyoid, anterior belly of the digastric, tensor tympani, and tensor palati.

113. What is the pathway by which sensation from the face reaches the cortex?
After cranial nerve V enters the brainstem, the afferent nerves split into two parts: those carrying dorsal-column-type information and those carrying spinothalamic-type information. The former goes to the ipsilateral chief sensory nucleus of V (mid-pons) → synapse → enters the contralateral trigeminal lemniscus (which lies medial to the medial lemniscus) → VPM nucleus of the thalamus → synapse → through the posterior limb of the internal capsule to the postcentral gyrus. The pain-carrying fibers become the spinal tract of V → descend from mid-pons to lower medulla → synapse in the spinal nucleus of V → cross diffusely to form the contralateral trigeminal lemniscus (at mid-pons) → VPM nucleus of the thalamus → synapse → through the posterior limb of the internal capsule to the postcentral gyrus.

114. What is the function of cranial nerve VI?
Cranial nerve VI, the abducens nerve, abducts the eye.

115. What is the function of cranial nerve VII?
Cranial nerve VII, the facial nerve, innervates the muscles of facial expression (special visceral efferent), innervates the lacrimal, submandibular, sublingual, and parotid glands (general visceral efferent), supplies taste sensation to the anterior two-thirds of the tongue (special visceral afferent), and supplies sensation to the external ear (general somatic afferent).

116. How does the nucleus for cranial nerve VII receive higher cortical input?
The innervation to the muscles of facial expression can be separated into the muscles of the upper part of the face and the muscles of the lower part of the face. The supranuclear input responsible for the movement of the upper facial musculature is a bilateral input from the cortex to the nucleus. The supranuclear input responsible for the movement of the lower facial musculature is only a contralateral input from the cortex to the facial nucleus.

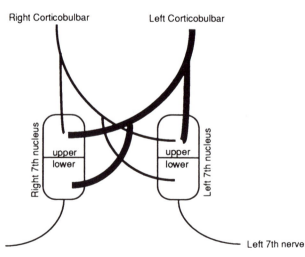

117. What is the difference between an upper motor neuron (central) and lower motor neuron (peripheral) facial weakness?
If the patient with a facial droop can move the upper facial muscles (i.e., wrinkle the forehead), then the lesion is supranuclear on the contralateral side. The lesion is somewhere in the contralateral corticobulbar tracts above the facial nerve nucleus (e.g., in the crus, in the genu of the internal capsule, etc.). If the patient cannot voluntarily move any muscle involved in facial expression, either upper or lower facial musculature, then the lesion is localized to the facial nucleus or the peripheral facial nerve on the ipsilateral side.

118. What is Mobius syndrome?
Mobius syndrome is congenital absence of both facial nerve nuclei, resulting in a facial diplegia. Patients may also have associated absence of the abducens nuclei.

119. What is the function of cranial nerve VIII?
Cranial nerve VIII, the vestibulocochlear nerve, has two functionally distinct sensory divisions: the vestibular nerve and the cochlear (or auditory) nerve. The vestibular nerve responds to position and movement of the head, serving functions often identified as equilibrium. The cochlear nerve mediates auditory functions.

120. What is the locus ceruleus? Where is it located?
The locus ceruleus is a paired irregular collection of pigmented (bluish hue) cells located near the central gray of the pons, just ventral to the fourth ventricle. The locus ceruleus is a major source of noradrenergic innervation to the diencephalon and cortex.

Medulla

121. Which nerves exit in the postolivary fissure?
The glossopharyngeal nerve (cranial nerve IX), vagus nerve (cranial nerve X), and the spinal accessory nerve (cranial nerve XI) exit the brainstem in the postolivary fissure.

122. What is the nucleus ambiguus?
It is a cigar-shaped nucleus that lies in the depths of the medulla that innervates the volitional muscles of the pharynx by way of both cranial nerves IX and X, and the larynx (for phonation) via cranial nerve X. The larynx and pharynx have bilateral cortical input.

123. What is pseudobulbar palsy?
Pseudobulbar palsy is paralysis of swallowing and phonation as a result of bilateral upper motor neuron innervation to the nucleus ambiguus.

124. What is the nucleus solitarius?
It is the nucleus in the medulla that receives afferent information from the larynx (via cranial nerve X) and posterior pharynx, and mediates the gag and cough reflexes (cranial nerves IX and X). Pain sensation from these areas enters the brainstem via cranial nerves IX and X, but terminates in the descending spinal tract of the trigeminal nerve.

125. What is the salivary nucleus?
The superior salivatory nucleus sends efferent autonomic fibers (general visceral efferent) via cranial nerve VII to innervate the lacrimal, submandibular, and sublingual glands, as well as the mucous membranes of the nose and hard and soft palate. The inferior salivatory nucleus sends efferent autonomic fibers via cranial nerve IX to innervate the parotid gland.

126. What is the gustatory nucleus?

The gustatory nucleus is the nucleus in the medulla that receives afferent sensory informaton for the sensation of taste. Taste from the anterior two-thirds of the tongue is innervated by the chorda tympani (cranial nerve VII), the posterior one-third of the tongue is innervated by cranial nerve IX, and the epiglottis is innervated by cranial nerve X.

127. Describe the function of cranial nerves IX and X (glossopharyngeal-vagal complex).

Cranial nerve IX (the glossopharyngeal nerve) and cranial nerve X (the vagus nerve) are usually considered together because of their overlapping functions. Both cranial nerves travel together intracranially and both exit the cranial vault via the jugular foramen. The nucleus ambiguus innervates the volitional muscles of the pharynx via both cranial nerves IX and X, and the larynx via cranial nerve X. Sensation from the larynx enters the medulla via cranial nerve X to terminate in the nucleus solitarius. Taste fibers from the posterior one-third of the tongue travel via cranial nerve IX, and taste from the epiglottis via cranial nerve X. They terminate in the gustatory nucleus. Cranial nerve IX also supplies parasympathetic innervation to the parotid, originating in the inferior salivatory nucleus. Branches of cranial nerve X, the vagus nerve, continue beyond the larynx to innervate the heart, lungs, and abdominal viscera, providing primarily parasympathetic input.

128. What is the function of cranial nerve XI?

Cranial nerve XI, the spinal accessory nerve, is a small nerve of about 3500 motor fibers that arises from the upper cervical and lower medullary anterior horn cells and supplies the sternocleidomastoid and trapezius muscles. It exits the cranial vault via the jugular foramen.

129. What is the jugular foramen syndrome?

Because cranial nerves IX, X, and XI exit the cranial vault through the jugular foramen, the jugular foramen syndrome is a constellation of symptoms arising from a lesion (typically a tumor) at the level of the jugular foramen that compromises the function of these cranial nerves. Symptoms include loss of taste to the posterior two-thirds of the tongue; paralysis of the vocal cords, palate, and pharynx; and paralysis of the trapezius and sternocleidomastoid (SCM) muscles.

130. If the left spinal accessory nerve were cut, which functions would be lost?

Because cranial nerve XI supplies the SCM and the trapezius, these muscles would be weakened. Because the left SCM is involved in turning the head to the right, a lesion of the left cranial nerve XI would result in an inability to turn the head to the right. The left trapezius would also lose function and the patient would not be able to shrug the left shoulder.

131. Which nerves exit in the preolivary fissure?

Cranial nerve XII, the hypoglossal nerve, exits the brainstem from the preolivary fissure.

132. If the left hypoglossal nucleus were injured, which way would the tongue deviate?

Lesioning the nucleus is similar to lesioning the peripheral nerve. The left hypoglossal nerve innervates the left tongue muscles, which, if acting alone, would push the tongue to the right. The right hypoglossal nerve innervates the right tongue muscles, which, if acting alone, would push the tongue to the left. Normally these muscles work in balance to push the tongue forward without deviation. If the left hypoglossal nucleus were lesioned, then the right hypoglossal muscles would be acting unopposed. The tongue would thus deviate to the left, or, in other words, the tongue deviates toward the affected side of the tongue.

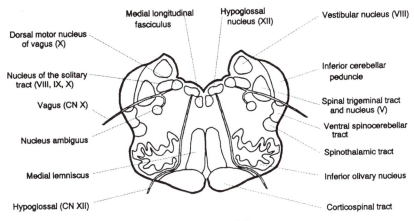

Anatomy of the medulla.

Breathing

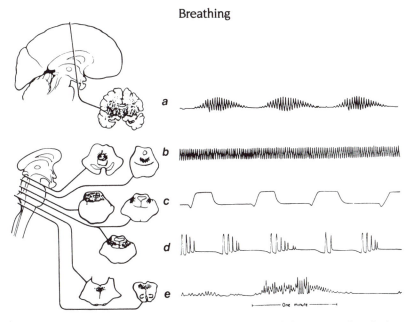

Diagram showing the location of lesions causing various characteristic patterns of respiration: a = Cheyne-Stokes; b = central neurogenic hyperventilation; c = apneustic; d = cluster; e = ataxic. (Reprinted with permission from Plum F, Posner J: The Diagnosis of Stupor and Coma, 3rd ed. Philadelphia, F.A. Davis, 1986, p 65.)

133. What is Cheyne-Stokes breathing? Where is the lesion that causes it?
Cheyne-Stokes is a crescendo-decrescendo pattern of periodic breathing in which phases of hyperpnea regularly alternate with apnea. Cheyne-Stokes respirations are seen most often with lesions affecting both cerebral hemispheres.

134. What is central neurogenic hyperventilation? What causes it?
It is a sustained, rapid, deep hyperpnea. Central hyperventilation is produced by lesions in the low midbrain to upper one-third of the pons.

135. What is apneustic breathing? What causes it?
Apneusis is a prolonged "respiratory cramp," a pause at full inspiration. Apneustic breathing may occur after damage to the mid or caudal pons.

136. What is cluster breathing? When does it occur?
Cluster breathing, a disorderly sequence of breaths with irregular pauses between the breaths, may result from damage to the lower pons or upper medulla.

137. What is ataxic breathing? Where is the lesion that causes it?
It is a completely irregular pattern of breathing in which both deep and shallow breaths occur randomly. The respiratory rate tends to be slow. The lesion that causes it is in the central medulla.

Posturing

138. What is decorticate posturing? What causes it?
Decorticate posturing is a stereotyped response to noxious stimuli. It consists, in the upper extremity, of flexion of the arm, wrist, and fingers, and, in the lower extremity, of extension, internal rotation, and plantar flexion. Decorticate posturing most often occurs in comatose patients with lesions below the thalamus but above the red nucleus.

139. What is decerebrate posturing? In whom does it occur?
Decerebrate posturing is a stereotyped response to noxious stimuli. It consists of extension, adduction, and hyperpronation in the upper extremity and extension with plantar flexion in the lower extremity. Comatose patients with lesions below the red nucleus but above the vestibular nucleus may have decerebrate posturing.

Vestibular Apparatus

140. What are the five receptors of the vestibular apparatus, and what do they sense?
Three semicircular canals that are oriented 90 degrees to each other sense rotational acceleration in all three planes. One horizontally oriented utricle and one vertically oriented saccule sense linear acceleration.

141. Where does the vestibular information synpase?
The vestibular nerve, carrying sensory data from the receptors, divides and synapses in four vestibular nuclei grouped together in the medulla: the superior, inferior, medial, and lateral vestibular nuclei.

142. What is the output from these nuclei?
The vestibulospinal tracts and the medial longitudinal fasciculus (MLF) are the two efferent tracts from the vestibular nuclei.

143. Where do the vestibulospinal tracts travel in the spinal cord?
The lateral vestibulospinal tract travels ventrolateral to the spinothalamic tract in the cord, whereas the medial vestibulospinal tract runs in the descending MLF.

144. Where do the vestibular nuclei project?
Vestibular nuclei project to (1) the oculomotor nuclei (cranial nerves III, IV, and VI), (2) cranial nerve XI, (3) cervical nuclei for head and neck position, (4) fastigial nuclei of the cerebellum, and (5) reticular formations of the brainstem.

145. What is the response of a normal person to cold water injected in the left ear?
Injecting cold water in to the left ear causes slow eye movements toward the left, followed by a quick phase of nystagmus back to the right.

146. What is the expected response of a comatose patient with an intact brainstem to cold water in the left ear?
The patient will have slow eye deviation toward the left ear. The fast phase component is absent.

147. What is vestibular neuronitis?
Vestibular neuronitis is a condition affecting primarily young adults, causing a sudden attack of vertigo without tinnitus or hearing loss. This benign disorder usually resolves within several days. The etiology is presumed to be a viral infection.

148. What is benign positional vertigo? How is it diagnosed?
Benign positional vertigo is a disorder characterized by paroxysms of vertigo and nystagmus upon assumption of certain positions of the head. Hearing tests are normal. The diagnosis is made by performing head maneuvers that elicit the patient's symptoms and nystagmus. The cause is calcification and dislocation of otoliths, which move freely in the semicircular canal, thus abnormally stimulating the hair cells within the semicircular canals.

Hearing

149. Which structures constitute the external ear? Middle ear? Inner ear?
The **external ear** is composed of the pinna, the external auditory canal, and the tympanic membrane. The **middle ear** is composed of the tympanic membrane, ossicles (malleus, incus, stapes), and oval window. The ossicles function as an impedance matching device between air and fluid during the travel of the sound wave. The **inner ear** is composed of part of the oval window, the cochlea, and the round window.

150. Which compartments of the cochlea are filled with perilymph?
- **Scala vestibuli.** It is separated from the scala tympani by Reissner's membrane.
- **Scala tympani.** It is separated from the scala media by the basilar membrane.
- **Scala media.** The third compartment is filled with endolymph and is located between Reissner's and the basilar membranes.

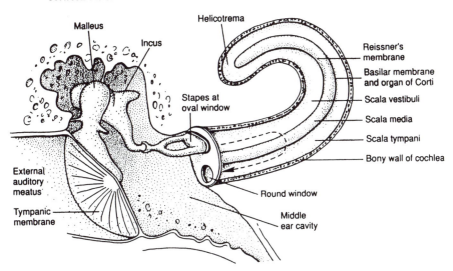

Anatomy of the hearing apparatus. (Reprinted with permission from Kandel E, Schwartz JH, Jessell TM (eds): Principles of Neuroscience, 3rd ed. New York, Elsevier, 1991, p 369.)

151. What is the pathway traveled by the cochlear fluid pressure wave initiated by a sound wave?

The stapes transmits the pressure to the round window and from it to the perilymph of the scala vestibuli, which, in turn, sets up vibrations of Reissner's membrane, resulting in a wave in the scala media. The basilar membranes move next and transmit the pressure to the scala tympani and from there to the oval window.

152. What is the arrangement of the neuroepithelial cells of the organ of Corti?

1. The outer hair cells (arranged in 3 rows) rest on the basilar membrane, with their stereocilia inserted into the tectorial membrane; these cells are able to contract and initiate the flow of endolymph toward the inner hair cells.

2. The inner hair cells (1 row) sit on the bone; they do not contract. These cells respond to the movement of endolymph and provide most of the afferent input to the spiral ganglion.

153. How does the organ of Corti serve as an audiofrequency analyzer?

The anatomic arrangement allows for frequency analysis of sounds:

1. The basilar membrane responds to high frequencies at its base and to low frequencies at its apex.

2. The hair cells in the base of the cochlear duct have short and fat stereocilia, which are stimulated by high frequencies.

3. The hair cells in the apex of the cochlea have long and thin stereocilia, which respond best to low frequencies.

154. What is the anatomy of the auditory pathway?

Spiral ganglion → auditory nerve (cranial nerve VIII) → dorsal and ventral cochlear nuclei at the junction of the medulla and pons → trapezoid body (at this point 50% of the axons cross over to the other side) → superior olivary nucleus → lateral lemniscus → inferior colliculus → medial geniculate body → transverse gyrus of Heschl (area 41, partly buried in the sylvian fissure).

155. Apart from the main auditory pathway, where else does acoustic information travel?

The alternate pathways, which mediate acoustic reflexes, include: (1) to cranial nerves V and VII, (2) from the inferior colliculus to the motor centers, and (3) to the reticular activating system.

156. At what level is there crossing of information between the left and right ascending tracts?

The crossing of axons occurs on every level from the trapezoid body to the medial geniculate body.

157. To produce unilateral deafness, where could the lesion be?

The lesion must be at the cochlear nucleus or more peripheral, because of multiple crossovers above the cochlear nucleus.

158. What is Weber's test?

A vibrating tuning fork is placed in the middle of the forehead. In patients with conduction deafness, the sound is localized to the affected ear (bone > air conduction). In patients with sensorineural deafness, the signal is localized to the healthy ear.

159. What is Rinne's test?

A vibrating tuning fork is placed on the mastoid bone; when the patient can no longer hear it, it is removed and placed next to the ear. In this way, bone conduction is compared to air conduction. In conduction deafness, bone $>$ air conduction. In sensorineural deafness, air $>$ bone conduction.

160. What is the innervation of the external ear canal?
The external ear canal is supplied by cranial nerves V3, VII, IX, and X.

161. Damage to which structures results in hyperacusis?
    1. **Facial nerve** (VII)—innervates the stapedius muscle, which retracts the stapes from the round window.
    2. **Trigeminal nerve** (V)—supplies the tensor tympani, which inserts into the malleus and tenses the tympanic membrane, thus preventing it from vibrating.

162. What is the pathway for the feedback loop?
When auditory input reaches the superior olive, it sends signals to the olivocochlear bundle via the VIII nerve, which then terminate on the outer hair cells or afferent fibers in the spiral ganglia.

163. What is Meniere's disease?
Meniere's disease causes the symptomatic triad of episodic vertigo, tinnitus, and hearing loss. It is caused by an increased amount of endolymph in the scala media. Pathologically, hair cells degenerate in the macula and vestibule.

Eye Movements

164. What is the paramedian pontine reticular formation (PPRF)?
The PPRF is a collection of cells lying in the pons adjacent to the nucleus of cranial nerve VI, and is an important center for horizontal gaze. Efferent fibers from the PPRF project to the ipsilateral abducens (VI) nucleus, and to the contralateral oculomotor (III) nucleus via the medial longitudinal fasciculus (MLF), stimulating both eyes to move horizontally.

165. What is the difference between saccades and smooth pursuit movements?
Saccades are fast conjugate eye movements under voluntary control. Saccades are generated in the contralateral frontal lobe (Brodmann's area 8). Smooth pursuits are slow involuntary movements of eyes fixed on a moving target. Pursuit movements to one side are generated in the ipsilateral occipital lobe (Brodmann's areas 18 and 19).

166. What is the pathway for saccades?
Fibers from the frontal eye field (Brodmann's area 8) pass through the genu of the internal capsule, decussate at the level of the upper pons, and synapse in the PPRF.

167. What is the pathway for smooth pursuit?
The pathway for smooth pursuit is not clearly defined but appears to arise in the anterior occipital lobe (Brodmann's areas 18 and 19) and travel to the ipsilateral PPRF.

168. What is the brainstem area for vertical gaze?
Near the superior colliculus, there are subtectal and pretectal centers that control vertical eye movements and project to cranial nuclei III, IV, and VI.

169. What are the pathways for voluntary vertical eye movements?
Vertical movements are driven symmetrically from both frontal lobes. When activated bilaterally, fibers from Brodmann's area 8 project via the frontopontine tract to act upon bilateral cranial nuclei III, IV, and VI, which then innervate their respective muscles.

CEREBELLUM

170. Describe the anatomic divisions of the cerebellum.
The cerebellum is anatomically divided into the two hemispheres, the midline vermis, and the flocculonodulus.

171. What are the functions of each cerebellar "lobe"?
The hemispheres are involved in appendicular control, the vermis is involved in axial control, and the flocculonodular lobe is involved in vestibular balance.

172. What are the three layers of the cerebellar cortex?
(1) The outermost molecular cell layer, (2) the middle Purkinje cell layer, and (3) the innermost granular cell layer.

173. What types of cells are located in each of these layers?
The **molecular layer** contains (1) stellate cells, (2) basket cells, (3) dendrites of Purkinje cells, (4) dendrites of Golgi type II cells, and (5) axons of granule cells. The **Purkinje layer** contains the cell bodies of Purkinje cells. The **granular layer** contains (6) granule cells, (7) Golgi type II cells, and (8) glomeruli (synaptic complexes that contain mossy fibers, axons and dendrites of Golgi type II cells, and dendrites of granule cells).

174. What is the afferent fiber from the inferior olives? Through which peduncle does it reach the cerebellum?
The afferent fiber from the inferior olives is the climbing fiber. It enters the cerebellum through the inferior cerebellar peduncle.

175. What is Molleret's triangle?
Molleret's triangle is a physiologic connection between the red nucleus, inferior olives, and dentate nucleus of the cerebellum. A lesion in this pathway can cause palatal myoclonus.

176. What are the deep nuclei of the cerebellum (medial to lateral)?
Medial to lateral, the cerebellar deep nuclei are: fastigial, globus, emboliform, and dentate.

177. What are the primary inputs and outputs of the cerebellum?
Cerebellar function can be conceptualized as a feedback loop, with input arriving from an origin, synapsing in a cerebellar nucleus, and then projecting back, often to the same origin.

Cerebellar Connections

CEREBELLAR PEDUNCLE	CONNECTED TO:	TRACTS THAT RUN IN THE PEDUNCLE			
Superior (SCP)	Midbrain	Dentatorubrothalamic (DRT) and ventral spinocerebellar (VSC)			
Middle (MCP)	Pons	Corticopontocerebellar			
Inferior (ICP)	Medulla	All other tracts to/from the cerebellum			

ORIGIN	INFLOW TRACT	INFLOW PEDUNCLE	CEREBELLAR NUCLEUS	OUTFLOW PEDUNCLE	OUTFLOW TRACT	DESTINATION
Precentral gyrus	CPC	MCP	Dentate	SCP	DRT	Precentral gyrus
Spinal cord	SC	ICP	Fastigial	ICP	—	Vestibular nucleus
Vestibular nucleus	VC	ICP	Vestibular	ICP	LVS (MLF)	Spinal cord

Superior cerebellar peduncle = SCP; middle cerebellar peduncle = MCP; inferior cerebellar peduncle = ICP; corticopontocerebellar = CPC; spinocerebellar = SC; vestibulocerebellar = VC; lateral vestibulospinal = LVS; and medial longitudinal fasciculus = MLF.

178. Where do the frontopontocerebellar fibers travel in the internal capsule?
They travel in the anterior limb of the internal capsule.

179. Where do the frontopontocerebellar fibers synapse?
The fibers synapse in the mid-pons prior to decussating.

180. What type of fiber originating in the cerebellar cortex is inhibitory on the deep cerebellar nuclei?
Purkinje fibers originate in the cerebellar cortex and synapse on the deep nuclei as an inhibitory neuron.

181. Where does the dentatorubrothalamic tract synapse?
These fibers synapse in the ventrolateral (VL) nucleus of the thalamus before ascending to the cortex.

BASAL GANGLIA

182. What are the basal ganglia?
The basal ganglia are a collection of nuclei, largely concerned with motor control, composed primarily of the corpus striatum, and the lenticular complex.

183. What are the parts of the corpus striatum?
The corpus striatum is composed of the putamen and caudate.

184. What is the lenticular complex?
The lenticular complex, or lentiform nucleus, is composed of the globus pallidus and putamen.

185. Which structure is the lateral border of the caudate?
The anterior limb of the internal capsule is the lateral border of the caudate.

186. What is the major outflow of the basal ganglia?
The major outflow of the basal ganglia projects from the medial globus pallidus as a fiber bundle known as the lenticular fasciculus (Forel's field H2). Another bundle from the medial globus pallidus loops around the internal capsule as the ansa lenticularis. It then merges in Forel's field H with the lenticular fasciculus and with fibers from the dentatorubrothalamic tract. These fibers then continue as the thalamic fasciculus (Forel's field H1) and synapse in the thalamic nuclei: centromedian, ventral lateral, and ventral anterior. These thalamic nuclei then relay information up to the motor cortex.

187. Is there any other output from the medial globus pallidus?
Yes. Apart from the lenticular fasciculus and the ansa lenticularis, a third fiber tract leaves the medial globus pallidus as the pallidotegmental tract and descends onto the pedunculopontine nucleus in the midbrain, where neurons help to regulate posture. This is the only descending tract from the basal ganglia.

188. Is there any output from the basal ganglia that does not originate in the medial globus pallidus?
The only other output is a small tract (pallidosubthalamic fibers) that leaves the lateral globus pallidus to synapse in the subthalamic nucleus.

189. What is the major input to the basal ganglia?
The major input is from the motor cortex and the thalamic nuclei. The basal ganglia function, simplistically, as a feedback loop: cerebral cortex → basal ganglia → thalamus → cerebral cortex.

THALAMUS

190. What structure lies lateral to the thalamus? Medial to the thalamus?
The posterior limb of the internal capsule is the lateral border of the thalamus. The third ventricle lies medial to the thalamus.

191. What are the anatomic structures encountered by going medial to lateral starting from the massa intermedia?
Massa intermedia → thalamus → posterior limb of the internal capsule → globus pallidus → putamen → external capsule → extreme capsule

192. What is the anatomy of the thalamus?
The intermedullary lamina divides the thalamus into an anterior, medial, and lateral group. The lateral group is further divided into a ventral and dorsal tier. Each group contains specific nuclei:

    I. Anterior group
       1. Anterior nucleus
   II. Medial group
       1. Dorsomedial nucleus (DM)
  III. Lateral group
       1. Dorsal tier
          a. Lateral dorsal nucleus (LD)
          b. Lateral posterior nucleus (LP)
          c. Pulvinar
       2. Ventral tier
          a. Ventral anterior nucleus (VA)
          b. Ventral lateral nucleus (VL)
          c. Ventral posterolateral nucleus (VPL)
          d. Ventral posteromedial nucleus (VPM)
          e. Lateral geniculate (LG)
          f. Medial geniculate (MG)

    Other nuclei that are often considered part of the thalamus include (1) **reticular nucleus**—a small group of neurons that projects to other thalamic nuclei and may help regulate cortical activity; (2) **midline nuclei**—diffuse neurons connected to the hypothalamus; and (3) **centromedian (CM)**—an intralaminar nucleus that is part of the reticular formation which activates the cortex.

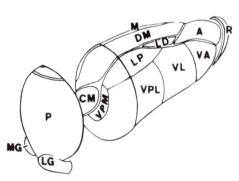

thalamic nuclei

R	reticular
M	midline
CM	centromedian
DM	dorsomedial (medial)
A	anterior
LD	lateral dorsal
LP	lateral posterior } dorsal tier
P	pulvinar
VA	ventral anterior
VL	ventral lateral
VPL	ventral posteriolateral
VPM	ventral posteriomedial } ventral tier
LG	lateral geniculate
MG	medial geniculate

Diagram of the major nuclei of the thalamus. (Reprinted with permission from Dunkerley GB: A Basic Atlas of the Human Nervous System. Philadelphia, F.A. Davis, 1975, p 89.)

193. What are the inputs and outputs to and from the main thalamic nuclei?

Connections of the Thalamic Nuclei

THALAMIC NUCLEUS	PRINCIPAL INPUT	PRINCIPAL OUTPUT	FUNCTION
LP	Parietal lobe	Parietal lobe	Sensory integration
LD	Cingulate gyrus	Cingulate gyrus	Emotional expression
Pulvinar	Association areas of cortex	Association areas of cortex	Sensory integration
DM	Amygdala, olfactory, and hypothalamus	Prefrontal cortex	Limbic
MG	Auditory relay nuclei (from inf. colliculus)	Auditory cortex– area 41,42	Hearing
LG	Optic tract	Visual cortex–area 17	Vision
Anterior	Mammillary body	Cingulate gyrus	Limbic
VA	Globus pallidus	Premotor cortex	Motor
VL	Cerebellum	Premotor and motor cortices	Motor
VPM	Trigeminal lemniscus	Post central gyrus	Somatic sensation (face)
VPL	Medial lemniscus and spinothalamic	Post central gyrus	Somatic sensation (body)
CM	Reticular formation, globus pallidus, hypothalamus	Basal ganglia (striatum)	Sensory integration, smell, limbic

194. What is the limbic "lobe"?
The limbic lobe is not a true lobe of the brain but rather a functional collection of structures that regulate higher activities such as memory and emotion. It is commonly said to include: (1) cingulate gyrus, (2) parahippocampal gyrus, (3) hippocampal gyrus, and (4) uncus.

195. What is Papez's circuit?
This is a route by which the limbic system communicates between the hippocampus, thalamus, hypothalamus, and cortex. It forms a circuit form the hippocampal formation → fornix → mammillary body → mammillothalamic tract → anterior group of thalamus → cingulate gyrus → cingulate bundle → hippocampus (**Note**: the amygdala is not part of the classic Papez circuit).

OLFACTION

196. What are the olfactory receptor cells?
The receptor cells are bipolar neurons that pass from the olfactory mucosa through the cribiform plate to the olfactory bulb. Collectively, the central processes of the olfactory receptor cells constitute cranial nerve I.

197. What is the anatomy of the olfactory pathway?
1. In the olfactory bulb, the axons of receptor cells synapse on dendrites of mitral and tufted cells (forming a "glomerulus").

2. The axons of mitral and tufted cells compose the olfactory tract, which soon divides into medial and lateral stria. Medial stria fibers cross to the contralateral side via the anterior commissure, while the lateral stria fibers terminate in the anterior perforated substance, amygdaloid complex and lateral olfactory gyrus (which is the primary olfactory cortex).

3. From the lateral olfactory gyrus (prepiriform area), fibers project to the entorhinal cortex, the medial dorsal nucleus of the thalamus, and the hypothalamus.

198. What is unique about the projection of olfactory information to the cerebral cortex?
Unlike other sensory modalities, olfaction reaches the cortex without relay through the thalamus.

199. What are the most common causes of anosmia?
1. Rhinitis/nasal congestion
2. Smoking
3. Head injury
4. Craniotomy
5. Subarachnoid hemorrhage
6. Meningiomas of the olfactory groove
7. Zinc and vitamin A deficiency
8. Hypothyroidism
9. Congenital (Kallmann's syndrome)
10. Dementing diseases (Alzheimer's, Parkinson's)
11. Multiple sclerosis

VISION

200. What is the arrangement of cones and rods in the retina?
The six million cones are concentrated toward the center and the 120 million rods are in the periphery of the retina. In the fovea, located centrally within the macula, each cone is served by a single ganglion cell, resulting in very high resolution. In the periphery, many rods project to a single ganglion cell, giving high sensitivity but lower resolution.

201. What are the primary functions of rods?
Rods are concerned with night vision and are most sensitive between the blue and green wavelengths.

202. What are the primary functions of cones?
Cones are concerned with color vision and daytime vision. The three types of cones are tuned, via visual pigments, to different frequencies in the blue, green, and red wavelength ranges.

203. What is the afferent pathway for the pupillary light reflex?
Retinal ganglion cells concerned with the light reflex travel with the optic nerve and tract and then break away to project down to the midbrain pretectal nucleus. From the pretectal nucleus, fibers project bilaterally, decussating via the posterior commissure to each Edinger-Westphal nucleus.

204. Which nucleus mediates pupil constriction?
The Edinger-Westphal nucleus, or preganglionic parasympathetic nucleus of cranial nerve III, mediates pupillary constriction.

205. What is the pathway for pupillary dilatation?
This pathway has three neurons. First-order fibers descend from the ipsilateral hypothalamus through the brainstem and cervical cord to T1–T2. They synapse on ipsilateral preganglionic

sympathetic fibers, exit the cord, travel up the sympathetic chain as second-order neurons to the superior cervical ganglion, and then synapse on postganglionic sympathetic fibers. The third-order neurons travel via the internal carotid artery to the orbit and innervate the radial smooth muscle of the iris.

206. What is Horner's syndrome?
Horner's syndrome is an interruption of the sympathetic supply to the eye, resulting in the classic triad of ptosis, miosis, and anhydrosis.

207. Describe the pharmacologic tests to diagnose Horner's syndrome.
Instill 2% cocaine solution in both eyes, which will dilate the pupils by preventing the reuptake of the sympathetic neurotransmitter norepinephrine. If one eye fails to dilate, then a diagnosis of Horner's syndrome can be made, since failure to dilate would mean there has been an interruption of the sympathetic supply (norepinephrine) to that eye. To further localize the lesion, one can use amphetamine in the affected eye, since this displaces norepinephrine from the nerve terminal and dilates the pupil. If the pupil dilates in response to this test, then the lesion is affecting the third-order neuron, causing denervation hypersensitivity. Otherwise, the lesion is in the first- or second-order neurons.

208. What is the anatomy of the lesion that causes an afferent pupillary defect?
An afferent pupillary defect means the pupil will not react to light. The lesion must be prechiasmal, and almost always involves the optic nerve.

209. What is the test for an afferent pupillary defect (Marcus Gunn pupil)?
The swinging flashlight test determines an afferent pupillary defect. Shine a light into the normal eye and the pupil constricts (the affected eye will also constrict consensually). Quickly move the light onto the opposite affected eye, and the pupil will be seen to dilate. Removing the light from the normal pupil causes it and the affected pupil, responding consensually, to dilate. The affected pupil will thus seem to be dilating when the swinging light hits it.

210. What is the value of the pupillary reflex for diagnosing third-nerve palsies?
Because the parasympathetic fibers travel along the outside of the third nerve, they are usually damaged by nerve compression, resulting in pupillary dilatation. Third-nerve palsies that cause pupillary dilatation are usually masses (tumors, aneurysms, etc.), whereas those palsies that do not involve the pupil are usually medical (ischemia, vasculitis, etc.).

211. What is the pathway for pupillary constriction that occurs with convergence?
The pathway begins in the occipital lobe (Brodmann's area 18) and projects to the Edinger-Westphal nucleus bilaterally. The details of how pupils constrict during convergence are poorly understood.

212. What is an Argyll Robertson pupil?
An Argyll Robertson pupil, one form of light-near dissociation, is an irregular pupil that does not constrict to light but does constrict to accommodation. This finding is quite specific for CNS syphilis. Light-near dissociation with a regular pupil can be found in many diseases and is not specific for CNS syphilis.

213. What is the pathway of the optic nerve?
The ganglion cells from the nasal half of the retina travel in the optic nerve, where they decussate in the optic chiasm and join the contralateral optic tract to the lateral geniculate

body. The ganglion cells from the temporal half of the retina travel in the optic nerve, stay in the ipsilateral optic tract, and project to the lateral geniculate body. In this way, the contralateral visual field is projected from each eye to the lateral geniculate body.

214. What thalamic nucleus is concerned with vision?
The lateral geniculate body is the thalamic nucleus that handles vision.

215.   What is the pathway of the optic radiation?
Second-order neurons from the lateral geniculate body project to the calcarine cortex (Brodmann's area 17). The superior visual field fibers wrap around the temporal horn on their way to the inferior lip of the calcarine fissure. The macular area is served by the most medial area of the calcarine cortex.

Visual Fields

216. Where is the lesion that causes a field defect in only one eye?
If only one eye is affected, the lesion must be prechiasmal.

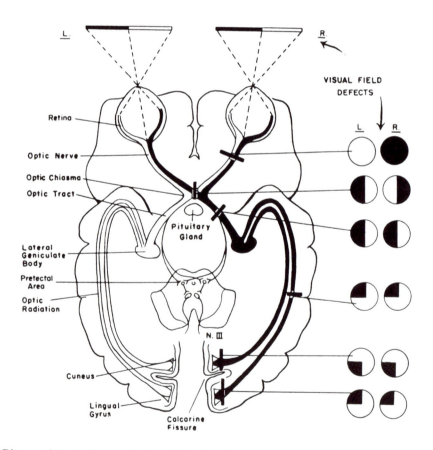

Diagram of the visual system showing the location of lesions responsible for the most common visual field defects. (Reprinted with permission from Gilman S, Newman SW: Manter and Gatz's Essentials of Clinical Neuroanatomy and Neurophysiology, 5th ed. Philadelphia, F.A. Davis, 1978, p 113.)

217. Where is the lesion that causes left homonymous hemianopsia? Bitemporal hemianopsia? Binasal hemianopsia?

Left homonymous hemianopsia can arise from the right optic tract, right lateral geniculate body, right optic radiations, or the right occipital cortex. **Bitemporal hemianopsia** is caused by midline chiasmal lesions such as pituitary lesions (from below) or craniopharyngeal tumors (from above). **Binasal hemianopsia** can be caused only by simultaneous lesions on the lateral optic nerves or chiasm, such as bilateral internal carotid artery aneurysms.

218. What is a junctional scotoma?

A junctional scotoma results from a lesion at the junction of the optic nerve and chiasm. It causes an ipsilateral central scotoma and a superior temporal defect in the other eye. It occurs because some optic nerve fibers from the inferior temporal retina, when they decussate in the chiasm, travel forward for a few millimeters in the contralateral nerve; they are thus affected by a lesion in that nerve.

219. Where is the lesion that causes superior quadrantanopsia?

Superior quadrantanopsia usually results from damage to the inferior optic radiations. This may occur in Meyer's loop, which is the bundle of inferior optic radiations that swings forward into the temporal lobe.

220. What visual field results from a right occipital lobe infarction?

A right occipital lobe infarction causes a left homonymous hemianopsia with macular sparing.

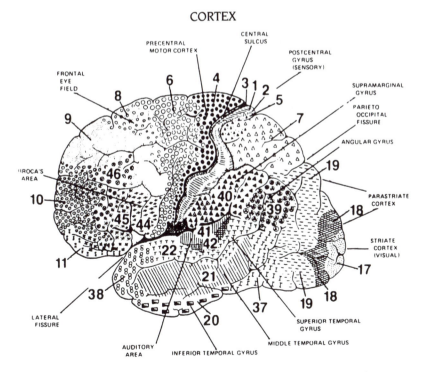

The superficial anatomy of the cerebral cortex showing Brodmann's areas. *(Continued on next page.)*

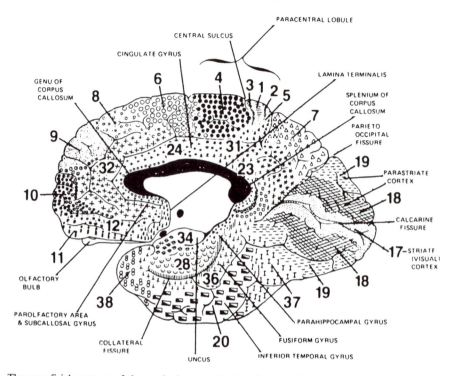

The superficial anatomy of the cerebral cortex showing Brodmann's areas *(Continued)*. (Reprinted with permission from Garoutte B: Survey of Functional Neuroanatomy, 2nd ed. Greenbrae, CA, Jones Medical Publications, 1992, p 144.)

221. What are the layers of the cerebral cortex?
The layers of the cerebral cortex are:

I. Molecular layer	IV. Inner granular layer
II. Outer granular layer	V. Inner pyramidal or ganglion layer
III. Outer pyramidal layer	VI. Multiform layer

Afferent fibers activated by various sensory stimuli terminate in layers IV, III, and II. These signals are then transmitted to adjacent superficial and deep layers through multiple interconnections. All the efferent fibers originate in layer V.

222. What is the columnar organization of the cortex?
Cortical neurons are arranged in cylindrical columns, each containing 100–300 neurons, which are heavily interconnected up and down through the cortical layers. Throughout the somatosensory system, cells responding to one modality are grouped together in the columns. All neurons in the column receive input from the same area and therefore comprise an elementary functional module of cortex.

223. What is the line of Gennari?
The fourth layer of the occipital cortex in area 17 is divided by a greatly thickened band of myelinated fibers, which is grossly visible and is called the line of Gennari. This stripe also gives the name of striate cortex to that area of the brain. Brodmann's areas 18 and 19 lack the line of Gennari.

224. In what cortical cell layer are the Betz cells located?
Betz cells give rise to efferent motor tracts (corticospinal fibers) and lie in cortical layer 5.

225. What is the function of the frontal lobe?
The frontal lobes (both right and left) are involved in voluntary eye movements, somatic motor control, planning and sequencing of movements, and emotional affect. The left frontal lobe is crucial for motor control of speech (Broca's area).

226. What is the function of the temporal lobe?
The temporal lobes (both right and left) handle auditory and visual perception, learning and memory, emotional affect, and olfaction. The dominant temporal lobe influences comprehension of speech (Wernicke's area). The nondominant temporal lobe mediates prosody and spatial relationships.

227. What is the function of the parietal lobe?
The parietal lobes (both right and left) handle cortical sensation, motor control, and visual perception. The dominant parietal lobe also handles ideomotor praxis. The nondominant parietal lobe controls spatial orientation.

228. What is the function of the occipital lobe?
The occipital lobes (both right and left) mainly handle visual perception and involuntary smooth pursuit eye movements.

229. In which lobe is visual-spatial information processed?
It is mainly processed in the nondominant parietal lobe.

230. Where is language processed?
Language is primarily processed in Broca's area (posterior inferior frontal gyrus, Brodmann's area 44) and Wernicke's area (posterior part of the superior temporal gyrus, posterior part of Brodmann's area 22), in the dominant hemisphere.

231. Where is the lesion that causes achromatopsia?
Achromatopsia results from a lesion of the dominant occipital lobe (Brodmann's area 18) and is a feature of the syndrome of alexia without agraphia.

232. What is Exner's area?
Exner's area lies superior to Broca's area, in Brodmann's area 8; if damaged, agraphia without aphasia results.

CIRCULATION

233. What is meant by the terms anterior and posterior circulation?
The anterior circulation refers to the common carotid and its distal ramifications, including the internal carotid, middle cerebral, and anterior cerebral arteries. The posterior circulation refers to the vertebral and basilar arteries and their branches, including the posterior cerebral artery.

234. Which vessels make up the circle of Willis?
1. The **anterior circulation**, composed of the middle cerebral arteries, anterior cerebral arteries, and the anterior communicating artery which connects the two anterior cerebral arteries.

2. The **posterior circulation**, composed of the posterior cerebral arteries.

3. The **posterior communicating artery**, which connects the middle cerebral with the posterior cerebral arteries, thus forming a true "circle."

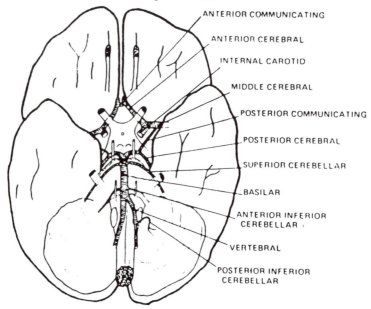

ANTERIOR COMMUNICATING

ANTERIOR CEREBRAL

INTERNAL CAROTID

MIDDLE CEREBRAL

POSTERIOR COMMUNICATING

POSTERIOR CEREBRAL

SUPERIOR CEREBELLAR

BASILAR

ANTERIOR INFERIOR CEREBELLAR

VERTEBRAL

POSTERIOR INFERIOR CEREBELLAR

Diagram of the blood vessels that form the circle of Willis at the base of the brain. (Reprinted with permission from Garoutte B: Survey of Functional Neuroanatomy, 2nd ed. Greenbrae, CA, Jones Medical Publications, 1992, p 15.)

235. If the right anterior cerebral artery is occluded proximally, how would the circle of Willis protect the patient from becoming symptomatic?

If the occlusion were slow enough for the blood flow to accommodate, the right anterior cerebral artery could receive blood from the contralateral internal carotid, via the left anterior cerebral and anterior communicating arteries.

236. What region is supplied by the anterior cerebral artery? Middle cerebral artery? Posterior cerebral artery?

The **anterior cerebral artery** supplies the medial (midline) cerebral hemispheres, superior frontal lobes, and superior parietal lobes. The **middle cerebral artery** supplies the inferior frontal, inferolateral parietal, and lateral temporal lobes. The **posterior cerebral artery** supplies the occipital lobes and medial temporal lobes.

237. What is the first intracranial branch off of the internal carotid artery?

The ophthalmic artery.

238. What is the origin of the anterolateral artery?

The anterolateral perforating vessels usually branch off of the middle cerebral artery, but sometimes they arise from the internal carotids.

239. What is the name of the artery that supplies the genu of the internal capsule?

The recurrent artery of Heubner, which is one of the named anteromedial lenticulostriate arteries, supplies the genu of the internal capsule.

240. Which artery is the first branch off of the basilar artery?
The anterior inferior cerebral artery (AICA).

241. What is the blood supply to the brainstem?
The brainstem receives its blood supply exclusively from the posterior circulation, including the vertebrals and basilar artery. The medulla receives its blood supply from the vertebrals via medial and lateral perforating arteries. The pons and midbrain receive their blood from the basilar via the medial and lateral perforating arteries.

242. What is the blood supply to the cerebellum?
The cerebellum receives its blood supply from the three cerebellar vessels:
1. Posterior inferior cerebellar artery (PICA), off of the vertebrals.
2. Anterior inferior cerebellar artery (AICA), the first branch off of the basilar.
3. Superior cerebellar artery (SCA), the last branch off of the basilar.

243. Which nerves exit the brainstem area between the posterior cerebral aretry and superior cerebellar artery?
Cranial nerve III exits between the vessels medially, whereas cranial nerve IV exits between them laterally. Aneurysms of these blood vessels may thus damage these cranial nerves.

244. What is the blood supply to the thalamus?
The thalamus receives its blood supply mainly from the posterior circulation. It is irrigated by the thalamogeniculate artery, posterior choroidal artery, and paramedian artery.

CEREBROSPINAL FLUID (CSF)

245. What anatomic structure or structures produce CSF?
The majority of CSF is produced by the choroid plexus. A small amount of CSF is also produced by the blood vessels in the subependymal region and pia.

246. Where is the choroid plexus located?
The choroid plexus is located within the ventricular system, mainly in the lateral and fourth ventricles.

247. What is the rate of CSF production?
The rate is approximately 25 cc/hr (approximately 500 cc/day).

248. How much CSF does an average adult normally have?
The average male adult has approximately 100–150 cc of CSF.

249. What is communicating hydrocephalus? Noncommunicating hydrocephalus?
Communicating hydrocephalus occurs when there is dilatation of the ventricles due to obstruction of CSF flow outside the ventricular system (i.e., distal to the foramen of Magendie), so the CSF communicates with the subarachnoid space. Noncommunicating hydrocephalus occurs when there is dilatation of the ventricles due to an obstruction of CSF flow within the ventricular system at or above the foramen of Magendie.

250. What is the route of CSF from production to clearance?
Choroid plexus → lateral ventricle → interventricular foramen of Monro → third ventricle → cerebral aqueduct of Sylvius → fourth ventricle → two lateral foramina of Luschka and one medial foramen of Magendie → subarachnoid space → arachnoid granulations → dural sinus → venous drainage.

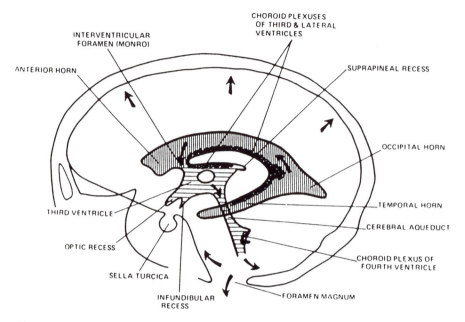

CHOROID PLEXUSES
OF THIRD & LATERAL
VENTRICLES

INTERVENTRICULAR
FORAMEN (MONRO)

ANTERIOR HORN

SUPRAPINEAL RECESS

OCCIPITAL HORN

TEMPORAL HORN

THIRD VENTRICLE

CEREBRAL AQUEDUCT

OPTIC RECESS

CHOROID PLEXUS OF
FOURTH VENTRICLE

SELLA TURCICA

INFUNDIBULAR
RECESS

FORAMEN MAGNUM

Diagram of cerebrospinal fluid. (Reprinted with permission from Garoutte B: Survey of Functional Neuroanatomy, 2nd ed. Greenbrae, CA, Jones Medical Publications, 1992, p 27.)

251. What space is invaded by a lumbar puncture?
During a lumbar puncture, the needle enters the subarachnoid space.

252. What is the ideal spinal level to do a lumbar puncture?
The ideal level for a lumber puncture is below the conus medullaris at approximately vertebral level L4–L5.

BIBLIOGRAPHY

1. Adams R, Victor M: Principles of Neurology, 4th ed. New York, McGraw-Hill, 1989.
2. Carpenter D: Human Neuroanatomy, 8th ed. New York, Macmillan, 1990.
3. Dunkerley GB: A Basic Atlas of the Human Nervous System. Philadelphia, F.A. Davis, 1975.
4. Garoutte B: Survey of Functional Neuroantomy, 2nd ed. Greeenbrae, CA, Jones Medical Publications, 1992.
5. Gilman S, Newman SW: Manter and Gatz's Essentials of Clinical Neuroanatomy and Neurophysiology, 8th ed. Philadelphia, F.A. Davis, 1992.
6. Kandel E, Schwartz JH, Jessell TM (eds): Principles of Neuroscience, 3rd ed. New York, Elsevier,
   1991.
7. Plum F, Posner J: The Diagnosis of Stupor and Coma, 3rd ed. Philadelphia, F.A. Davis, 1986.
8. Tindall B: Aids to the Examination of the Peripheral Nervous System. London, W.B. Saunders,
   1990.

2. APPROACH TO THE PATIENT WITH NEUROLOGIC DISEASE

Loren A. Rolak, M.D.

1. What is the first question to be answered in any patient with neurologic disease?
Where is the lesion? The neurologist, unlike most other physicians, approaches patients from an anatomic perspective, leaving issues of physiology and etiology to be addressed later. The first step when evaluating patients with neurologic symptoms is to localize the lesion to a specific part of the nervous system.

2. What is the best way to localize a lesion?
The history and physical examination accurately localize most lesions of the nervous system. The brain is unique among organs for its high degree of specialization. Because each part of the peripheral nerves, spinal cord, and brain have such specialized functions, damage to each region produces unique clinical deficits. Identification of specific signs and symptoms therefore permits localization, sometimes within a millimeter, to discrete parts of the nervous system. Pioneer neurologists of the past century referred to the brain as "eloquent"—it speaks directly to the clinician.

3. What are the most important regions for anatomic localization?
For clinical purposes, the great complexity of neuroanatomy can be simplified to a few major regions. Lesions should be localized to one of these regions:
1. Muscle
2. Neuromuscular junction
3. Peripheral nerve
4. Root
5. Spinal cord
6. Brainstem
7. Cerebellum
8. Subcortical brain
9. Cortical brain

4. How are symptoms localized to these neuroanatomic regions?
The history is the most important part of the neurologic evaluation of a patient. Although precise localizing information can be gleaned from the neurologic physical examination, asking the proper questions during the history accurately localizes most neurologic lesions.

A helpful system for diagnosis is to begin distally and ask patients questions about each part of the neurologic anatomy, working proximally through the muscle, neuromuscular junction, peripheral nerve, root, spinal cord, cerebellum, brainstem, subcortex, and ending with the cortex of the brain. By sequentially asking about each of these areas, the patient can be "examined" thoroughly. If localization of the lesion is still not clear after a careful history directed at each anatomic region, do not begin the physical examination yet—go back and take a better history!

5. Which clinical features of muscle disease can be elicited by history?
Muscle disease (myopathy) causes proximal symmetric weakness without sensory loss. Questions should therefore elicit these symptoms.
1. **Proximal leg weakness:** Can the patient get out of a car, off of the toilet, or up from a chair without using his hands?
2. **Proximal arm weakness:** Can the patient lift or carry objects such as grocery bags, garbage bags, young children, school books, or briefcases?
3. **Symmetric weakness:** Does the weakness affect both arms or both legs? (Although generalized processes such as myopathies are often slightly asymmetric, weakness confined to one limb or one side of the body is seldom caused by a myopathy.)

4. **Normal sensation:** Is there numbness or other sensory loss? (Although pain and cramping may occur in some myopathies, actual sensory changes should not occur with any disease that is confined to the muscle.)

6. After a history of muscle disease is elicited, what findings can be expected on physical examination?
The examination should show proximal symmetric weakness without sensory loss. The muscles are usually normal in size, without atrophy or fasciculations, and muscle tone is usually normal or mildly decreased. Reflexes are also normal or mildly decreased.

7. Which clinical features of neuromuscular junction disease can be elicited by history?
Fatigability is the hallmark of diseases affecting the neuromuscular junction. Although these disorders resemble myopathies, causing proximal symmetric weakness without sensory loss, the weakness worsens with use and recovers with rest. Because strength improves with rest, fatigability does not usually manifest itself as a steadily progressive decline in function, but rather it presents as waxing and waning weakness. When the muscles fatigue, the patient must rest, leading to recovery of strength, which permits further use of the muscles, causing fatigue, which necessitates rest and recovery again, etc. This worsening with use and recovery with rest produces a variability or fluctuation in strength that is highly characteristic of neuromuscular junction diseases.

8. After a history of neuromuscular junction problems is elicited, what findings can be expected on physical examination?
Examination should show fatigable proximal symmetric weakness without sensory loss. Repetitive testing weakens the muscles, which regain their strength after a brief period of rest. Sustained muscular activity may also lead to fatigability, such as the development of ptosis with persistent upward gaze. The weakness is often extremely proximal, involving muscles of the face, eyes, and jaw. The muscles are normal in size, without atrophy or fasciculations, with normal tone and reflexes. There is no sensory loss.

9. Which clinical features of peripheral neuropathies can be elicited by history?
Unlike myopathies and neuromuscular junction disease, weakness caused by peripheral neuropathies is often distal rather than proximal. It is also often asymmetric and accompanied by atrophy and fasciculations. Sensory changes almost always accompany neuropathies. The history should elicit these symptoms.
    1. **Distal leg weakness:** Does the patient trip, drag his feet, or wear out the toes of his shoes?
    2. **Distal arm weakness:** Does the patient frequently drop things or have trouble with his grip?
    3. **Asymmetric weakness:** Are the symptoms confined to one localized area? (Some neuropathies cause a symmetric stocking-and-glove weakness and numbness, especially those due to metabolic conditions such as diabetes. However, most neuropathies are asymmetric.)
    4. **Denervation changes:** Is there a wasting or shrinkage of the muscle (atrophy) or quivering and twitching within the muscle (fasciculations)?
    5. **Sensory changes:** Has the patient felt numbness, tingling, or paresthesias?

10. After a history of peripheral neuropathy is elicited, what findings can be expected on physical examination?
Examination should reveal distal, often asymmetric weakness with atrophy, fasciculations, and sensory loss. Muscle tone may be normal but is often decreased. Reflexes are usually diminished. Because involvement of autonomic fibers frequently occurs in peripheral

neuropathies, there may be trophic changes as well, such as smooth, shiny skin, vasomotor changes such as swelling or temperature dysregulation, and loss of hair or nails.

11. Which clinical features of root diseases (radiculopathies) can be elicited by history?
Pain is the hallmark of root disease. Otherwise, radiculopathies often resemble peripheral neuropathies because of their asymmetric weakness with evidence of denervation (atrophy and fasciculations) and sensory loss. The weakness, while asymmetric, may be either proximal or distal, depending upon which roots are involved. (The most common radiculopathies in the legs affect the L5 and S1 roots, causing distal weakness, whereas the most common radiculopathies in the arms affect the C5 and C6 roots, which innervate proximal regions.) The history should therefore elicit symptoms similar to a neuropathy with the added component of pain. The pain is usually described as sharp, stabbing, hot, and electric, and it typically shoots or radiates down the limb.

12. After a history of a radiculopathy is elicited, what findings can be expected on physical examination?
As is the case with a peripheral neuropathy, the physical examination will show asymmetric muscle weakness with atrophy and fasciculations. Tone is normal or decreased, and the reflexes in the involved muscles are diminished or absent. Weakness is confined to one myotomal group of muscles, such as those innervated by the C6 root in the arm or the L5 root in the leg. Similarly, sensory loss occurs in a dermatomal distribution. Maneuvers that stretch the root often aggravate the pain, such as straight leg raising, or neck rotation.

13. Which clinical features of spinal cord disease can be elicited by history?
Spinal cord lesions usually cause a triad of symptoms:
   1. **A sensory level is the hallmark of spinal cord disease.** Patients usually describe a sharp line or band around their abdomen or trunk, below which there is a decrease in sensation. The symptom of a sensory level is essentially pathognomonic for spinal cord disease.
   2. **Distal, symmetric, spastic weakness.** The muscle, neuromuscular junction, nerves, and roots all make up the peripheral nervous system, but the spinal cord is in the central nervous system and so has special motor properties. Damage to the spinal cord produces upper motor neuron lesions, affecting the pyramidal (or corticospinal) tract. However, the weakness mimics that of a peripheral neuropathy, because it is distal more than proximal. In actual clinical practice, almost all processes affecting the cord are symmetric. Upper motor neuron lesions cause spasticity, but this increase in tone may cause few noticeable symptoms—it is best extracted from the history by asking about stiffness in the legs.
   3. **Bowel and bladder problems.** Sphincter dysfunction commonly accompanies cord lesions because of involvement of the autonomic fibers within the cord.

14. Which questions should be asked during the history to elicit the symptoms of spinal cord disease?
   1. **Distal leg weakness:** Does the patient drag his toes or trip?
   2. **Distal arm weakness:** Does the patient drop things or have trouble with his grip?
   3. **Symmetric symptoms:** Does the process involve the arms and/or legs approximately equally?
   4. **Sensory level:** Is a sensory level present? Patients often describe this as a band, belt, girdle, or tightness around their trunk or abdomen.
   5. **Sphincter dysfunction:** Is there retention or incontinence of the bowel or bladder? (The bladder is usually involved earlier, more often, and more severely than the bowel in spinal cord lesions.)

15. After a history of spinal cord disease is elicited, what findings can be expected on physical examination?

The physical examination in a patient with spinal cord disease usually shows a sensory level below which all sensory modalities are diminished. The sensory (and motor) tracts in the spinal cord are somatotopically organized, meaning that there is a distinctive anatomic layering and lamination to the pathways that result in fibers from the legs and lower part of the body suffering the most damage in the majority of spinal cord lesions. Because most leg fibers lie laterally and are easily compressed, spinal disease usually affects the legs more than the arms. Also, because of this organization, the level of the symptoms detected clinically does not always correspond to the true anatomic site of the damage. For example, a mass pressing on the spinal cord may cause a sensory level and weakness any place at or below the actual anatomic level of the lesion.

The patient may also have urinary retention or incontinence, and may lose superficial reflexes, including the anal wink, bulbocavernosus, and cremasteric reflexes. The examination shows evidence of upper motor neuron damage:

1. Weakness that is distal greater than proximal
2. Weakness of extensors and antigravity muscles greater than flexors
3. Increased tone (spasticity)
4. Increased reflexes
5. Clonus
6. Extensor plantar responses (positive Babinski signs)
7. Absent superficial reflexes
8. No significant atrophy or fasciculations

16. Which clinical features of brainstem disease can be elicited by history?

Cranial nerve symptoms characterize brainstem disease. The brainstem is essentially the spinal cord with cranial nerves embedded in it, so brainstem lesions cause many of the symptoms of spinal cord disease accompanied by symptoms of cranial nerve impairment.

Like the spinal cord, the brainstem contains "long tracts," a term given to the pathways that extend from the brain down through the spinal cord. The major long tracts are the pyramidal (corticospinal) tract for motor function, the spinothalamic tract carrying pain and temperature sensations up to the thalamus, and the dorsal columns carrying position and vibration sense up to the thalamus. Because of the decussation of these tracts, lesions in the brainstem do not produce a horizontal motor or sensory level as they do in the spinal cord, but rather produce a vertical motor or sensory level—that is, a hemiparesis or hemianesthesia affecting one side of the body.

Lesions affecting the cranial nerves in the brainstem often produce symptoms referred to as the "Ds":

Symptoms of Cranial Nerve Damage

CRANIAL NERVE	SYMPTOMS
III	Diplopia
IV	Diplopia
V	Decreased facial sensation
VI	Diplopia
VII	Decreased strength and drooping of the face
VIII	Deafness and dizziness
IX	Dysarthria and dysphagia
X	Dysarthria and dysphagia
XI	Decreased strength in neck and shoulders
XII	Dysarthria and dysphagia

17. Which questions are asked to elicit symptoms of combined cranial nerve and long tract dysfunction?

1. **Long tract signs:** Does the patient have hemiparesis or hemisensory loss?

2. **Cranial nerve signs:** Does the patient have diplopia, dysarthria, dysphagia, dizziness, deafness, or decreased strength or sensation over the face?

3. **Crossed signs:** Because the long tracts cross but the cranial nerves generally do not, brainstem lesions often produce symptoms on one side of the face and the opposite side of the body. For example, a lesion in the pons that affects the pyramidal tracts and the facial (VII) nerve will cause weakness of that side of the face and the opposite, crossed side of the body. Brainstem disease often produces bilateral or crossed findings.

18. After a history of brainstem disease is elicited, what findings can be expected on physical examination?

The physical examination in brainstem disease is almost like a mathematical equation: cranial nerves + long tracts = brainstem disease.

Examination of the cranial nerves may reveal ptosis, pupillary abnormalities, extraocular muscle paralysis, diplopia, nystagmus, decreased corneal and blink reflexes, facial weakness or numbness, deafness, vertigo, dysarthria, dysphagia, weakness or deviation of the palate, decreased gag reflex, or weakness of the neck, shoulders, or tongue.

Long tract abnormalities may include hemiparesis, which will show an upper motor neuron pattern of distal extensor weakness with hyperreflexia, spasticity, and a positive Babinski sign. Hemisensory loss may occur to all modalities.

19. Which clinical features of cerebellar disease can be elicited by history?

Cerebellar disease causes incoordination, clumsiness, and tremor, because the cerebellum is responsible for smoothing out and refining voluntary movements. Questions should therefore focus on these symptoms:

1. **Clumsiness in the legs:** Does the patient have a staggering, drunken walk? (Most laymen describe cerebellar symptoms in terms of alcohol and drunkenness, probably because drinking alcohol impairs the cerebellum. The characteristic ataxic, wide-based, staggering gait of the person intoxicated by alcohol is a reflection of his cerebellar dysfunction.)

2. **Clumsiness in the arms:** Does the patient have difficulty with targeted movements, such as lighting a cigarette or placing a key in a lock? (Cerebellar tremor is worse with voluntary, intentional movements that require accurate placement.)

3. **Brainstem symptoms:** Are brainstem symptoms present? (Because the cerebellar inflow and outflow must pass through the brainstem, and the blood supply to the cerebellum arises from the same vessels that supply the brainstem, cerebellar disease is almost always accompanied by some brainstem abnormalities as well, and vice versa.)

20. After a history of cerebellar disease is elicited, what findings can be expected on physical examination?

The patient's gait will be staggering, wide-based, and ataxic, causing difficulties especially with tandem walking. Patients may require support to avoid falling. Fine coordinated movements of the legs are impossible, such as sliding a heel down a shin or tracing patterns on the floor with the foot. The cerebellar tremor is most visible in the upper extremities, which waver and wobble when attempting to touch a specific target, such as the examiner's finger or the patient's own nose. Rapid alternating movements are irregular in rate and rhythm.

21. How can the history determine whether disease of the brain is subcortical or cortical?

The history can differentiate subcortical from cortical disease by focusing upon four major areas:

1. The presence of specific cortical deficits
2. The pattern of motor and sensory deficits
3. The type of sensory deficits
4. The presence of visual field deficits

22. What specific deficits are seen with cortical lesions?
The most useful symptom of cortical disease in the dominant (usually left) hemisphere is aphasia. The history should therefore focus on any difficulties with language functions, including not only speech but also writing, reading, and comprehension. A lesion affecting the left side of the brain that does not affect language function is unlikely to be cortical.

In the nondominant (usually right) hemisphere, cortical dysfunction is more subtle but usually causes visual-spatial problems. Patients with nondominant cortical lesions often have neglect and denial, including inattention to their own physical signs and symptoms. This can be a difficult finding to elicit on history, however, and sometimes depends upon the physical examination.

23. How does the pattern of motor and sensory deficits differentiate cortical from subcortical involvement?
The motor homunculus in the primary and supplemental motor strips is spread upside-down over a vast expanse of gray matter. Neurons controlling the lower extremities reside between the two hemispheres, in the interhemispheric fissure, whereas neurons moving the trunk, arms, and face are draped upside-down over the superficial cortex. Cortical lesions therefore often involve the face, arm, and trunk, but spare the legs, which are "protected" in the interhemispheric fissure. Cortical lesions thus cause an incomplete hemiparesis, affecting the face and arm but not the leg.

Of course, fibers to the leg descend and merge with those to the face and arm as the pyramidal tract forms deep within the brain, subcortically, to run in the internal capsule, cerebral peduncles, and the pyramids themselves. Therefore, even a small subcortical lesion can affect all of these conjoined fibers. Subcortical lesions thus will cause a compelte hemiparesis, affecting face, arm, and leg.

The sensory homunculus has a similar somatotopic arrangement that results in an analogous pattern of localization.

24. How does the type of sensory deficit differentiate cortical from subcortical lesions by history?
Most of the primary sensory modalities reach "consciousness" in the thalamus and do not require the cortex for their perception. A patient with severe cortical damage can still feel pain, touch, vibration, and position. A history of significant numbness or sensory loss therefore suggests a subcortical lesion.

Cortical sensory loss is more refined and usually involves complicated sensory processing such as two-point discrimination, accurate localization of perceptions, stereognosis, and graphesthesia. These symptoms can be difficult to elicit by history alone.

25. How do visual symptoms differentiate cortical from subcortical disease by history?
Visual pathways run subcortically for most of their length. Visual impulses in the optic nerves may cross in the chiasm and run through the optic tracts, lateral geniculate bodies, and optic radiations before synapsing in the occipital cortex. Cortical lesions, such as those affecting the motor strip, sensory strip, language areas, etc., are too superficial to affect these visual fibers, and thus do not cause visual field deficits. Subcortical lesions often affect the visual fibers, producing visual field cuts. Therefore, a history of visual field loss suggests a subcortical lesion. (Of course, a strictly cortical lesion in the occipital lobes will produce visual symptoms, but it will not affect motor, sensory, or other functions and so will not cause confusion with the typical picture of a subcortical lesion.)

26. After a history of cortical or subcortical disease is elicited, what findings can be expected on physical examination?

Physical examination findings parallel the historical deficits.

1. **Cortical dysfunction:** The patient may show aphasia or visual-spatial dysfunction.

2. **Motor involvement:** Physical examination shows upper motor neuron weakness affecting the face and arm in a cortical lesion, and the face, arm and leg in a subcortical lesion.

3. **Sensory dysfunction:** In subcortical disease, the examination shows problems with primary sensory modalities, such as decreased pinprick and vibration, but in cortical disease it shows relatively normal sensation with impaired higher sensory processing, such as graphesthesia and astereognosis.

4. **Visual dysfunction:** Patients with subcortical disease may have visual field cuts, but patients with cortical disease will not.

27. How accurate is the history and physical examination for diagnosing neurologic disease?

The clinical examination is very accurate in localizing neurologic disease. Once a localization has been made to one of these broad anatomic regions, an etiology usually suggests itself. For example, if a lesion can be localized to the peripheral nerve, it is usually easy to develop a differential diagnosis for peripheral neuropathies (such as diabetes, alcoholism, etc.) and develop a diagnostic plan (blood testing, nerve conduction studies, etc.). The anatomy usually implies an etiology.

Organized questioning and examination of the nervous system in this fashion are an excellent way to approach the neurologic patient.

BIBLIOGRAPHY

1. Caplan L: The Effective Clinical Neurologist. Cambridge, Blackwell Scientific Publications, 1990.
2. Haerer A: Dejong's The Neurologic Examination, 5th ed. Philadelphia, J.B. Lippincott, 1992.

3. MYOPATHIES

Yadollah Harati, M.D., FACP

1. What conditions are covered under the myopathies?
Myopathies are diseases of the muscle that cause acute, subacute, and chronic weakness, myalgia, muscle spasms and stiffness, asthenia and fatigue, or myoglobinuria.

2. What are the most important myopathies?
- Muscular dystrophies: Duchenne's, myotonic, etc.
- Congenital myopathies: Kearns-Sayre, central-core, etc.
- Inflammatory myopathies: polymyositis, dermatomyositis, etc.
- Toxic myopathies: alcohol, zidovudine, etc.
- Endocrine myopathies: hypothyroidism, hypoadrenalism, etc.
- Infectious myopathies: trichinosis, AIDS, etc.

3. What is a motor unit?
A motor unit consists of a motor neuron, its single axon and terminal axon branches, and the many muscle fibers that they supply. Muscle fibers belonging to a single motor unit are all of the same histochemical type.

4. What is the embryonic origin of skeletal muscles?
Muscles develop from mesodermal cell populations arising in the somite. The connective tissues around the muscles have a different embryologic origin and are derived from the somatopleural mesoderm.

5. What is a myoblast, a myotube, and a myofiber?
A **myoblast** is a postmitotic, mononucleated cell capable of fusion and contractile protein synthesis. **Myotubes** are long, cylindrical, multinucleated (syncytial) cells formed from the fusion of myoblasts. When their central nuclei are shifted to a subsarcolemmal position in the later stages of development, they are called **myofibers.** The appearance of central nuclei within an otherwise normal adult muscle is a useful sign of muscle regeneration. Each adult myofiber is packed with numerous **myofibrils,** largely composed of hexagonal arrangements of thick and thin contractile filaments. Myosin is the major constituent of the thick filaments, whereas actin is the contractile protein of the thin filaments.

6. What are the most valuable tests for evaluating patients with suspected muscle disease?
A diagnosis can often be established by supporting the clinical findings with results from three key tests: (1) serum creatine kinase (CK) levels, (2) electromyography (EMG), and (3) muscle biopsy.

7. In a quick survey of motor function in a patient with a suspected myopathy, what are the minimum maneuvers the patient must perform?
1. Arise from a chair with arms folded.
2. Walk the length of the examining room on toes, on heels, and tandem.
3. Hop on either foot.
4. Bend and arise in deep knee bends.
5. Step on a step.
6. Horizontally abduct arms and reach the vertex of the head.
7. Lift up head from table.
8. Arise from supine position with hands over head.
9. Lift head and shoulders, and extend the neck while in a prone position.

8. How many fiber types are recognized by muscle histochemistry?

Type 1 = slow-twitch, red fibers. Type 2 = fast-twitch, white fibers. Type 2 fibers are also divided into subgroups, the two major ones being type 2A and 2B.

9. What is the differential diagnosis of a myopathy with elevated serum CK levels in an adult?

Myopathies with increased CK levels include:
- Inflammatory myopathies (e.g., polymyositis-dermatomyositis)
- Alcoholic myopathy
- Drug-induced myopathies (clofibrate, aminocaproic acid, lovastatin and similar drugs)
- Infectious myopathies (AIDS, trichinosis, toxoplasmosis)
- Hypothyroid myopathy
- Metabolic myopathies (acid-maltase deficiency, late-onset myophosphorylase or phosphofructokinase deficiency)
- Genetic myopathies (e.g., Becker's muscular dystrophy, limb-girdle muscular dystrophy)

10. During an EMG study, the slightest movement of the needle evokes prolonged waxing-and-waning trains of high-frequency spikes and positive waves. What are these discharges called? In which conditions are they characteristically seen?

These are myotonic discharges. They occur because the muscle fibers continue to fire repetitively after stimulation. Myotonic discharges occur in myotonia congenita, paramyotonia congenita, myotonic dystrophy, Schwartz-Jampel syndrome, myopathy with infantile and adult forms of acid maltase deficiency, and hyperkalemic periodic paralysis. Of these, myotonia congenita is due to abnormal chloride channel function, whereas paramyotonia congenita, hyperkalemic periodic paralysis, and Schwartz-Jampel syndrome are caused by abnormal sodium channel function. Myotonia in myotonic dystrophy and acid maltase deficiency are caused by other, not fully understood, membrane defects.

11. Your elderly patient had a left cerebral infarction with right hemiplegia 1 month ago. For some reason he had an EMG of all limbs, the report of which indicates moderate numbers of fibrillation potentials in muscles of the right extremities. Do you believe this report?

You should not. Fibrillation potentials are not found when muscle atrophy or weakness is a result of a disease of the central nervous system.

12. For several years a 35-year-old man has had transient painless slowing of hand movements following clenching and unclenching of his fists ("my fingers won't open"). Percussion with a hammer does not induce myotonia, and immersion of the forearm in cold water does not influence the stiffness. Insertion of an EMG needle into the thenar and hypothenar muscles is "silent," and no myotonic discharges are seen. What does this patient have?

The patient has Lambert-Brody or Brody's syndrome, first described by Lambert in 1957 as impaired muscle relaxation and "silent myotonia," and later by Brody, who demonstrated a markedly reduced calcium uptake by isolated sarcoplasmic reticulum. All reported patients were male and had inherited the condition through an autosomal recessive or X-linked recessive mode.

Lambert-Brody symptoms develop during the first decade of life and consist of progressive exercise-induced stiffness and cramping in most arm and leg muscles. EMG shows no abnormalities, and muscle biopsy shows only mild, nonspecific, type 2 fiber atrophy with a normal ultrastructural appearance. There is severe reduction in calcium-ATPase, which is responsible for calcium reaccumulation by sarcoplasmic reticulum in type

2 muscle fibers. This explains why impaired relaxation is noted only after phasic exercise when primarily type 2 (fast twitch) motor units are recruited.

Karpati G, et al: Myopathy caused by a deficiency of calcium-adensine triphosphate in sarcoplasmic reticulum (Brody's disease). Ann Neurol 20:33–49, 1986.

13. A 19-year-old male with a history of exercise-induced severe muscle cramps and exercise intolerance was forced by his trainer in a military camp to run up 50 flights of stairs. A few hours later, he noted a dark (Coca-Cola colored) urine, and had fever, chills, and severe muscle soreness. A CBC showed a normal WBC count, mild anemia, and an increased reticulocyte count. What is the differential diagnosis in this patient?

The patient most likely has muscle phosphofructokinase (PFK) deficiency (type VII glycogenolysis, or Tarui's disease). He could have McArdle's disease, but hemolytic anemia with an elevated reticulocyte count strongly favors the former diagnosis. Normally, erythrocyte PFK is composed of both muscle (M) type and RBC (R) type subunits. Patients with PFK deficiency lack the M subunit. The inheritance pattern in most cases of PFK deficiency is autosomal recessive, and reduced erythrocyte PFK activity may be demonstrated in otherwise asymptomatic parents. Muscle PFK deficiency results in blockage of glycolysis. Clinical manifestations of PFK deficiency closely resemble those of McArdle's disease, and include exercise intolerance that develops soon after vigorous activity and causes muscle fatigue, stiffness, and pain; it resolves at rest within a few minutes to several hours.

14. What is the differential diagnosis of the adult form of acid-maltase deficiency?

This condition (type II glycogenosis) is caused by a genetically determined deficiency of the lysosomal enzyme alphaglycosidase (acid maltase) and produces dissimilar diseases in infants (Pompe's disease) and adults. The adult form, presenting in the third and fifth decade of life with insidious painless limb-girdle weakness, is frequently misdiagnosed as polymyositis, motor neuron disease, myotonic dystrophy, or limb-girdle muscular dystrophy. The respiratory muscles are disproportionately affected. Because there is usually a mildly elevated CK and the EMG findings may resemble those found in polymyositis, a muscle biopsy is most helpful in the diagnosis. Characteristically, there are muscle fibers with vacuoles filled with PAS-positive material with a prominent acid phosphatase activity. Similar vacuoles also occur in chloroquine myopathy.

15. What is the treatment for McArdle's disease?

The treatment of McArdle's disease begins with counseling about the risks of exercise-induced rhabdomyolysis. Patients should be instructed to adjust their lifestyles to avoid strenuous exercise, and to seek prompt medical attention and treatment if myoglobinuria develops. Treatments aimed at bypassing the biochemical block by supplying the muscle with a glycolytic intermediate (i.e., glucose, fructose) appear to increase work capacity in some patients, but their long-term use results in undesirable weight gain and usually proves disappointing. Injection of glucagon to promote hepatic glycogenolysis and to increase blood glucose concentration has inconsistent results, and its repeated injection is objectionable for prolonged treatment. High-fat and low-carbohydrate diets have no demonstrable effect. However, diets high in amino acids (especially alanine) may be beneficial. In vivo P31-NMR spectroscopy and exercise performance are partially normalized by a high-protein diet, but are unaffected by intravenous amino acid infusion. This finding suggests that intramuscular protein stores are providing an alternative energy substrate and are capable of partially correcting the metabolic deficits.

16. How is a forearm ischemic exercise test performed?

This simple provocative test, the forearm ischemic exercise test for lactate production, is used to diagnose McArdle's disease and similar conditions producing a metabolic block anywhere along the glycogenolytic or glycolytic pathway.

The ischemic exercise test is easy to perform. While the patient is at rest, blood is drawn for the "baseline" levels of ammonia and lactate. A blood pressure cuff is then placed over the upper arm and inflated to a pressure greater than systolic, rendering the forearm ischemic. The patient immediately begins repetitive, rapid grip exercises. With strong encouragement, normal subjects are able to tolerate ischemic exercise for as long as 180 seconds before pain and fatigue cause discontinuation of the test. Patients with disorders of glycogen metabolism seldom exercise more than 60 seconds. When the patient fatigues, the blood pressure cuff is released and 1 minute later blood is drawn from the exercised arm. Similar samples are drawn again at 2, 4, 6, 10, and 14 minutes following the end of exercise. Normal subjects exhibit a three- to fivefold increase in lactate levels within 5 minutes after the end of exercise, with a full return to baseline level in about 30 minutes. Failed lactate production suggests a metabolic block.

The venous level of ammonia also rises during ischemic exercise; failure of the two to rise together suggests an inadequate test. Normal lactate but impaired ammonia production suggests myoadenylate deaminase deficiency or a related disorder of purine nucleotide metabolism.

17. Provide a classification for muscle disorders causing complaints of "muscle cramp" and pain.

Muscle Disorders That Cause Muscle Cramp and Pain

    I. Disorders Resulting from Deficient Muscle Fuel Utilization
       "Muscle cramp" resulting from glycogen metabolism abnormalities
          Myophosphorylase deficiency (type V glycogenosis)
          Phosphofructokinase deficiency (type VII glycogenosis)
          Phosphorylase b kinase deficiency (type VIII glycogenosis)
          Phosphoglycerate kinase deficiency (type IX glycogenosis)
          Muscle phosphoglycerate mutase deficiency (type X glycogenosis)
          Lactate dehydrogenase deficiency (type XI glycogenosis)
       "Muscle cramp" resulting from lipid metabolism abnormalities
          Carnitine palmityltransferase 1 deficiency
          Carnitine palmityltransferase 2 deficiency
       Myalgia resulting from purine nucleotide metabolism
          Myoadenylate deaminase deficiency

   II. Disorders Resulting from Other Muscle Dysfunctions
       "Muscle cramp" resulting from dysfunction of sarcoplasmic reticulum
          Lambert-Brody syndrome
       Myalgia associated with other muscle dysfunctions
          Myalgia associated with tubular aggregates
          Myalgia with intracellular acidosis
          Myalgia with abnormal structure or function of mitochondria
          Myalgia with low myosin ATPase and phosphocreatine content
          Myalgia with type 2 muscle fiber predominance

  III. Myotonic Disorders

Myotonia congenita	Hypokalemic
Thomsen's disease (autosomal dominant)	Normo- or hyperkalemic
Recessive type	(adynamia episodica)
With painful cramps (autosomal dominant)	Schwartz-Jampel syndrome
Myotonic dystrophy (autosomal dominant)	Acquired myotonia
Paramyotonia congenita	Drug-induced
(autosomal dominant)	Associated with malignancy
Periodic paralysis (autosomal dominant)	

18. A patient with AIDS on AZT is complaining of myalgia and weakness. What is wrong?
The exact diagnosis in this setting is often difficult. Myalgia and increased CK is frequently encountered in patients with AIDS, and some patients have a symmetric and predominately proximal muscle weakness. EMG findings are those usually seen in polymyositis. Many patients have typical muscle biopsy findings of polymyositis (necrotic fibers, with perimysial, endomysial, and perivascular lymphocytic infiltration). Zidovudine (AZT) therapy is also associated with myopathy, which is chiefly characterized by muscle wasting and proximal weakness, and tends to occur in individuals who have been treated with high doses of the drug for more than 6 months. Muscle biopsy, however, may show changes suggestive of a mitochondrial disorder. Numerous "ragged-red" fibers, indicative of abnormal mitochondria, may be seen. Rods (nemaline) and cytoplasmic bodies may also be seen. Both the myopathy and the biopsy abnormalities improve with the discontinuation of AZT. It is thought that AZT causes inhibition of the mitochondrial DNA polymerase, which causes depletion of mitochondrial DNA, resulting in myopathy.
    Dalakas MC, et al: Mitochondrial myopathy caused by long-term zidovudine therapy. N Engl J Med 322:1098–1105, 1990.

19. Describe the salient features of the Duchenne's muscular dystrophy gene.
The gene is large (2.5×10^6 base pairs), located in the short arm of the X-chromosome, and is expressed in skeletal, cardiac and smooth muscle cells, neurons, glia, and myotubes. It is by far the largest gene characterized to date, occupying approximately 1% of the human X chromosome. The size of the gene makes it a very large target for random mutational events. Mutations within it cause Duchenne's muscular dystrophy (DMD), Becker's muscular dystrophy (BMD), X-linked myoglobinuria, and quadriceps myopathy. In about two-thirds of cases of DMD-BMD, the gene, which codes for a structural protein called dystrophin, has a major mutation, 90% being deletions and 10% duplications.

20. What are the characteristics of the myotonic dystrophy gene?
The mutation in myotonic dystrophy is an expansion of a trinucleotide (CTG) repeat in the protein kinase gene on the long arm of chromosome 19. In normal individuals, the number of repeats is less than 37, whereas in myotonic dystrophy it ranges from 50 to a few thousand. The size of the expanded repeat closely correlates with the severity and age of onset of myotonic dystrophy, and generally increases in successive generations within a family, providing a molecular basis for the clinically observed phenomenon known as "anticipation" (progressively earlier onset of the disease in successive generations). The exact consequences of the mutation at the molecular level are currently under investigation.

21. What are the muscular manifestations of sarcoidosis?
Patients with sarcoidosis may have focal or generalized myopathies. Many patients (about 65%) have asymptomatic granuloma of muscles, but less than 1% of patients have any progressive muscle weakness or elevated CK. Calf muscles may be enlarged or tender. The EMG may show myopathic changes. In both symptomatic and asymptomatic patients, muscle biopsy shows typical sarcoid granuloma. The presence of such granulomatous changes may be the earliest or the only manifestations of sarcoidosis. Most patients respond to moderate doses of corticosteroids.

22. What are the most important congenital myopathies?
1. Central-core disease
2. Nemaline myopathy
3. Centronuclear myopathy
4. Congenital fiber type disproportion
5. Reducing-body myopathy
6. Myopathy associated with tubular aggregates
7. Fingerprint-body myopathy
9. Sarcotubular myopathy
8. Multi-core myopathy
10. Trilaminar myopathy
11. Cytoplasmic body myopathy
12. Familial myopathy with lysis of myofibril in type I fibers

All the above myopathies have a number of common clinical characteristics. Their presentation in infancy is associated with hypotonia. Early muscle weakness is the main clinical manifestation, although in some the onset of weakness may be delayed into adulthood. Some are also associated with discrete skeletal deformities or other somatic features, such as scoliosis, elongated faces, and high-arched palate.

23. Is there a relation between malignant hyperthermia and central-core disease?

Central-core disease is a congenital myopathy. Malignant hyperthermia is a reaction to general anesthetics. Both conditions are transmitted by an autosomal dominant pattern of inheritance. Some patients with central-core disease are susceptible to malignant hyperthermia, and the genes for both diseases are located next to each other on chromosome 19 (19 q12–q13.2). Patients with central-core disease and their family members must be cautioned about the possibility of malignant hyperthermia reactions to anesthetics.

24. What are the most important factors when performing a muscle biopsy for histochemical studies?

1. **Selection of a muscle for biopsy.** This is the most important aspect of a muscle biopsy. The selected muscle must be mild to moderately weak, free of previous trauma (e.g., EMG needle, injection, previous biopsy), unaffected by other unrelated processes, and not subject to heavy work (e.g., gastrocnemius muscle). The three commonly selected muscles for biopsy are biceps, vastus lateralis, and deltoid.

2. **Biopsy procedure.** This procedure must be done by a surgeon or a trained neuromuscular specialist who understands the need for the careful and gentle handling of tissue sample and avoids conditions that can generate artifacts. Muscle specimens should be removed in strips (1–2 cm long and 0.5 cm wide), with the center of the specimen untouched, and then placed on a lightly saline-moistened gauze. The specimen must arrive at the laboratory no later than 30–60 minutes after the biopsy. Immediately flash-frozen sections may be submitted to the laboratory from long distances in a proper container of dry ice.

3. **Processing the specimen.** Paraffin sections are not suitable for histochemistry. Properly prepared frozen sections are required for this purpose, although ice-crystal artifacts may occur.

25. Which conditions are associated with muscle hypertrophy?

1. Duchenne's muscular dystrophy
2. Becker's muscular dystrophy
3. Limb-girdle dystrophy
4. Myotonia congenita
5. Chronic spinal muscular atrophy
6. Cysticercosis
7. Amyloidosis
8. Childhood type of acid maltase deficiency
9. Myopathy of congenital hypothyroidism (Kocher-Debre-Semelaigne)
10. Hereditary motor-sensory neuropathy
11. Chronic relapsing inflammatory polyneuropathy
12. Focal mononeuropathy (focal hypertrophy)
13. Radiculopathy (focal hypertrophy)

26. What is myokymia?

Myokymia is the continuous undulation of a group of muscle fibers caused by the successive spontaneous contraction of motor units. On EMG, they appear as groups of 2–10 potentials, firing at 5–60 Hz, recurring regularly at 0.2–10-second intervals. Myokymia, frequently observed in facial muscles, occurs in a number of brainstem diseases, especially multiple sclerosis, radiation-induced nerve damages, chronic peripheral nerve disorders, and Isaacs' syndrome.

27. What are "ragged-red" fibers?
A muscle fiber that shows an increased red-staining at the subsarcolemmal and intermyofibrillar region on staining with modified Gomori's trichorome stain is called a ragged-red fiber. The red-stained material is mitochondria. The mitochondria usually are abnormal in size and structure when seen by electron microscopy. Collections of glycogen and lipid are conspicuous in the ragged-red fibers. Although ragged-red fibers are typically seen in mitochondrial myopathies, they may also occur in a number of other conditions and in the muscle biopsies of normal-aged individuals as an isolated, nonspecific finding.

28. What are the most important myopathies due to point mutations in mitochondrial DNA?
   1. Myoclonic epilepsy with ragged-red fibers (MERRF)
   2. Mitochondrial encephalomyopathy with lactic acidosis and stroke (MELAS)
   3. Some myopathies with cardiomyopathy

29. What does this muscle biopsy photograph signify?

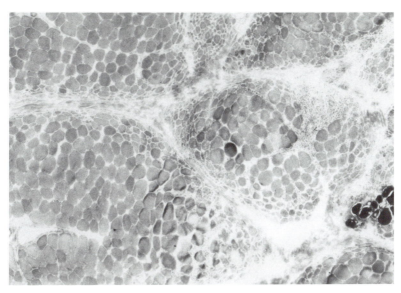

This is the typical finding of "perifascicular atrophy." The muscle fibers at the periphery of the muscle fascicles are smaller, whereas the fibers in the deepest part of the fascicle are of normal size. This type of atrophy is generally recognized to be a conspicuous feature of childhood dermatomyositis, and, to a lesser extent, adult dermatomyositis. Even in the absence of inflammation, this biopsy is characteristic. This pattern of atrophy is probably due to capillary changes and involves mainly muscle fibers near the perimysial connective tissue, because these fibers are less likely to have collateral circulation.

30. How are the polymyositis and dermatomyositis syndromes classified?
   I Adult polymyositis and dermatomyositis
  II Childhood and juvenile dermatomyositis
  III Dermatomyositis associated with other diseases (connective tissue disorders, malignancy)
  IV Polymyositis associated with other diseases (connective tissue diseases, malignancy)
  V Inclusion-body myositis (myopathy)

31. What are the major pathologic changes on light microscopy in the muscle biopsies of patients with polymyositis (PM), dermatomyositis (DM), and inclusion-body myopathy (IBM)?

Both PM and DM have:
1. Inflammatory infiltrate
   Perivascular (more in DM)
   Endomysial or perimysial (more in DM)
2. Fiber necrosis, phagocytosis
3. Perifascicular atrophy (especially in DM of childhood)
4. Variation and rounding of muscle fibers; occasional angular and atrophic fibers
5. Capillary loss or necrosis (in DM)
6. Eosinophilic cytoplasmic inclusions and rimmed vacuoles, denervation changes, and interstitial infiltration (in IBM)

32. What is the differential diagnosis of a patient who presents with chronic bilateral distal leg weakness?

1. Neurogenic causes:
   Distal chronic spinal muscular atrophy
   Neuronal forms of Charcot-Marie-Tooth disease
   Motor neuropathies
2. Myopathic causes:
   Myotonic dystrophy
   Inclusion-body myopathy
   Nemaline myopathy
   Central-core disease
   Centronuclear myopathy
   Welander's myopathy (distal arm weakness begins earlier than leg weakness)

Most myopathies have an unexplained predilection for proximal muscles, and a myopathy presenting with distal muscle weakness is considered rare.

33. What is armadillo disease?

It is another name for Isaacs' syndrome.

34. What is Isaacs' syndrome (neuromyotonia)?

Isaacs' syndrome has been described under several other names, including myokymia with impaired muscle relaxation, neuromyotonia, pseudomyotonia, quantal squander, armadillo disease, and continuous muscle fiber activity. The onset is typically during the second or third decade of life, both sexes are affected equally, and complaints include muscle stiffness, intermittent cramping, and difficulty chewing, speaking, and even breathing. Ocular muscles and sphincters function normally, and sensation is not affected.

The most remarkable feature of Isaacs' syndrome is myokymia. In Isaacs' syndrome the skeletal muscles, especially of distal limbs, are in continuous, although variable, myokymia. Repetitive passive limb movement leads to increasing resistance and pain, but repetitive voluntary activity tends to increase muscle mobility, although temporarily. The cramps and myokymic movements persist during sleep. Some patients display marked hyperhidrosis, muscle hypertrophy, or elevated CK. Detailed laboratory and cerebrospinal fluid evaluations typically are normal.

The etiology of this syndrome remains unknown. Recently, it has been suggested that the syndrome may be caused by an antibody directed against the presynaptic nerve terminals' ion channels.

EMG studies of Isaacs' syndrome show spontaneous and continuous long, irregularly-occurring trains of variably formed discharges that originate in the proximal parts of nerves. Fasciculation, doublets, or multiplets, firing at intervals of about 20 msec, may also be present. Because of the clinical and electrophysiologic similarities of Isaacs' syndrome to hyperventilation-induced tetany, it is essential that all patients suspected to have Isaacs' syndrome have calcium, phosphorus, and blood gas studies, as well as investigations of clinical and electrophysiologic effects of hyperventilation.

Successful symptomatic treatment has been achieved with phenytoin (300–400 mg/day) or carbamazepine (200 mg TID, QID). Some patients may respond favorably to plasma exchange. Diazepam, clonazepam, and baclofen are of no benefit. Patients often remain well on therapy over many years, leading normal lives, as demonstrated by Isaacs' own 10-year follow-up report of his original cases.

35. What is eosinophilia-myalgia syndrome (EMS)?
EMS is a clinically heterogeneous syndrome characterized by myalgia and fatigue, associated with a variable combination of the following: eosinophilia, eosinophilic pneumonia, edema, fasciitis, alopecia, sclerodermatous skin changes, myopathy, arthralgia, and neuropathy. Some patients suffer from chronic myalgia, muscle cramps, and fatigue with the variable presence of cardiac, neurologic, hematologic, dermatologic, and pulmonary complications.

EMS occurred as a transient epidemic in 1989 and 1990, affecting more than 1500 users of L-tryptophan. The epidemic has been linked with the use of a single manufacturer's product that contained several contaminants: the exact toxin and its mechanism of action remain undefined. EMS shares many features with the Spanish "toxic oil syndrome," and both appear to be chronic, contaminant-induced immune-mediated disorders.

36. What are the three major symptoms of the periodic paralysis?
(1) Transient attacks of weakness, (2) myotonia (symptomatic only in potassium-sensitive periodic paralysis), and (3) interattack weakness, which may be progressive.

37. How are the different types of periodic paralysis classified?
1. Primary: hypokalemic, hyperkalemic, or normokalemic.
2. Secondary: potassium depletion, potassium retention, thyrotoxic (hypokalemic), hypernatremia with defective thirst in hypothalamic lesions, or barium poisoning.

This, or similar clinical classifications, however, may undergo significant changes in the near future as the understanding of the genetic basis of these conditions is further enhanced. For example, current evidence suggests that the potassium-sensitive periodic paralyses, and the myotonic disorder paramyotonia congenita, are the result of single-base-pair changes in the alpha subunit of the skeletal muscle sodium channel gene. The gene abnormalities result in single amino acid substitutions in highly conserved regions of the sodium channel. The clinical variations of the diseases associated with the sodium channel gene, therefore, may be explained by a number of different allelic mutations.

38. What is the treatment for periodic paralysis?
Acetazolamide, a carbonic anhydrase inhibitor, is effective in some patients with each form of periodic paralysis. Its effect on the prevention of attacks of hypokalemic periodic paralysis, which is usually provoked by measures that lower the plasma potassium level, is particularly dramatic. Another carbonic anhydrase inhibitor, dichlorphenamide, may be more effective than acetazolamide in preventing the attacks and reducing interattack weakness. Patients who are intolerant of carbonic anhydrase inhibitors may benefit from potassium-sparing diuretics such as spironolactone and triamterene. A low-carbohydrate and low-sodium diet is generally recommended for patients with hypokalemic periodic paralysis. In hyperkalemic periodic paralysis, inhalation of albuterol, a beta-adrenergic agonist, may prevent the attack in some patients. Ingestion of a high-carbohydrate, low-postassium diet may also alleviate the attacks.

39. What is the approach to evaluating a persistent but incidental elevation of serum creatine kinase?

  1. Determine the origin of the enzyme by isoenzyme testing: MB (cardiac), BB (brain), or muscle (MM).

  2. If MM, consider the following:
  • Acquired myopathy (metabolic, inflammatory)
  • Drugs (cholesterol-lowering agents, alcohol, licorice)
  • Muscle trauma (needle injection, EMG, surgery, ischemia, vigorous exercise, or contusion)
  • Neurogenic disease (motor neuron disease)

  3. Perform an EMG if symptoms of weakness, myalgia, cramps, or tenderness are present.

  4. If EMG is abnormal, perform a muscle biopsy.

  5. If biopsy shows a specific disease (e.g., myositis, glycogen-storage disease, or dystrophy), treat accordingly.

  6. If the EMG is normal and the elevation of CK persists, but the history and physical examinations are completely normal, follow the patient periodically. A muscle biopsy in this circumstance rarely yields useful information.

40. What are the clinical features of myopathic carnitine deficiency?

Carnitine deficiency causes a slowly progressive limb, neck, and trunk muscle weakness beginning in early childhood or mid-adult life. Cardiomyopathy (sometimes fatal) and a peripheral neuropathy may also be seen, but myalgias and muscle cramps do not occur. The muscle, but not serum or liver, carnitine level (free and acyl) is usually reduced, and there is an excess of lipid globules in muscle fibers. Treatment with regular oral intake of carnitine usually results in improvement of muscle strength.

41. What are the most important myotoxic drugs?

  1. Clofibrate and other cholesterol-lowering agents
  2. Chloroquine
  3. Emetine
  4. Ethanol
  5. Epsilon-amino-caproic acid
  6. D-penicillamine
  7. Phenformin
  8. Zidovudine

42. Which drugs cause an inflammatory myopathy?

A painful inflammatory myopathy develops in some patients treated with D-penicillamine or procainamide.

BIBLIOGRAPHY

1. Brooke M: A Clinician's View of Neuromuscular Disease, 2nd ed. Baltimore, Williams & Wilkins, 1986.
2. Engel AG, Banker BQ: Myology. New York, McGraw-Hill, 1986.
3. Harati Y, McKinley K: Cramps and myalgias. In Jankovic J, Tolosa E (eds): Movement Disorders. Baltimore, Williams & Wilkins, 1993.
4. Walton J: Disorders of Voluntary Muscle, 4th ed. Oxford, Churchill Livingstone, 1988.

4. NEUROMUSCULAR JUNCTION DISEASES

Tetsuo Ashizawa, M.D.

ANATOMY AND PHYSIOLOGY

1. What are the presynaptic events of neuromuscular transmission?
When the action potential reaches the presynaptic nerve terminal, voltage-gated calcium channels open, allowing Ca^{2+} influx. This triggers release of acetylcholine from presynaptic vesicles into the synaptic cleft.

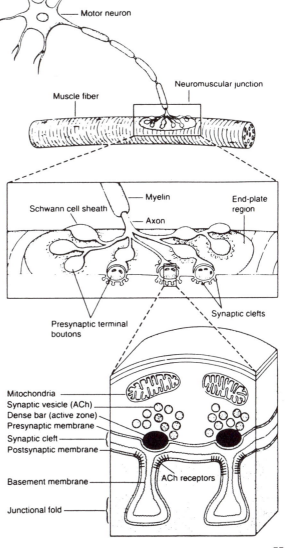

Diagram of the neuromuscular junction. (Reprinted with permission from Kandel ER, Schwartz JH, Jessel TM (eds): Principles of Neural Science. New York, Elsevier, 1991, p 136.)

2. What are the events in the synaptic cleft during neuromuscular transmission?
After acetylcholine molecules are released, diffusion of the molecules allows some of them to reach the postsynaptic membrane and bind the acetylcholine receptors. Acetylcholine esterase in the neuromuscular junction then catalyzes the hydrolysis of acetylcholine into choline and acetic acid. Choline is subject to uptake by the presynaptic nerve terminal and used for the synthesis of new acetylcholine, regulated by the enzyme choline acetyltransferase.

3. What are the postsynaptic events of neuromuscular transmission?
Binding of acetylcholine to the acetylcholine receptor opens a channel within the receptor molecule, allowing Na^+ influx and generating endplate potentials at the postsynaptic membrane. The amplitude of the endplate potential is proportional to the number of the receptors activated. When a sufficient number of acetylcholine receptors are activated at the same time, the endplate potential becomes large enough to trigger an action potential. The action potential then propagates along the muscle sarcoplasmic membrane to the T-system, leading to the release of Ca^{2+} from the sarcoplasmic reticulum and muscle contraction.

4. What is the active zone?
The active zone is a specialized area of the presynaptic nerve terminal membrane, visualized by freeze-fracture technique as a structure consisting of particles aligned in two rows in parallel. The particles are thought to represent L-type voltage-gated Ca^{2+} channels.

Engel AG, Fukuoka T, Lang B, et al: Lambert-Eaton myasthenic syndrome IgG: Early morphologic effects and immunolocalization at the motor endplate. Ann NY Acad Sci 505:333–345, 1987.

MYASTHENIA GRAVIS

5. What neuromuscular diseases demonstrate autoimmunity directed against constituents at the neuromuscular junction?
Myasthenia gravis (MG) and Lambert-Eaton myasthenic syndrome (LEMS) are the two diseases in which autoantibodies play a key pathogenic role at the neuromuscular junction. Recent studies also suggest the presence of autoimmune reactions at the neuromuscular junction in amyotrophic lateral sclerosis (ALS).

Smith RG, Hamilton S, Hofmann F, et al: Serum antibodies to L-type calcium channels in patients with amyotrophic lateral sclerosis. N Engl J Med 327:1721–1728, 1992.

6. What are the neuromuscular manifestations of MG?
Patients with MG often have variable degrees of weakness and easy fatigability of skeletal muscles. Skeletal muscle weakness may or may not be present at rest but increases after sustained or repetitive exercise. The exercise-induced weakness improves rather dramatically after short rest. Extraocular muscles, bulbar muscles, and limb muscles often exhibit fatigability that is easily detectable on clinical examination.

7. What are the epidemiologic characteristics (incidence, sex differences, age of onset, familial occurrences, mortality, and remission rate) of MG?
The incidence of MG is approximately 1 in 20,000. The disease afflicts more women than men by a ratio of about 3:2. Although the onset may be at any age from neonatal to late adult life, women in the third decade and men in the fifth decade have the peak incidence. Five to seven percent of cases are familial; however, no mendelian inheritance pattern is demonstrated. One study found a spontaneous remission rate of about 10%. Although mortality may reach 35% without treatment, nowadays death due to MG is uncommon thanks to modern medical facilities (i.e., intensive care units) and treatments. Maximum symptoms usually occur within 3 years of onset.

8. What are the HLA types associated with MG?

HLA-A1, B8, and DR3 are frequently found in young Caucasian women with MG; older men tend to have A3, B7, and DRw2. In American Blacks, A1, B8, and DR5 are associated with MG. In Chinese and Japanese, none of these is increased. Genetic susceptibility to experimental autoimmune MG (EAMG) has also been associated with certain histocompatibility types. Autoimmunity in MG may be under some genetic control via major histocompatibility types.

Compston DA, Vincent A, Newsom-Davis J, Batchelor JR: Clinical, pathological, HLA antigen and immunological evidence for disease heterogeneity in myasthenia gravis. Brain 103:579–601, 1980.

9. What experimental evidence suggests that antibodies against the acetylcholine receptor cause MG?

Animals immunized with acetylcholine receptor develop serum antibodies against the receptor and exhibit clinical and electrophysiologic findings resembling human MG (experimental autoimmune myasthenia gravis, or EAMG). Passive transfer of human MG IgG to animals results in development of EAMG in the animals. Immunocytochemical studies have demonstrated IgG at the postsynaptic membrane of motor endplates in myasthenic skeletal muscles. Additionally, the antibodies decrease the number of available acetylcholine receptors in cultured muscle cells in vitro.

10. What clinical evidence suggests that antibodies against the acetylcholine receptor cause MG?

Greater than 90% of patients with MG have circulating antibodies against the nicotinic acetylcholine receptor. Removal of the antibodies by plasmapheresis often improves the symptoms and signs of MG. The severity of the disease in a given individual with MG generally correlates with the titer of antiacetylcholine receptor antibodies. Favorable responses to immunotherapies are consistent with the antibody-mediated autoimmune pathogenesis of MG.

11. What are the immunopathologic mechanisms by which antiacetylcholine receptor antibodies cause MG?

The antibodies decrease the number of available nicotinic acetylcholine receptors in the postsynaptic membrane by several mechanisms:

1. The binding of the antibodies causes pharmacologic blockade of the cholinergic binding sites.

2. The antibodies cross-link adjacent receptors and increase the rate of internalization and subsequent degradation of the receptors.

3. The antibodies bound to the receptors activate the cascade of complement reactions, which damages the postsynaptic membrane, leading not only to further receptor loss but also widening of the synaptic cleft, which increases the diffusion of released acetylcholine and decreases the chance of acetylcholine molecules to reach the postsynaptic membrane.

4. The antibodies bound to the receptors also change the ion channel properties of the receptors.

Ashizawa T, Appel SH: Immunopathologic events at the endplate in myasthenia gravis. Spring Semin Immunopathol 8:177–196, 1985.

12. What is the concept of a safety margin in the context of synaptic transmission at the motor endplate?

Normally, the presynaptic nerve terminal releases a successively decreasing amount of acetylcholine on repetitive nerve stimulation at a slow rate, resulting in a successive decrease in the amplitude of endplate potentials at the postsynaptic membrane. At the normal neuromuscular junction, however, the endplate potentials are still large enough to trigger action potentials. Thus, the amplitude of compound muscle action potentials does not change with repetitive stimulation.

In MG, this safety margin is decreased because of the decreased number of acetylcholine receptors. Because fewer acetylcholine receptors are activated, the endplate potentials are smaller. These smaller potentials decline even further with repetitive stimulation, and an increasing number of endplate potentials fail to trigger an action potential in successive stimulations. This successively decreasing number of action potentials results in successively smaller compound muscle action potentials.

13. What is the structure of the binding sites of the nicotinic acetylcholine receptor for acetylcholine and myasthenic autoantibodies?

The human acetylcholine receptor is a pentameric protein (molecular weight of 250,000) consisting of two alpha subunits and one each of beta, epsilon (or gamma in fetal form), and delta subunits. Acetylcholine binds to the main extracellular domain of the alpha subunit close to the N-terminal. Acetylcholine molecules must bind both alpha subunits of a receptor to open the channel within the receptor. The majority of myasthenic autoantibodies also bind to the main extracellular domain of the alpha subunit.

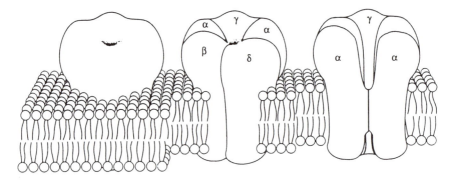

Diagram of the molecular structure of the acetylcholine receptor at the neuromuscular junction. (Reprinted with permission from Kandel ER, Schwartz JH, Jessel TM (eds): Principles of Neural Science, 3rd ed. New York, Elsevier, 1991, p 146.)

Ashizawa T, Oshima M, Ruan KH, Atassi MZ: Autoimmune recognition profile of the alpha chain of human acetylcholine receptor in myasthenia gravis. Adv Exp Med Biol 303:255–261, 1991.

14. What is the Mary Walker phenomenon?

Fatigue and weakness of the forearm muscles develop in myasthenic patients during ischemic exercise testing, when the forearm muscles are exercised with a cuff around the upper arm, inflated above systolic pressure. After the cuff is deflated, a dramatic deterioration of myasthenic manifestations in the rest of the body may occur in some patients. This phenomenon, designated the Mary Walker phenomenon, has been reproduced by several investigators and is also present in the myasthenic dog. Although some experts doubt that this is a true biologic phenomenon, others attribute it to the effect of released lactic acid from the exercised muscle. Lactic acid binds calcium and reduces ionized and total serum calcium. Lactate infusions do produce increased weakness in MG patients much more than in control patients.

Walker MB: Myasthenia gravis: A case in which fatigue of the forearm muscles could induce paralysis of the extraocular muscles. Proc Roy Soc Med 31:722, 1938.

15. Which tumors are associated with MG?

Approximately 15% of MG patients have a thymoma. The majority of thymomas are epithelial rather than lymphocytic in origin and are often invasive. Thymic hyperplasia is seen in about 50% of MG patients.

16. What are the diagnostic tests for thymoma?

Antiskeletal muscle antibodies, especially against citric acid (CA) extracted antigens, are detectable in the majority of MG patients with thymoma. Both the sensitivity and specificity of anti-CA antibodies for thymoma in MG patients are 94%. The sensitivity and specificity of CT scan of the chest for thymoma are 85% and 99%, respectively. Most MG patients undergo thymectomy anyway, so these tests may be most valuable in patients who have a marginal benefit/risk ratio for thymectomy or have a possible recurrence of thymoma.

Aarli JA, Gilhus NE, Matre R: Myasthenia gravis with thymoma is not associated with an increased incidence of non-muscle autoimmune disorders. Autoimmunity 11:159–162, 1992.

Ellis K, Austin JH, Jaretzki A: Radiologic detection of thymoma in patients with myasthenia gravis. AJR 151:873–881, 1988.

17. What are the data suggesting that the thymus plays a major role in the pathogenesis of MG?

1. The majority of MG patients have a histologic abnormality in the thymus, such as hyperplasia or thymoma.

2. Removal of the thymus improves MG.

3. Thymic B-lymphocytes produce antiacetylcholine receptor antibodies disproportionally more than other antibodies.

4. Addition of thymic cells to myasthenic B-lymphocytes in vitro enhances the production of antiacetylcholine antibodies but not other antibodies.

5. All subunits of the acetylcholine receptor, particularly the fetal type, are expressed in non-neoplastic MG thymuses. In contrast, MG thymomas do not appear to express any subunit but rather a protein epitope that cross-reacts with the alpha subunit.

6. Transplantation of MG thymus tissue to mice with severe combined immunodeficiency produces persistently elevated titers of antiacetylcholine receptor antibodies in serum and human IgG deposits at skeletal muscle endplates, whereas passive transfers of dissociated MG thymocytes show only a transient increase of antiacetylcholine receptor antibodies.

7. Myoid cells are present in the thymus, and the thymus is the site of T-lymphocyte maturation with acquisition of immunologic tolerance.

Geuder KI, Marx A, Witzemann V, et al: Pathogenetic significance of fetal-type acetylcholine receptors on thymic myoid cells in myasthenia gravis. Dev Immunol 2:69–75, 1992.

Schonbeck S, Padberg F, Hohlfeld R, Wekerle H: Transplantation of thymic autoimmune microenvironment to severe combined immunodeficiency mice: A new model of myasthenia gravis. J Clin Invest 90:245–250, 1992.

Lisak PP, Levinson AI, Zweiman B: Autoimmune aspects of myasthenia gravis. In Cruse JM, Lewis RE Jr (eds): Concepts in Immunopathology: Organ-based Autoimmune Diseases, vol 2. Karger, Basel, 1985, pp 65–101.

18. What is the myoid cell?

The myoid cells are musclelike cells found mainly within the medulla of the thymus. Although their number is few, they bear nicotinic acetylcholine receptors. Because antibodies against nicotinic acetylcholine receptors play the major pathogenic role in MG patients, the myoid cells may provide the primary antigens involved in the autoimmune response of MG. Myasthenic thymuses contain DR-positive lymphoid cells that may be able to present these antigens to T-lymphocytes, allowing for sensitization.

19. What is the role of thymectomy in the treatment of MG?

Although prospective randomized controlled trials have never been conducted to evaluate the efficacy of thymectomy in MG, the beneficial effects appear overwhelming. Whether patients have thymoma, thymic hyperplasia, or an apparently normal thymus, early thymectomy frequently improves MG. Over 75% of MG patients benefit, and many eventually experience remission. In general, a thymectomy is recommended for patients with generalized MG who are not high surgical risks. Congenital myasthenic syndromes do not respond to thymectomy, and neonatal MG improves without thymectomy. Thymectomy is usually not performed on patients with strictly ocular MG. Most experts prefer a transsternal approach over a transcervical approach because the chance of complete resection is better with the former. Recently, thoracoscopic thymectomy, a less invasive procedure, has shown promising results.

20. What is neonatal myasthenia gravis?

Approximately 12% of neonates born to mothers with MG are "floppy" babies who have difficulty breathing and sucking. The disease is transient, typically lasting for a few weeks and not exceeding 12 weeks. Passive transfer of maternal antibodies to the infant through the placenta is probably the major pathophysiologic mechanism. However, the severity and duration of the maternal disease do not necessarily correlate with the occurrence of neonatal MG. Many infants born to severely affected mothers may have high antiacetyl-choline antibody titers but few develop neonatal myasthenia. In contrast, some infants of mothers in remission may develop the disease. The rate of destruction of the passively transferred antibodies in the child may influence the development of the illness. Analysis of the subclasses of antibodies suggests that infants with neonatal MG may also produce their own antibodies distinct from the maternal antibodies. Thus, elucidation of the exact pathophysiology of neonatal MG requires further investigation.

21. What are the congenital myasthenic disorders?

Congenital myasthenic disorders are characterized by neonatal or infantile onset of extraocular, facial, bulbar, and limb weakness and fatigability, which persist into adult life. Electrophysiologic findings suggest defective neuromuscular transmission. Unlike in neonatal MG, in congenital myasthenic disorders the mother shows no evidence of the disease, acetylcholine receptor antibodies are not detectable in plasma, and the disease is not transient. The patients do not respond to a thymectomy or other treatments directed to the immune system.

There are different mechanisms for the defective neuromuscular transmission in each of the congenital myasthenic disorders. Familial infantile myasthenia gravis, for example, is an autosomal recessive disease with depleted synaptic vesicles. Other congenital myasthenic disorders include:

1. Congenital endplate acetylcholinesterase deficiency
2. Slow channel syndrome
3. Congenital endplate acetylcholine receptor deficiency
4. Congenital paucity of synaptic vesicles and reduced quantal release
5. High-conductance fast-channel syndrome
6. Abnormal acetylcholine receptor interaction with acetylcholine
7. Acetylcholine receptor deficiency with short channel-open time

Engel AG: Congenital myasthenic syndromes. J Child Neurol 3:233–246, 1988.
Engel AE, Walls TJ, Nagel A, Uchitel O: Newly recognized congenital myasthenic syndromes: I. Congenital paucity of synaptic vesicles and reduced quantal release. II. High-conductance fast-channel syndrome. III. Abnormal acetylcholine receptor (AChR) interaction with acetylcholine. IV. AChR deficiency and short channel open-time. Prog Brain Res 84:125–137, 1990.

22. What are the diagnostic tests for MG?

The diagnosis of MG may be suspected from the clinical observation of skeletal muscle weakness increased by exercise and relieved by rest. To confirm the diagnosis of MG, the following features should be sought:

1. Improvement of weakness and fatigability by anticholinesterases (e.g., edrophonium [Tensilon] or neostigmine test)
2. Electrophysiologic evidence for defective neuromuscular transmission by repetitive stimulation or single-fiber EMG

3. The presence of circulating antibodies against acetylcholine receptors

Thymic pathology may also confirm the diagnosis, although it cannot serve as a primary diagnostic means.

23. What is the rationale for the edrophonium (Tensilon) test?

Edrophonium is a rapid and short-acting anticholinesterase drug. The defective neuromuscular transmission in MG can be improved by anticholinesterase medications, which increase the concentration of acetylcholine in the synaptic cleft by inhibiting the breakdown of acetylcholine. The increased concentration of acetylcholine improves the chance that each acetylcholine receptor will encounter acetylcholine molecules, allowing more receptors to be activated. Intravenous administration of edrophonium produces immediate and dramatic improvement in the signs of MG and therefore is a valuable diagnostic test.

24. How is the edrophonium test performed?

After noting the baseline degree of weakness and fatigue, administer a test dose of 1 mg of edrophonium intravenously to verify that adverse effects do not occur. Keep a crash cart in the immediate vicinity in case of untoward cholinergic effects. Then, inject up to 10 mg of edrophonium intravenously. Most subjects, including nonmyasthenic patients, may experience some degree of flushing, palpitation, and tearing with this dose. (In children, dosage depends on body weight, to a maximum of 10 mg.) After administering the drug, document the level of weakness and fatigue again to determine any change. When there are ocular and bulbar signs, objective assessment is not difficult. However, when fatigue is demonstrable only in limb muscles, quantitative measurement of strength and fatigability is important, since relying on patient's and examiner's impression can be misleading. Double-blind testing using normal saline as a control may be useful. If the test unequivocally demonstrates improvement of weakness and fatigability, it is diagnostic of MG.

25. Which electrophysiologic findings are diagnostic for MG?

A decrement of greater than 10% in the amplitude of the evoked compound action potential recorded from the skeletal muscle upon low-frequency (typically 3 per second) repetitive stimulation of the motor nerve is diagnostic of MG. The first muscle response has normal amplitude, but the subsequent responses show a reduction in amplitude before reaching a plateau in the fourth to sixth responses. The decrement at 3 per second is determined first in the rested muscle and then in the same muscle after it has been exercised. The decrement should be correctable in MG by administration of anticholinesterase medications such as edrophonium.

26. What is single-fiber electromyography (SFEMG)?

SFEMG involves simultaneous recordings of evoked responses from two muscle fibers belonging to the same motor unit. The motor unit discharge is elicited by either submaximal voluntary contraction of the muscle or repetitive submaximal stimulation of the nerve to that muscle. Recording from a normal muscle shows two evoked responses from the two muscle fibers firing with a minimum fluctuation of the interval between the two. The fluctuation is called "jitter." In myasthenia gravis, the jitter is increased and may be associated with an occasional lack of response from one of the muscle fibers ("blocking"). These changes have been attributed to the variably decreased amplitude of the endplate potentials. Increased jitter can also occur in LEMS and diseases in which nerve sprouting exists.

27. What is pyridostigmine (Mestinon)? Why is it the most widely used anticholinesterase medication in MG?

Pyridostigmine is slightly longer acting (with a half-life of 4 hours) and has fewer cholinergic side effects than neostigmine bromide and other anticholinesterase preparations.

Unlike physostigmine, pyridostigmine does not have unwanted CNS effects because it does not cross the blood-brain barrier. However, some cases of MG may be refractory to pyridostigmine but respond to other anticholinesterases.

28. What are the chronic adverse effects of anticholinesterases on the neuromuscular junction?

In addition to the acute event of cholinergic crisis, excess acetylcholine can cause chronic changes at the postsynaptic membrane, resembling the endplate seen in MG itself. Postsynaptic junctional folds are simplified and the number of acetylcholine receptors is decreased. The postsynaptic effects of excess acetylcholine add an additional damage to the already existing changes caused by MG antibodies.

29. What is Mestinon Timespan?

The bedtime dose of pyridostigmine may not last throughout the night. MG patients may complain of difficulty in swallowing their medication the next morning. A slow-release tablet of 180 mg of pyridostigmine (Timespan) may alleviate this problem, although the release rate of this preparation is somewhat unpredictable.

30. What is the dose of parenteral pyridostigmine that is equivalent to the standard 60-mg oral pyridostigmine pill?

A parenteral dose of 2 mg is equivalent to an oral dose of 60 mg.

31. What are the drugs to be used with caution in MG?

The list of the drugs that may adversely affect MG is long and they should be used with caution.

I. Antibiotics

  A. Aminoglycosides
    Neomycin
    Streptomycin
    Kanamycin
    Gentamicin
    Tobramycin

  B. Other Peptide Antibiotics
    Polymyxin B
    Colistin

  C. Other Antibiotics
    Oxytetracycline
    Rolitetracycline
    Lincomycin
    Clindamycin
    Erythromycin
    Ampicillin

II. Neuromuscular Blockers

III. Cardiac Drugs
    Quinine
    Quinidine
    Procainamide
    Trimethaphan
    Licocaine
    Beta-adrenergic blockers

IV. Other Drugs
    Phenytoin   Oxytocin
    Chloroquine   Aprotinin
    Trimethadione   Propanidid
    Lithium carbonate Diazepam
    Mg^{2+} Ketamine
    Meglumine diatrizoate D-penicillamine
    Methoxyflurane Carnitine

The aminoglycosides, including neomycin, streptomycin, kanamycin, gentamicin, and tobramycin, and two other peptide antibiotics, polymyxin B and colistin, may have adverse effects both pre- and postsynaptically. Oxytetracycline and rolitetracycline, lincomycin, clindamycin, erythromycin, and ampicillin may also show adverse effects in MG. Many drugs used for cardiac diseases, such as quinine, quinidine, procainamide, trimethaphan, lidocaine, and beta-adrenergic blockers, may also exacerbate MG. Chloroquine and phenytoin may aggravate or unmask MG. Lithium carbonate may interfere with neuromuscular transmission by compromising pre- and postsynaptic Na^+ influx. Neuromuscular blocking agents, magnesium salts, and anticholinesterases require close monitoring when administered to MG patients. A CT scan contrast material, meglumine diatrizoate, has been reported to cause an acute exacerbation in MG patients. An anesthetic, methoxyflurane, may unmask subclinical MG. Oxytocin, aprotinin, propanidid, diazepam, and ketamine have been reported to prolong postoperative recovery in MG. Among these, the aminoglycosides, the peptide antibiotics, oxprenolol, practolol, trimethaphan, phenytoin, trimethadione, D-pencillamine, and carnitine have been reported to induce MG without the presence of underlying MG.

32. What precautions are necessary when treating MG with corticosteroids?

In addition to the usual side effects of corticosteroids, MG patients may become weaker 1–3 weeks after initiation of oral prednisone therapy, usually followed by a gradual but marked improvement. Gradually increasing doses of oral prednisone, from 25 mg PO every other day to 100 mg PO every other day, may alleviate this phenomenon. During the initial weakness associated with the introduction of prednisone, respiratory functions should be carefully monitored. With prednisone-induced improvement, the sensitivity of MG patients to anticholinesterase drugs may increase and the doses of anticholinesterase often need to be reduced or discontinued. Patients may require maintenance doses of prednisone for up to 2 years before its discontinuation, since recurrences are common. Reducing the doses of prednisone must be done carefully, because relapses often result from reducing the doses too fast or too soon.

33. What causes drug-induced autoimmune myasthenia gravis?

Approximately 1% of patients taking D-penicillamine for the treatment of rheumatoid arthritis or Wilson's disease develop clinical myasthenia. The disease afflicts women six times more frequently than men, and is associated with HLA A1 and B8, which are frequent HLA types in spontaneously occurring MG. The disease first strikes the ocular muscles and then becomes generalized. Patients with D-penicillamine-induced MG have autoantibodies against acetylcholine receptors. The disease and the autoantibodies slowly disappear after discontinuation of D-penicillamine. An anticonvulsant, trimethadione, may also induce myasthenia via autoimmune mechanisms because the myasthenia is associated with high titers of antimuscle antibodies and antinuclear factor, and clinically resembles systemic lupus erythematosus.

Dawkins RL, Christiansen FT, Garlepp MJ: Autoantibodies and HLA antigens in ocular, generalized, and penicillamine-induced myasthenia gravis. Ann NY Acad Sci 377:372–383, 1981.

34. What is a myasthenic crisis?

Myasthenic crisis is an acute exacerbation of MG with respiratory and bulbar dysfunction. Respiratory care to maintain adequate ventilation is the most important factor in the treatment. Mortality of MG was drastically decreased with the introduction of ICUs even prior to the introduction of steroids as a treatment of MG. Life-threatening respiratory failure can be prevented by close monitoring of pulmonary functions, especially forced vital capacity and FEV_1, which decline before blood gases deteriorate. Early endotracheal intubation with mechanical ventilatory support is lifesaving in myasthenic crisis.

Anticholinesterase medications may be useful. However, when cholinergic crisis cannot be excluded as the cause of the clinical exacerbation, discontinuation of anticholinesterases under respiratory support is recommended. A few days later, an anticholinesterase can be started at a low dose and the dose gradually increased as needed. High-dose oral prednisone therapy and intravenous glucocorticoids often provide improvement. If the patient is refractory to these medications, intravenous gamma globulin may be tried, followed, if needed, by plasmapheresis. Immunosuppressive agents such as cyclophosphamide, cyclosporine A, azathioprine, and methotrexate are often needed. If the patient has not had a thymectomy, it should be performed as soon as the patient can tolerate the surgery.

35. What is a cholinergic crisis?

Overdosing a patient with anticholinesterase may result in excess acetylcholine in the synaptic cleft, causing depolarization block of acetylcholine receptors. The end result is defective neuromuscular transmission similar to a myasthenic crisis. Fasciculations are common. Establishing an airway, supporting respiration, and withholding anticholinesterase medications are the mainstays of treatment.

36. What is the value of the edrophonium test to differentiate myasthenic crisis from cholinergic crisis?

The edrophonium (Tensilon) test improves myasthenic crisis but aggravates cholinergic crisis. However, interpretation of the result is often difficult and misleading because one group of muscles may deteriorate while others improve. Securing the respiration and discontinuing all anticholinesterase drugs in a protected environment in the ICU offers a safer and more practical solution.

LAMBERT-EATON MYASTHENIC SYNDROME

37. What are the primary manifestations of Lambert-Eaton myasthenic syndrome (LEMS)?

In LEMS, weakness and fatigability of proximal muscles, especially in the thighs and pelvic girdle, with depressed or absent tendon reflexes are the primary manifestations. Muscle strength may increase for a short while after exercise (postexercise facilitation). Although ptosis may be present in LEMS, extraocular and bulbar muscles are otherwise spared as a rule. Autonomic dysfunction may be prominent in LEMS.

38. What tumor is associated with LEMS?

Over 90% of patients with LEMS have small-cell carcinoma of the lung. This tumor plays an important role in the pathogenesis of LEMS.

39. What experimental evidence suggests an autoimmune pathogenesis of LEMS?

Passive transfers of IgG from patients with LEMS to animals produce electrophysiologic defects characteristic of LEMS. The LEMS IgG contains autoantibodies against voltage-gated calcium channels.

40. What is the autoimmune pathophysiology involved in LEMS?

The primary antigen for the LEMS antibodies appears to be present in the small-cell carcinoma of the lung that is often associated with LEMS. The LEMS antibodies cross-react with N type and L type voltage-gated Ca^{2+} channels and with synaptotagmin. The antibody action does not involve complement-mediated membrane lysis. The decreased number of the voltage-gated Ca^{2+} channels with the resulting decrease in miniature endplate potential (MEPP) frequency and the morphologic changes at the active zone have been attributed to the actions of LEMS antibodies.

Vincent A, Lang B, Newsom-Davis J: Autoimmunity to the voltage-gated calcium channel underlies the Lambert-Eaton myasthenic syndrome, a paraneoplastic disorder. Trends Neurosci 12:496–502, 1989.

41. What is the mechanism of incremental response on the repetitive stimulation test in LEMS?

In LEMS the decreased Ca^{2+} influx into the presynaptic nerve terminal upon depolarization of the presynaptic membrane results in insufficient release of acetylcholine from the presynaptic nerve terminal. With repetitive stimulation, the release of acetylcholine may be facilitated by an accumulation of presynaptic calcium, causing an increased number of acetylcholine quanta to be released. This explains the incremental response of the muscles to repetitive stimulation of the nerve in this disease.

42. What are the morphologic changes at the neuromuscular junction in LEMS?
On light microscopy, there are proliferation and enlargement of the secondary synaptic clefts in LEMS, in contrast to the widened and simplified postsynaptic folds in MG. The proliferative and hypertrophic postsynaptic membranes are considered to be a response to repeated degeneration and regeneration of presynaptic membranes. At the electron microscopic level, the freeze-fracture technique shows that the active zone protein particles are decreased and disorganized.

43. What is the treatment for LEMS?
Release of acetylcholine from the presynaptic nerve terminal is facilitated by guanidine hydrochloride, 4-aminopyridine, and 3,4-diaminopyridine. Because the latter two may decrease the seizure threshold, guanidine hydrochloride, 20–30 mg/kg/day, in divided doses is the recommended treatment. Anticholinesterases may also improve symptoms. When an associated neoplasm is resectable, tumor removal may reverse the syndrome. Glucocorticoids and plasmapheresis have been useful, but other immunosuppressive agents may accelerate growth of the carcinoma. Improvement after intravenous gamma globulin treatment has also been reported.

44. What precautions must be taken for surgical procedures that require general anesthesia in MG and LEMS?
A thoracotomy for resection of the lung cancer in LEMS and a thymectomy in MG are often necessary procedures. Precautions include:
    1. A delayed recovery from the effect of neuromuscular blocking agents must be anticipated in both LEMS and MG. Give a short-acting neuromuscular blocker of the minimum dose necessary for the surgical procedure.
    2. If the patient has been on glucocorticoids, give greater than equivalent doses intravenously before, during, and after the surgery until the original oral glucocorticoid therapy can be reinstated.
    3. Anticholinesterase therapy is usually unnecessary during surgery but is started postoperatively as needed when the patient regains consciousness. The differences between parenteral and oral doses of anticholinesterase should be recognized (see question 30).
    4. Maintain normal serum electrolytes, calcium, and magnesium.
    5. Avoid unnecessary medications to minimize drug-related complications.
    6. Avoid medications that may worsen the defective synaptic transmission at the neuromuscular junction (see question 31).

OTHER NEUROMUSCULAR JUNCTION DISEASES

45. What are the clinical characteristics of botulism?
Two to 48 hours after ingesting improperly prepared canned or bottled foods contaminated with *Clostridium botulinum*, ocular and bulbar muscle paralysis begins, with difficulty in convergence of the eyes, diplopia, ptosis, weakness of the jaw muscles, dysphagia, and dysarthria. Nausea, vomiting, and diarrhea may precede these symtpoms. Constipation, urinary retention, and nonreactive dilation of the pupils may occur because of autonomic dysfunction. Subsequently, the paralysis spreads and causes respiratory failure and total limb paralysis without abnormalities in mental status or sensation.

In infants, the initial manifestations are poor sucking and difficulty with feeding, weak cries, loss of head control, and bilateral ptosis, which subsequently result in generalized flaccid paralysis. Rapid respiratory failure due to botulism may account for as many as 10% of pathologically unexplained sudden infant deaths.

The course depends on the amount of toxin absorbed. In severe cases, death usually occurs within 4–8 days. If only a small amount of the toxin is absorbed, the symptoms are mild and recovery may be complete.

46. What is the infectious process in botulism?

Botulinum toxin is an exotoxin of *Clostridium botulinum*. The presence of common bacteria inhibit the growth of *Clostridium botulinum*, but infection occurs when the victim ingests improperly prepared canned or bottled foods in which the common bacteria are killed but the more resistant Clostridium spores are spared. In infants, the intestinal bacterial flora may not effectively inhibit the growth of *Clostridium botulinum*. Human botulism is usually caused by exotoxin produced by types A, B, and E.

47. What is the pharmacologic action of black widow spider venom?

Black widow spider venom promotes release of acetylcholine from the presynaptic nerve terminal and depletes presynaptic acetylcholine. The venom also inhibits choline uptake. Clinically, this causes painful muscle spasm followed by weakness.

48. What is the pharmacologic action of curare?

Curare is a classic antagonist of nicotinic acetylcholine receptors and competes with acetylcholine for the binding site. Curare therefore has been used as a neuromuscular blocking agent (nondepolarizing blocker) for general anesthesia.

49. What snake venom causes a neuromuscular disease? What is its importance in experimental studies of MG?

Pharmacologically, alpha-bungarotoxin blocks acetylcholine binding to the receptor, causing defective neuromuscular transmission similar to MG. This toxin comes from the binding of alpha-bungarotoxin to the receptor at multiple sites on the alpha subunit. Alpha-bungarotoxin has a high affinity for the alpha subunit of the nicotinic acetylcholine receptor, which makes this toxin a useful marker for acetylcholine receptors in both in vivo and in vitro experiments. Experiments on the purification, characterization, and localization of the receptor, as well as detection of serum autoantibodies against the receptor, have all used alpha-bungarotoxin.

50. What are the autoimmune abnormalities demonstrated at the neuromuscular junction in amyotrophic lateral sclerosis (ALS)?

Antibodies against L-type voltage-gated Ca^{2+} channels have been found in 75% of ALS patients, although the antibodies have also been found in patients with LEMS, Guillain-Barré syndrome, and some control subjects. The titer of the antibodies in ALS correlates with the rate of disease progression. The pathogenic importance of the autoimmunity in ALS needs to be further investigated.

   Smith RG, Hamilton S, Hofmann F, et al: Serum antibodies to L-type calcium channels in patients with amyotrophic lateral sclerosis. N Engl J Med 327:1721-1728, 1992.

BIBLIOGRAPHY

1. Brooke MH (ed): A Clinician's View of Neuromuscular Diseases, 2nd ed. Baltimore, Williams & Wilkins, 1986.
2. Drachman DB (ed): Myasthenia gravis: Biology and treatment. New York, Ann NY Acad Sci 505: 1-909, 1987.
3. Grob D (ed): Myasthenia gravis: Pathophysiology and management. New York, Ann NY Acad Sci 377:1-898, 1981.
4. Raine CS (ed): Advances in Neuroimmunology. Ann NY Acad Sci, vol. 540, 1988.
5. Vincent A, Wray D (eds): Neuromuscular Transmission: Basic and Applied Aspects. Manchester, England, Manchester University Press, 1990.
6. Walton J (ed): Disorders of Voluntary Muscle, 5th ed. Edinburgh, Churchill Livingstone, 1988.

5. PERIPHERAL NEUROPATHIES

Yadollah Harati, M.D., FACP

1. What are the most common diseases affecting the peripheral nerve?

The most important neuropathies can be classifed by the mnemonic DANG THE RAPIST:

D	Diabetes	T	Trauma	R	Rheumatic (collagen vascular)
A	Alcohol	H	Hereditary	A	Amyloid
N	Nutritional	E	Environmental	P	Paraneoplastic
G	Gullain-Barré		toxins and drugs	I	Infections
				S	Systemic disease
				T	Tumors

2. What are the patterns of peripheral nerve damage?

The nerve can be damaged by injury to the myelin, the axon, the cell body, or the vasa nervorum.Three basic pathologic mechanisms underlie nerve injury:

   1. **Wallerian degeneration:** This develops after injury to the axon and myelin, as in transection of the nerve. Distal to the transection, the myelin and the axon degenerate, and within a week there will be a conduction block. The axon may regrow within the architecture provided by the basement membrane of Schwann cells, but the degree and efficiency of regrowth depend on good approximation of the nerve ends.

   2. **Segmental demyelination:** This develops after damage to the myelin sheath. Because the muscle is not denervated, no atrophy develops, in contrast to wallerian degeneration, in which the axon is also damaged and the muscle degenerates. Prognosis for complete recovery is good.

   3. **Axonal degeneration:** Damage to the cell body of the neuron results in distal dying of the axon. Subsequently, myelin loss occurs. Once the distal nerve dies, there is denervation of the muscle, and hence muscle atrophy develops. Reinnervation of the denervated muscle occurs from surrounding nerves, but there may not be total recovery.

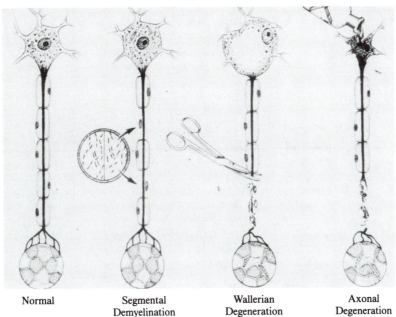

| Normal | Segmental Demyelination | Wallerian Degeneration | Axonal Degeneration |

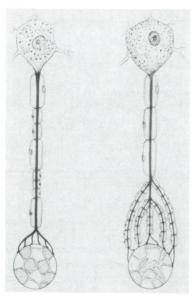

Following segmental demyelination there may be segmental remyelination. The remyelinated segments are shorter and have a smaller diameter. Axonal regeneration is associated with the formation of clusters of small and thinly myelinated fibers.

Regeneration after   Regeneration after
Segmental Demyelination   Axonal Degeneration

3. What is the most common form of treatable peripheral neuropathy in the world?
Leprosy. There are approximately 10–20 million cases of leprosy in the world.

4. What are the clinical tests for the common root syndromes?

Clinical Tests for Common Root Syndromes

ROOT	MUSCLE TESTED	EXAMINATION	REFLEX
C5	Deltoid	Shoulder abduction: push down on arms abducted to 90°	
C6	Biceps Brachioradialis	Flexion at elbow: pull outward at wrist with elbows flexed at 90°	Biceps Brachioradialis
C7	Triceps Pronator teres	Extension at elbow: push down on elbow with arm in extension and supination	Triceps
C8	Finger flexors	Finger flexion: "squeeze my finger"	
T1	Intrinsic hand muscles	Finger abduction and adduction: fingers are spread out—try squeezing them inward	
L1–L2	Iliopsoas	Hip flexion: while sitting, patient flexes at hip. Push hip down with pressure at knee	Cremasteric
L2–L3	Adductors	Hip adduction: try to push legs inward	
L3–L4	Quadriceps	Extension of leg at knee	Knee reflex
L5	Anterior tibial	Dorsiflexion of foot	
S1	Gastrocnemius	Plantarflexion of foot	Ankle jerk

5. Which peripheral neuropathies may have cranial nerve involvement?

Peripheral Neuropathies with Cranial Nerve Involvement

NEUROPATHY	MOST COMMONLY INVOLVED CRANIAL NERVES	LESS COMMONLY INVOLVED CRANIAL NERVES
Diphtheria	IX	II, III
Sarcoid	VII	I, III, IV, VI
Diabetes	III*	IV, VI, VII
Guillain-Barré syndrome (GBS)	VI, VII	
Miller-Fisher variant of GBS	III, IV	
Lupus	V	
Polyarteritis nodosa	VIII	
Porphyria	VII, X	III, IV, V, XI, XII
Refsum's disease	I, VIII	
Amyloidosis	V	
Syphilis	III	IV, V, VII, VIII
Arsenic neuropathy	V	

* Pupil is usually not affected.

6. Which neuropathies begin proximally rather than distally?
Most neuropathies begin distally; however, a few may begin proximally:

1. Sensory neuropathies: porphyria and rare cases of Charcot-Marie-Tooth and Tangier disease.

2. Motor neuropathies: Guillain-Barré syndrome, chronic inflammatory demyelinating neuropathy, diabetes, and idiopathic acute brachial plexus neuropathy.

7. Which neuropathies begin in the arms rather than the legs?
Most often, neuropathies present with symptoms in the feet. Once the symptoms in the lower extremities proceed to the middle of the calf, the neuropathy will begin to appear in the hands. Although this generally holds, some neuropathies may start initially in the upper extremity:

1. Guillain-Barré syndrome
2. Lead neuropathy
3. Porphyria
4. Vitamin B12 deficiency
5. Some cases of Charcot-Marie-Tooth disease
6. Bilateral carpal tunnel syndrome

8. Which neuropathies are often predominantly motor?
Guillain-Barré syndrome, diphtheric neuropathy, dapsone-induced neuropathy, and porphyria.

9. What are the causes of a predominantly sensory polyradiculopathy-polyganglionopathy?
Pyridoxine intoxication, doxorubicin, Sjogren's syndrome, diphtheria, malignant inflammatory sensory polyganglionopathies (secondary to malignancies), idiopathic nonmalignant inflammatory sensory polyganglionopathies, and the sensory form of acute inflammatory-demyelinating polyneuropathy (AIDP).

10. In which conditions are the peripheral nerves palpably hypertrophic?

1. Hereditary neuropathies of Charcot-Marie-Tooth disease and Dejerine-Sottas syndrome
2. Amyloidosis
3. Refsum's disease
4. Leprosy
5. Acromegaly
6. Neurofibromatosis

11. What is an "onion-bulb" formation?
"Onion-bulb" formation is the pathologic hallmark of the hypertrophic neuropathies, in which repeated segmental demyelination and remyelination have occurred. As viewed in

transverse sections, onion-bulb formations are multiple concentric layers of intertwined, attenuated Schwann cell processes surrounding the remaining nerve fibers. The Schwann cell processes are separated from each other by layers of collagen fibers. The onion-bulb formations may be seen in any condition in which there is chronic segmental demyelination and remyelination, but are frequently seen in Charcot-Marie-Tooth disease, Dejerine-Sottas syndrome, Refsum's disease, and chronic relapsing idiopathic (inflammatory) demyelinating neuropathy.

12. What is Refsum's disease?

Refsum's disease is a multisystem illness manifesting with polyneuropathy, retinitis pigmentosa, ichthyosis, ataxia, deafness, and cardiomyopathy. Levels of cerebrospinal fluid (CSF) protein may be elevated. The disease is also called heredopathia atactica polyneuritiformis and is caused by the accumulation of dietary-derived phytanic acid in tissues. Phytanic acid is a branched long-chain fatty acid that requires alpha oxidation. A diet free of phytanic acid may result in substantial clinical improvement. Plasmapheresis may enhance the recovery.

13. What are fasciculations?

Fasciculations are irregular contractions of muscle fibers that are innervated by the same motor unit. Fasciculations are visible through the skin. They are caused by irregular firing of anterior horn cells or by an irritative focus in the peripheral nerve. Hence they are seen in a wide variety of diseases, including:

1. Motor neuron disease
2. Acute phase of poliomyelitis
3. Root disease (such as spondylotic radiculopathy)
4. Thyrotoxicosis
5. Severe hyponatremia
6. Hypomagnesemia
7. Generalized polyneuropathies
8. Drugs (anticholinesterase, lithium)

14. Who is the least likely to be diagnosed as having thoracic outlet syndrome and undergo surgery?

Patients who do not have private insurance or workers' compensation insurance. Medicaid patients almost never undergo surgery.

Cherington M, Cherington C: Thoracic outlet syndrome: Reimbursement patterns and patient profiles. Neurology 42:943, 1992.

15. Which diabetic neuropathies are painful?

- Third cranial nerve neuropathy
- Acute thoracoabdominal neuropathy
- Acute distal sensory neuropathy
- Acute lumbar radiculoplexopathy
- Chronic distal small-fiber neuropathy

16. What are the different types of Lyme neuropathies?

Lyme disease, a multisystem illness caused by a tick-borne spirochete, *Borrelia burgdorferi*, may cause many varieties of peripheral neuropathies, including cranial neuropathies (especially Bell's palsy), radiculitis, plexopathies, multiple mononeuropathies, a Guillain-Barré-like illness, and, more frequently, a symmetric sensory-motor neuropathy. In endemic areas, Lyme disease accounts for about two-thirds of pediatric cases of facial palsy and as many as one-fourth of adult cases. Involvement of other cranial nerves usually occurs in the setting of a lymphocytic meningitis. Radiculitis may be indistinguishable from a compression-induced radiculopathy. Such radiculopathies usually occur in the lower limbs, and CSF pleocytosis is common. Unilateral or bilateral lumbosacral or brachial plexopathies are rarely observed. The symmetric distal sensory-motor neuropathy is usually mild and occurs in many patients with chronic Lyme disease.

17. Which kinds of peripheral neuropathies are seen in association with HIV infection?

Up to 50% of patients with HIV infection develop a peripheral neuropathy, which may take one or a combination of the following forms:

1. Distal symmetric neuropathy (the most common form)
   Painful sensory type
   Sensory-motor type (mild or minimal motor involvement)
2. Inflammatory demyelinating polyneuropathy (both acute and chronic forms, usually with elevated CSF cell counts)
3. Mononeuropathy multiplex
4. Cytomegalovirus and herpes zoster radiculoneuropathy
5. Cranial neuropathy
6. Autonomic neuropathy
7. Nutritional, vitamin deficiency neuropathy
8. Drug-induced neuropathy

18. What is POEMS syndrome?

POEMS stands for polyneuropathy, organomegaly, endocrinopathy, M-protein, and skin changes. Patients typically have a chronic progressive sensory-motor polyneuropathy, peripheral edema, ascites, hypertrichosis, diffuse hyperpigmentation and thickening of the skin, hepatomegaly, lymphadenopathy, gynecomastia, impotence, or amenorrhea. The monoclonal protein is usually of the IgG or IgA type and almost always contains lambda light chains. POEMS syndrome is believed to be a variant of osteosclerotic myeloma with peripheral neuropathy.

19. What are the features of neuropathies secondary to monoclonal gammopathies?

Neuropathies are often seen in association with serum monoclonal gammopathies. In 63% of such patients, no cause of gammopathy is delineated (idiopathic monoclonal gammopathy, or IMG), but 12% have multiple myeloma, 9% amyloidosis, 5% lymphoma, and 3% leukemia. In many patients with IMG, an identifiable cause emerges with follow-up: the risk of developing an identifiable cause is 17% at 10 years and 33% at 20 years. Hence, it is important to follow these patients indefinitely. Clinically, patients with IMG and neuropathy are generally over 50 years of age, and develop a symmetric sensory (early) and motor (late) neuropathy or polyradiculopathy which affects the legs more than arms. There is no involvement of cranial nerves. CSF protein levels are elevated in 83% of patients. IgM is more common than IgG- or IgA-associated neuropathy. The treatment of patients with IMG-induced neuropathy is difficult; however, both prednisone and immunosuppressive-chemotherapeutic agents have been of some benefit. Plasma exchange provides significant symptomatic improvement in patients with IgG and IgA but not in IgM gammopathy.

20. What other plasma cell dyscrasias are associated with a peripheral neuropathy?

Other plasma cell dyscrasias associated with a peripheral neuropathy include nonmalignant IgG, IgA and IgM monoclonal gammopathies, multiple myeloma, Waldenström's macroglobulinemia and amyloidosis. The polyneuropathy associated with plasma-cell dyscrasias is mainly of the demyelinating type, in which pain and autonomic involvement are rare. It is important to evaluate the presence of plasma-cell dyscrasia in any patient presenting with unexplained peripheral neuropathy. In tertiary care centers, up to 10% of all patients with a peripheral neuropathy have an underlying plasma-cell dyscrasia. Detailed hematologic and radiographic studies as well as urine collections for Bence-Jones proteins are necessary to exclude multiple or osteosclerotic myeloma. In patients with osteosclerotic myeloma, tumoricidal radiation often results in resolution of the neuropathy.

The pathogenesis of the nerve damage in plasma-cell dyscrasia is unclear, but some patients with IgM monoclonal gammopathy have an antibody against a glycoprotein associated with M-protein on the myelin sheaths (anti-MAG antibody). Patients who have IgG and IgA paraproteins respond more satisfactorily to corticosteroids, cytotoxic drugs, or plasma exchanges than those with IgM paraprotein. Uncontrolled trials suggest a beneficial effect of high-dose intravenous gammaglobulin as well.

Miralles GD, O'Fallon JR, Talley NJ: Plasma-cell dyscrasia with polyneuropathy. N Engl J Med 327:1919–1923, 1992.

Dyck PJ, Low PA, Windebank AJ, et al: Plasma exchange in polyneuropathy associated with monoclonal gammopathy of undetermined significance. N Engl J Med 325:1482–1486, 1991.

21. What are the most important industrial agents causing peripheral neuropathy?

1. **Acrylamide:** Only direct skin exposure to the monomer of acrylamide is neurotoxic to peripheral nerves, resulting in symptoms of numbness, gait unsteadiness, mild weakness, palmar hyperhidrosis, and skin peeling. The neuropathy is caused by impairment of axoplasmic transport mechanisms, particularly retrograde transport. Withdrawal from exposure to acrylamide usually results in a slow recovery.

2. **Carbon disulfide:** Low-level prolonged inhalation of this agent, used in the production of cellophane films and rayon fibers, results in distal axonopathy. With higher levels or longer duration of exposure, encephalopathic and psychotic abnormalities may develop. Removal of the agent causes a slow and frequently incomplete recovery.

3. **Dimethylaminopropionitrile (DMAPN):** Inhalation of this agent, used in the manufacturing of polyurethane foam, results in urologic dysfunction (urinary hesitancy, decreased urine stream, incontinence, and sometimes impotence) followed by distal symmetric and predominantly sensory polyneuropathy, with a characteristic sensory loss in the sacral dermatomes. Removal from exposure results in gradual recovery.

4. **Ethylene oxide:** At high levels of exposure, this gas causes a symmetric, distal polyneuropathy, sometimes with encephalopathic symptoms. Prolonged low-level exposure among hospital sterilizer workers and patients receiving long-term hemodialysis is claimed to cause a subclinical neuropathy. Withdrawal from exposure results in gradual improvement.

5. **Hexacarbons (n-hexane, methyl n-butyl ketone):** Industrial use of these solvents in a poorly ventilated environment and the practice of inhalant abuse by teenagers (glue sniffing) are the major causes of hexacarbon neuropathy. Both n-hexane and methyl-n-butyl ketone (MBK) are metabolized to 2.5-hexanedione, the agent responsible for the neurotoxicity. The neurotoxic effect is caused by the interruption of the retrograde axoplasmic flow, resulting in symmetric distal sensory neuropathy with loss of ankle reflexes. In more severe cases, there is mild to moderate distal muscle weakness. Some patients may also manifest symptoms of autonomic neuropathy. The nerve conduction velocity is usually slow. In patients with a history of excessive abuse of solvents, the course of the illness may be more rapid; in industrial cases, the progression is usually slow. When the offending agent is stopped, the neuropathy characteristically progresses for another few months. In about 1 year, however, most patients with mild to moderate involvement recover completely. Nerve biopsies of patients with hexacarbon neuropathy show focally swollen axons (giant axons) with 10-nm neurofilaments and axonal degeneration.

6. **Methyl bromide:** Chronic exposure to high to moderate levels of methyl bromide results in the symptoms of distal sensorimotor neuropathy that gradually resolve following the withdrawal from the exposure. Pyramidal tract signs and cerebellar dysfunction may also be prominent. Whether the neuropathy is due to an axonopathy, myelin sheath disease, or both is not known. Methyl bromide has found use as a fumigant, fire extinguisher, refrigerant, and insecticide.

7. **Organophosphorus esters:** A number of organophosphorus esters, including tri-o-cresylphosphate (TOCP), leptophos, mipafox, chlorphos, and trichlorfon, cause a delayed distal axonopathy after a single or prolonged exposure. These esters are used as insecticides, petroleum additives, and modifiers of plastic. Their toxic effect on the peripheral nerves is

not due to their inhibition of acetylcholinesterase but may involve inhibition of a neuropathy target esterase (NTE). With the progression of neuropathy, pyramidal tract signs and spasticity may also develop. The prognosis in mildly affected individuals is good, but in severe cases there is varying degree of residual peripheral and central nervous system dysfunction.

8. **Trichlorethylene:** Industrial exposure to this agent results in a peculiar syndrome manifesting as sensorimotor trigeminal neuropathy, facial neuropathy, oculomotor dysfunction, and optic nerve dysfunction. The agent is used in dry cleaning, degreasing, and rubber production. The reason for the selective predilection of this agent for the cranial nerves is not known.

9. **Vacor:** When accidentally ingested, this rodenticide causes severe destruction of the pancreatic beta cells and severe axonal and autonomic neuropathy. The agent is thought to impair fast anterograde axoplasmic flow.

22. What is critical-illness polyneuropathy?

Critical-illness polyneuropathy develops in 50% of patients who have been in a critical care unit for more than 2 weeks. The neuropathy occurs irrespective of the illness that precipitated the admission to intensive care, although most patients have evidence of multiple past or current infections. Attention is initially brought to the neuropathy by weakness of respiratory muscles, and hence difficulty in weaning the patient off the ventilator. With severe neuropathy, marked sensory loss and weakness set in. Electrophysiologic studies reveal an axonal neuropathy, and nerve biopsies confirm predominantly axonal loss. Muscle biopsy reveals neurogenic atrophy. The severity of the neuropathy is proportional to the length of stay in the hospital. If patients do not die from the illness that necessitated intensive care admission, most patients who develop critical-illness polyneuropathy recover.

23. Which tests on physical examination can be used to aid in the diagnosis of carpal tunnel syndrome?

Carpal tunnel syndrome (CTS) is the most common peripheral nerve entrapment syndrome, affecting 1% of the population. Typical symptoms consist of dysesthesias, especially worse at night, weakness, and decreased sensation. On examination, numbness envelops the median nerve innervation of the hand (the radial aspect of the palm and the thumb, the index and middle fingers, and the radial half of the ring finger), with weakness of the abductor pollicis brevis. Other muscles innervated by the median nerve that show some weakness include the lateral two lumbricals, opponens pollicis, and flexor pollicis brevis. Certain physical tests aid in the diagnosis of CTS:

1. **Median Nerve Percussion Test:** Tapping the area over the median nerve at the wrist. The test is positive when this procedure can produce paresthesias in a median nerve distribution.

Sensitivity: 44%   Specificity: 94%

2. **Carpal Tunnel Compression Test:** Apply pressure over the carpal tunnel for 30 seconds. If this duplicates the patient's sensory symptoms, the test is considered positive.

Sensitivity: 87%   Specificity: 90%

3. **Phalen Wrist Flexion Test:** Fully flex the wrist for 60 seconds. If it produces the patient's symptoms, it is positive.

Sensitivity: 71%   Specificity: 80%

24. Which conditions are associated with bilateral CTS?

1. Pregnancy
2. Hypothyroidism
3. Acromegaly
4. Hereditary amyloidosis
5. Mucopolysaccharidosis
6. Repetitive wrist motion

25. What are the causes of multiple mononeuropathy (mononeuritis multiplex)?

1. Trauma or compression
2. Diabetes
3. Vasculitis, with or without connective tissue diseases
4. Leprosy
5. Lyme disease
6. Sarcoidosis
7. Sensory perineuritis
8. Tumor infiltration
9. Lymphoid granulomatosis
10. Demyelinating paraproteinemic neuropathies (rare)
11. Hereditary liability to pressure palsies

26. Many neuropathies are treated with corticosteroids. What are the risks of oral steroids? How can these risks be prevented?

Generally, patients are started on 60–100 mg/day for 2–3 weeks, and then switched to 60–100 mg alternate-day therapy over 6–8 weeks. Patients are kept on this dose until maximum therapeutic efect is achieved (usually 4–6 months). It is critical for the physician to discuss the side effects of steroids with the patient. It is also imperative that steps be taken to prevent these side effects. Some recommendations are as follows:

1. **Ulcer:** Patients should be started on antacids (Maalox, Amphogel, etc.) and a histamine receptor blocker (Pepcid, 20 mg PO QHS). Maalox, which contains aluminum and magnesium, may lead to loose stools, whereas Amphogel can lead to constipation.

2. **Hypokalemia:** This may be prevented by having the patient take 30 mEq/day of oral K supplement or eat one or two bananas a day.

3. **Glucose intolerance:** This can occur in patients with latent diabetes or with a family history of diabetes. Efforts should be made to control the problem with dietary modification, but hypoglycemic agents may be required.

4. **Hypertension:** A low-sodium diet is essential. Patients may need antihypertensive drugs, such as diuretics.

5. **Osteopenia:** Older women are particularly susceptible to osteopenia. Patients should be started on calcium carbonate (Os-Cal, 500 mg PO BID). Tums is also a source of calcium (300 mg/tablet) and hence may be used as a source of calcium and as an antacid.

6. **Weight gain:** Patients must be placed on a low-calorie, low-carbohydrate, low-salt and high-protein diet.

7. **Cataracts and glaucoma:** Ophthalmologic evaluations need to be carried out every few months.

8. **Myopathy:** Steroid myopathy is suspected if the patient's weakness seems to increase while muscle enzymes and EMG remain unchanged. Women seem to be more susceptible to steroid myopathy. It is usually sufficient to reduce the dose of the steroid therapy, and, if improvement follows, one can assume that weakness was from the drug. A muscle biopsy shows type II fiber atrophy. The onset of steroid-induced myopathy partly depends on the dosage and duration of the steroid; however, there is considerable variation in individual susceptibility and the onset can occur in weeks rather than months.

27. Do pupillary responses aid in the diagnosis of autonomic neuropathy?

Absolutely! The pupillary aperture is under both sympathetic and parasympathetic control. The sympathetic stimulus originates from the intermediolateral horn cells at the level of T1 in the spinal cord and synapses in the superior cervical ganglion. Acetylcholine is the neurotransmitter. Second-order fibers originate from the cervical ganglion and ascend to innervate the radial fibers in the iris. Norepinephrine is the neurotransmitter here. Sympathetic stimulation leads to contraction of the radial muscles of the iris, which dilates the pupil. Damage to the sympathetic system causes a Horner's syndrome of ptosis, miosis, and anhydrosis. Parasympathetic fibers originate in the Edinger-Westphal nuclei and then synapse in the ciliary ganglion. Postganglionic fibers pass via the ciliary nerve and innervate the circular muscles of the iris, thereby causing pupillary constricton. Acetylcholine is the neurotransmitter at the postganglionic synapse. In patients with autonomic neuropathy, either or both systems can be affected, and a variety of drugs applied to the eye can aid in the diagnosis.

Drug	Normal Pupil	Autonomic Neuropathy: Pupil
4% Cocaine	Dilates	No dilation with a sympathetic lesion
1% Hydroxyamphetamine	Dilates	No dilation with a sympathetic lesion
1% Epinephrine	No change	Dilation (from denervation hypersensitivity) with a sympathetic lesion
2.5% Methacholine or .125% Pilocarpine	No change	Ptosis (from denervation hypersensitivity) with a parasympathetic lesion

28. What is the relationship between connective tissue diseases and trigeminal sensory neuropathy?

Trigeminal sensory neuropathy, a slowly progressive unilateral or bilateral facial numbness or paresthesia, may be the presenting symptom of progressive systemic sclerosis or mixed connective tissue disease. It has also been reported in Sjogren's syndrome, systemic lupus erythematosus, and dermatomyositis. The sensory symptoms often begin periorally in a localized patch and expand over weeks or months. The trigeminal sensory neuropathy is thought to be caused by vasculitis or fibrosis of the gasserian ganglion. The recognition of trigeminal neuropathy may lead to the diagnosis and treatment of the underlying connective tissue disease.

Lecky BF, Hughes RC, Murray NF: Trigeminal sensory neuropathy. Brain 110:1463–1485, 1987.

29. What are the three most common neurogenic causes of winging of the scapula?

1. **Long thoracic nerve palsy.** The long thoracic nerve innervates the serratus anterior muscle. Serratus anterior weakness leads to the most pronounced winging at rest. The medial border of the scapula is closer to the midline, and the inferior angle is medially rotated and so appears to be lower than the unaffected opposite scapula. The winging is decreased by abduction of the arms and accentuated by forward flexion of the arms.

2. **The spinal accessory nerve innervates the trapezius muscle.** Trapezius muscle weakness leads to mild winging of the scapula at rest. The medial border of the scapula is farther away from the midline, but the inferior angle is medially rotated. The winging is accentuated by arm abduction to 90 degrees and decreased by forward flexion to 90 degrees. Because of atrophy of the trapezius muscle, the shoulder is lower on the affected side.

3. **The dorsal scapular nerve innervates the rhomboid muscle.** Weakness of this muscle produces minimal winging at rest. The medial border is farther away from the midline, and the inferior angle is laterally displaced. The winging is accentuated by slowly lowering the arm from the forward overhead position and decreased by elevation of the arms overhead.

It is important to note that there are many non-neurogenic causes of winging of scapula, including myopathies and muscular dystrophy.

30. What is the most commonly used nerve for biopsy?

The best nerve to use is the sural nerve, a purely sensory nerve, located lateral to the lateral malleolus. The nerve can be biopsied at this level or at a higher level between the heads of the gastrocnemius muscles.

31. What are the indications for sural nerve biopsy?

The sural nerve biopsy is most helpful when the underlying condition is multifocal and asymmetric, and has produced multiple mononeuropathies. A diagnosis of leprosy, vasculitis, amyloidosis, or hereditary liability to pressure palsies requires a nerve biopsy. Storage diseases such as metachromatic leukodystrophy may also be diagnosed by a nerve biopsy. Metabolic and toxic causes of peripheral neuropathies are not usually diagnosed by a sural nerve biopsy.

With teased nerve fiber preparation segmental demyelination (figure A), remyelination (figure B), or axonal degeneration (figure C) is identified. In segmental demyelination the diameter of demyelinated segment is reduced. In remyelination, there is variation in the internodal length. Axonal degeneration causes breakdown of myelin into "ovoids and balls."

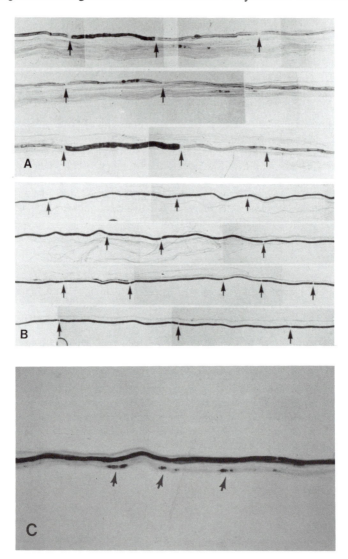

32. What is the outcome of the evaluation of patients with "peripheral neuropathy of undetermined etiology" when referred for a second opinion to a peripheral nerve expert at a tertiary referral center?

In 42% of such patients a hereditary neuropathy is found, in 21% an inflammatory neuropathy is identified, and in 13% other conditions are discovered. In 24% of cases, even after extensive evaluation, no etiology for the neuropathy is identified.

Dyck PJ, Oviatt KF, Lambert EH: Intensive evaluation of referred unclassified neuropathies yields improved diagnosis. Ann Neurol 10:222–226, 1981.

33. What are the major criteria for the diagnosis of chronic idiopathic inflammatory polyneuropathy (CIDP)?

The diagnosis of CIDP depends upon the subacute onset of muscle weakness and sensory symptoms, elevated CSF protein, slowed nerve conduction velocity, and the sural nerve biopsy finding of segmental demyelination.

34. What is the treatment of CIDP?

The treatment of CIDP is often difficult. **Prednisone** is considered the treatment of first choice. Most patients who respond to prednisone demonstrate a positive effect within 3–6 weeks of therapy. Patients who require prolonged treatment with high doses of prednisone, those who fail to respond to prednisone, or those in whom complications of corticosteroid therapy develop are candidates for alternate or additional therapies. **Azathioprine** in several small studies has proved beneficial. It may be useful in patients who fail to respond to corticosteroids and in those who are intolerant of the side effects of corticosteroids. **Cyclophosphamide** may be employed in patients unresponsive to initial therapies; further studies are necessary before final conclusions about risk-benefit ratios can be made. An uncontrolled study of a small number of CIDP patients refractory to corticosteroids, azathioprine, and plasma exchange has shown an excellent to moderate response to cyclosporine A. Total lymphoid irradiation has also been tried in refractory cases, but with limited success.

35. What is the role of plasma exchange in CIDP?

Plasma exchange (PE) may result in immediate short-term improvement in up to 30% of patients. The role of long-term intermittent PE in CIDP is currently under study. Approximately 20% of patients with CIDP become refractory to all other and multiple immunosuppressive therapies and will become dependent on long-term intermittent PE or intravenous immunoglobulin. Unfortunately, there are no predictors of outcome for treatment of CIDP. At present, PE is most commonly used in (1) the subgroup of patients with disability requiring a treatment with immediate effectiveness while prednisone therapy is being initiated, (2) patients with intermittent acute exacerbations, and (3) as alternative therapy in patients who are refractory or intolerant of other immunosuppressive therapies.

36. What is the role of intravenous immunoglobulin in CIDP?

Intravenous immunoglobulin (IVIG) is the most recent addition to the treatment of CIDP, and several reports of small series of patients suggest its usefulness. IVIG is usually administered intravenously in a dose of 0.4 gm/kg of body weight per day for 3–5 days. Benefits are often short-lived (2–9 weeks) but can be remarkable. A single dose of 1 gm/kg is as effective as a 5-day treatment. The best response is observed in patients with symptoms of recent onset (less than 1 year). IVIG therapy, if it is proved effective in controlled trials, may offer several potential advantages to chronic immunosuppressive or chronic plasmapheresis therapy. Future research will clarify its comparative effectiveness to PE or prednisone.

GUILLAIN-BARRÉ SYNDROME

37. What is the typical presentation of Guillain-Barré syndrome?

A typical patient with Guillain-Barré syndrome (GBS) reports a numb or tingling sensation in the arms and legs, followed by rapidly progressive ascending symmetric muscle weakness. Symptoms often begin 1–3 weeks after a viral upper respiratory or gastrointestinal infection, immunization, or surgery. Paralysis is maximal by 1 week in more than 50% of the patients, and by 1 month in more than 90%. A patient with a severe case of GBS may present with flaccid quadriplegia and an inability to breathe, swallow, or speak (due to oropharyngeal and respiratory paresis). Ten to twenty percent of patients require artificial respiration. Over 50% of patients develop facial weakness and 10% have extraocular muscle paralysis. Hyporeflexia or areflexia is invariably present. Preservation of reflexes in a severely weakened patient should seriously challenge the diagnosis of GBS. The patient may have mild impairment of distal sensation, but significant sensory loss is not seen. Many patients also have symptoms of autonomic dysfunction.

38. What are the typical laboratory findings in GBS?
About a week after the onset of symptoms, CSF protein content begins to rise in most patients and peaks in 4–6 weeks. The CSF cell count does not increase. Nerve conduction velocities are slowed in GBS but may be normal early in the course of the disease (first 2 weeks). EMG evidence of muscle denervation (fibrillations) may appear later in the disease.

39. What are the predictors of severe disease and poor outcome in patients with GBS?
1. Old age
2. Rapid onset of symptoms
3. Need for artificial ventilation
4. Severely decreased compound muscle action potentials (<20% of normal)
5. Acute axonal form of the disease
6. Preceding illness with *Campylobacter jejuni*

40. What is the significance of *Campylobacter jejuni* infection in GBS?
Patients with GBS and a preceding *Campylobacter jejuni* infection manifest a significantly more severe form of the disease. Not all patients with serologic evidence of *C. jejuni* have had GI symptoms before the onset of GBS. A higher incidence of autoantibodies against glycoconjugates such as GM1 and GD1a is found among these patients. There is cross-reactivity between antigens from *C. jejuni* and the P2 protein of peripheral nerve myelin, which may explain the pathogenetic connection between the infection and GBS.

41. What percent of patients with GBS suffer a relapse or second episode of the same illness?
About 3% of patients with GBS will have a relapse or second episode.

42. How is GBS treated?
Plasma exchange is of proven benefit in GBS, and IVIG may also be useful. Steroids are not indicated!

MOTOR NEURON DISEASES

43. What is the most common condition affecting the motor neurons?
Amyotrophic lateral sclerosis (ALS) is chronic, progressive deterioration of the upper motor neurons (pyramidal tract) and the lower motor neurons. It produces muscular weakness, spasticity, Babinski sign, and hyperreflexia (upper motor neurons), as well as flaccidity, atrophy, fasciculations, and hyporeflexia (lower motor neurons). The deficits are strictly motor, without significant sensory loss, ataxia, dementia, etc. For unexplained reasons, motor neurons controlling eye movements and sphincter function are usually spared as well. The disease, which usually begins in the sixth or seventh decade of life, generally progesses to death within 3–5 years from aspiration or respiratory paralysis.

44. How can the diagnosis of ALS be confirmed?
The clinical picture is usually characteristic. The EMG shows widespread denervation and reinnervation (fasciculations and polyphasic, high-amplitude muscle potentials). Muscle biopsy shows neurogenic atrophy (small, angulated fibers). Although serum CPK levels are sometimes mildly elevated, other tests are usually normal.

45. What causes ALS?

Approximately 8–10% of patients have a family history of the disease, usually in an autosomal dominant pattern. A gene for superoxide dismutase type 1 has been localized in chromosome 21, but the specific contribution of this gene to sporadic cases of ALS has not been worked out yet. Toxins have also been implicated in the cause of ALS, following the discovery of substances capable of selectively damaging motor neurons, such as lathyrism (chick peas) and BMOA (Guamanian nuts). Although the cause remains elusive, increasing evidence suggests an autoimmunal mechanism. ALS is associated with other autoimmune diseases, and inflammatory cells are present in the spinal cord. Recently antibodies have been found directed against voltage-gated calcium channels on the presynaptic terminal of the motor neurons.

Smith RG, et al: Serum antibodies to L-type calcium channels in patients with amyotrophic lateral sclerosis. N Engl J Med 327:1721–1728, 1992.

Rosen DR, et al: Mutations in Cu/Zn superoxide dismutase gene are associated with familial amyotrophic lateral sclerosis. Nature 362:59, 1993.

46. What is the differential diagnosis of ALS?

Other conditions that can affect the pyramidal tract and the lower motor neurons include: cervical spondylosis, paraneoplastic disease, hyperparathyroidism, metachromatic leukodystrophy, and hexosaminidase A deficiency.

47. What other conditions can affect the lower motor neuron (anterior horn cell)?

The differential diagnosis of deficits confined to the anterior horn cell includes polio and post-polio syndrome, Werdnig-Hoffmann disease (in infants), Kugelberg-Welander disease, and progressive spinal muscular atrophy.

48. What is primary lateral sclerosis?

It is a form of motor neuron disease in which only signs of corticospinal tract disease are seen (the Babinski sign, however, is usually absent). These signs may persist for many years unchanged. These patients rarely develop any bulbar or lower motor neuron signs.

49. Who was Lou Gehrig?

Lou Gehrig, whose name is now given to ALS, played first base for the New York Yankees from 1923–1939, usually hitting after Babe Ruth in the batting order. He had a lifetime batting average of .340 with 23 grand slams (a record) and was the first modern player to hit 4 home runs in one game. He is best known as the "Ironman" who played 2,130 consecutive games, a record that has never been approached. A kind, conscientious, thoughtful, hard-working, shy, and courteous man, Lou Gehrig, who died of ALS, was a true sports hero.

50. Name six other famous people who suffer(ed) from ALS?

1. David Niven, actor
2. Jacob Javits, senator
3. Ezzard Charles, heavyweight boxer
4. Stephen Hawking, physicist
5. Eliot Porter, photographer
6. Dmitri Shostakovich, composer

BIBLIOGRAPHY

1. Aminoff MJ: Electrodiagnosis in Clinical Neurology, 2nd ed. New York, Raven Press, 1990.
2. Dyck PJ (ed): Peripheral Neuropathy, 2nd ed. Philadelphia, W.B. Saunders, 1992.
3. Dyck PJ (ed): Peripheral neuropathy: New concepts and treatments. Neurol Clin 10:601–881, 1992.

6. RADICULOPATHY AND DEGENERATIVE SPINE DISEASE

Steven B. Inbody, M.D.

1. What is the most common cause of disability in patients under the age of 45?
Lumbar spine disorders cause enormous disability. It has been estimated that between 8 and 10 million individuals seek treatment each year for back pain. Six to eight million individuals in this country are said to claim permanent disability for this reason.

2. What are the clinical features of pain arising from nerve root compression?
The features of nerve root compression include pain, weakness, reflex change, and sensory loss. The pain is usually described as electrical, stinging, burning, searing, shooting, or sharp. It is distributed uniquely within the territory of the affected root and may radiate down (never up) the limb. The pain may be constant but worsens instantaneously from any act that abruptly increases intraspinal pressure, such as coughing or sneezing. Sensory loss is usually incomplete with respect to its density and its extent within the root territory.

3. What are the clinical features of mechanical pain associated with lumbar instability?
The pattern of pain seen with spinal instability occurs in lumbar spine diseases such as spondylosis, in which pain radiates from the center of the back toward the hip and flank on spinal movement. As the spondylitic process extends to involve more lateral portions of the spine, including the facets, pain extends into the lower limbs, usually along the back of the thigh to the popliteal space. This referred pain usually spreads gradually and is of moderate severity. These pain referral patterns usually indicate involvement of one of the lower three lumbar vertebrae, especially L4 or L5. Less commonly, the upper two vertebrae may be affected, causing pain primarily referred to the upper thigh anteriorly, just below the inguinal ligament. When severe or long-lasting, pain may extend to the back of the heel but not to the toes. The pain may be unilateral or bilateral and can shift from side to side. Patients are likely to retain full flexion and extension but display limited rotation, tilting, and squatting. There may be paravertebral or sacroiliac tenderness. Pain provocation may be related to either posture (extension) or movement (walking), and is characteristically relieved by a change in position or the pattern of movement.

Horenstein S: Clinical evaluation of patients with low back pain. Semin Neurol 6:390–402, 1986.

4. Which spinal disorders cause both back pain and disturbances of neurologic function?
Three syndromes are recognized in which spinal disorders cause both back pain and neurologic dysfunction:

1. **A herniated disc causing a single nerve root compression.** Clinical features include positive straight leg raising and radicular pain in the limb disproportionate to that in the spine. Loss of strength, reflex, and sensation occurs in that root's territory.

2. **The lateral recess syndrome.** Single or multiple nerve roots on one or both sides become compressed. Pain in the limb is usually equal to or greater than that in the spine. Symptoms are brought on by either walking or standing and are relieved with sitting. Testing by straight leg raising may be negative.

3. **Spinal stenosis.** Multiple nerve roots are involved, and the pain in the spine is significantly greater than that in the limb. Symptoms develop when standing or walking. Impairment in the bowel, bladder, or sexual function may occur.

5. What are the different patterns of root symptoms and signs in L4, L5, and S1 radiculopathies?

Compression of the L4 root produces pain radiating to the hip, anterior thigh, knee, and medial calf. Sensation is impaired over the medial calf and the territory of the saphenous nerve. L5 root compression produces pain radiating to the posterolateral buttock, lateral posterior thigh, and lateral leg. Sensory loss is most likely in a triangular wedge involving the great toe, second toe, and adjacent skin on the dorsum of the foot. S1 root compression causes pain to radiate to the posterior buttock, thigh, posterior calf, and lateral foot. Sensory loss occurs along the lateral aspect of the foot, especially the third, fourth, and fifth toes.

Weakness is rarely complete in unoperated patients. Muscle weakness due to L4 root compression is difficult to establish owing to the heavy overlap of root innervation. The quadriceps, abductor longus, gluteus medius, and tibialis anterior muscles may be weak. Weakness from an L5 root compression is most commonly found in the extensor hallucis longus, extensor digitorum brevis, and peroneus longus muscles. It is most easily identified in the extensor hallucis longus. It is difficult to identify weakness from involvement of the first sacral root. It is most easily found in the flexor hallucis brevis, but the hamstrings and gastrocnemius may also be affected.

The reflex changes may be relative or absolute. A reduced patellar reflex is seen in an L4 root compression, but because of overlapping innervation, there may be minimal change. There is ordinarily no reflex abnormality associated with L5 root compression. The ankle jerk is consistently reduced or absent in an S1 root compression, as are the hamstring reflexes, especially the semimembranosus.

6. What is the pathophysiologic process of spinal spondylosis?

Essential to the understanding of pathologic lesions that cause spondylosis (degenerative spine disease) is a knowledge of the anatomy of the spinal canal. At every level the spine rests on three supports, the so-called three joint complex, which consists of the superior joints, the intervertebral disc, and the posterior apophyseal joints (facets). The function of these three supports, or joints, is so intimately linked that changes in any one affect the other two. Often, pathologic changes start in one support (such as a disc or posterior joint) and by itself may cause symptoms. Later, the interplay between the changes in the three supports results in combined three-joint complex degeneration. As a result of these pathologic changes in the three-joint complex at one intervertebral level, mechanical changes occur that affect the levels above and below, resulting in multilevel spondylosis. The diagram of the L4–L5 vertebral bodies shows the various measurements.

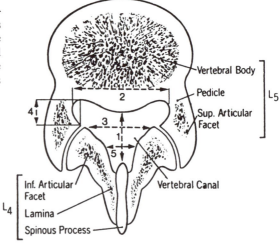

Yong-Hing K, Kirkaldy-Willis WH: The pathophysiology of degenerative disease of the lumbar spine. Orthop Clin North Am 14:491–504, 1983.

7. What are the spondylitic changes affecting the posterior joints?
Synovitis is the earliest demonstrable change in the posterior joints, which are composed of articular cartilage, a synovial membrane, and a capsule. Later, articular cartilage destruction occurs. The joint capsule becomes lax as a result of the thinning of the articular cartilage, producing instability and eventual subluxation in the joints. The two posterior joints may be unequally affected, resulting in a rotatory component. Eventually, osteophytes form around the articular processes, narrowing both the lateral recess and the central canal.

8. What are the spondylitic changes affecting the nucleus pulposus?
The earliest changes in the nucleus pulposus and anulus fibrosus are probably biochemical and may be part of aging. Trauma superimposed on these changes accelerates the degeneration. The layers of the anulus separate and form circumferential tears. Several of these circumferential tears may coalesce to form a radial tear, through which nuclear material may extrude, producing the typical disc herniation or prolapse. Even if a disc herniation does not occur, the multiple tears produce weakening and circumferential bulging of the anulus with loss of disc height. Further disc narrowing results from aging of the nucleus pulposus, which changes from a gelatinous consistency in childhood to a fibrotic consistency in adulthood.

9. What are the clinical features of lumbar stenosis?
Most patients are more than 50 years of age and have had symptoms referable to lumbar spinal stenosis for 1 or more years. Neurogenic intermittent claudication or pseudoclaudication is the most common presenting and constant symptom in lumbar spinal stenosis. Symptoms are usually bilateral, with one leg more involved than the other, but may be unilateral. Although most patients describe their leg symptoms as painful, it should be emphasized that the pain is distinctively different from the radicular type of pain seen with an acutely and laterally herniated intervertebral disc. The pain is usually of a dull, aching quality. The whole lower extremity is generally affected. The pain is provoked by walking and, in many patients, merely by standing. It is quickly relieved by sitting or leaning forward. In some patients the pain is accompanied by numbness of the affected leg that is usually described as a sensation of deadness rather than a tingling sensation. About half of the patients report weakness in the affected leg "as though it might at any moment give way." Low back pain with various degrees of severity is present in about 65% of patients with lumbar spinal stenosis. Back pain is most common during that stage of the disease in which the joint capsules and anulus have become lax, permitting transverse and rotatory movements of the involved vertebrae. Back pain frequently improves when osteophyte formation stabilizes the motion segment. Radicular pain is the least common manifestation of spinal stenosis.

10. What is the lateral recess syndrome?
The lateral recess syndrome, also known as the facet syndrome, produces radicular pain in the setting of spinal stenosis. The underlying cause is osteophyte formation on the superior articular facet, which intrudes into the nerve root canal, trapping the nerve root. The symptoms usually include unilateral or bilateral pain or paresthesias in the distribution of the L5 or S1 dermatome. Although quite similar to the symptoms of radiculopathy related to a herniated intervertebral disc, pain in the lateral recess syndrome is brought on by standing and walking and relieved by sitting, which is the opposite to what happens in discogenic disease. Additional differences include the failure of coughing or sneezing to aggravate symptoms, and negative straight leg raising in lateral recess syndrome radiculopathy.

Ciric I, Mikhael MA: Lumbar spinal-lateral recess stenosis. Neurol Clin 7:417–424, 1989.

11. What is the mechanism that causes symptoms in lumbar spinal stenosis?
Symptoms are related to the increase in lordotic posture provoked by standing or walking. Myelographic studies have shown that in lordosis, the cross-sectional area of the spinal canal narrows because of anterior encroachment by bulging discs, posterior encroachment by shortening and thickening of the ligamentum flavum and lateral approximation of the articular facets. In flexion (as in sitting), all these encroachments reverse with a resultant increase in the cross-sectional area of the spinal canal.

12. What are the most frequent causes of spinal stenosis?
Although more than 25 causes of spinal stenosis have been described, four conditions account for the majority of the cases:

1. Idiopathic (developmental) spinal stenosis is the result of shorter than normal pedicles, thickened convergent lamina, and a convex posterior vertebral body. Idiopathic spinal stenosis rarely becomes symptomatic on its own but rather predisposes to normal degenerative changes, eventually becoming symptomatic.

2. Degenerative spinal stenosis accounts for approximately half of all cases. Degenerative changes affect the facets posteriorly and the disc anteriorly. As the facets become lax, allowing instability and subluxation, osteophytes form and narrow both the nerve root and central canal. Simultaneously, disc degeneration, characterized by tears in the circumferential anular fibers, allows the disc to bulge into the nerve root and central canal.

3. Degenerative spondylolisthesis occurs when the facets degenerate, allowing slippage of the upper vertebra forward over the lower vertebra.

4. Postoperative spinal stenosis occurs after laminectomy or spinal fusion. Stenosis is produced by bone formation and scar tissue.

13. What are the indications for surgical treatment of lumbar spinal stenosis?
Specific indications for surgery include (1) persistent intolerable pain; (2) limitation of walking distance or standing endurance to a degree that compromises necessary activities; or (3) severe or progressive muscle weakness or disturbed bladder or sexual function. The surgical treatment consists of removal of spinal lamina and articular facets to the extent necessary to decompress the central canal, the nerve root canal, or both. Multilevel laminectomy is usually required. If spondylolisthesis is also present, spinal fusion may be necessary. Because the back pain associated with lumbar stenosis originates primarily from degenerative disc and joint disease, which is not corrected by surgery, many patients report little change in pain after the operation.

14. What is the relationship of spondylosis, spondylolysis, and spondylolisthesis?
Spondylosis refers to osteoarthritis involving the articular surfaces (joints and discs) of the spine, often with osteophyte formation and cord or root compression. Spondylolysis refers to a separation at the pars articularis, which permits the vertebrae to slip. The pars defect may be unilateral or bilateral. Spondylolisthesis may occur as a result of bilateral pars defects or may be due to degenerative disc disease. Spondylolisthesis is defined as the anterior subluxation of the suprajacent vertebra, often producing central canal stenosis; it is the slipping of one vertebra forward on the one below. When symptomatic, all three conditions cause pain in the lower back after motion or lifting. Splinting with contraction of the lumbar paraspinal muscles is frequent. The three disorders are confirmed radiographically, with flexion/extension spine films often demonstrating segmental instability.

15. What is the difference between a bulging disc and a herniated disc?
The bulging disc is so common after the age of 30 that it should be considered normal. The bulging disc appears rounded and symmetric and does not extend beyond the disc space, whereas the herniated disc appears angular and asymmetric and extends outside the disc space. Because the bulging disc is unlikely to cause nerve root compression, the nerve root

appears normal in size, whereas in the herniated disc the nerve root often appears widened in its distal part.

16. What is the role of plain radiographs in the evaluation of spinal disorders?

Plain radiography plays a role in the initial evaluation of the chronic pain patient by excluding traumatic, congenital, or pathologic fractures as a cause of the pain syndrome. If abnormalities are seen, plain x-rays can be followed by more sophisticated imaging such as MRI or post-myelogram CT. Plain radiographs are also useful in the evaluation of curvature of the spine, in which predisposing spinal disorders such as scoliosis or kyphosis can be recognized. Additionally, reversal of the normal lordotic curve in the cervical or lumbar region may suggest significant muscular spasm. The most useful application of plain radiographs is with flexion and extension views, in which spinal segmental instability can be identified and quantitated. This represents one of the few studies available for dynamic imaging of the spine.

17. What is the role of MRI of the spine?

With advancing technology, the accuracy of MRI is quickly approaching that of the post-myelogram CT. The relative strengths of MRI over conventional post-myelogram CT include better delineation of soft tissue abnormalities such as tumor, hematoma, or epidural scar formation. Epidural scar formation, in particular, makes MRI with gadolinium enhancement the radiographic evaluation of choice in the postoperative spine, where postsurgical scarring will enhance. The MRI scan below shows a herniated disc at L5 on sagittal (left) and axial (right) views.

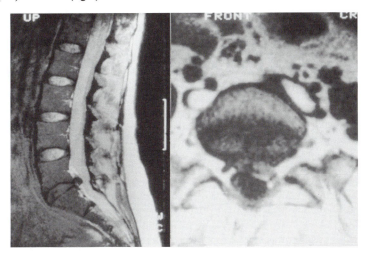

18. What are the major limitations of lumbar myelography without post-myelogram CT imaging?

Lumbar myelography is insensitive at the L5/S1 interspace, where the epidural space is often so deep that even large central disc herniations fail to cause indentation of the thecal sac. Additionally, far lateral disc herniations may be missed with myelography alone. Post-myelogram CT corrects these limitations and remains the gold standard in imaging spinal disorders.

19. What is the imaging study of choice for discitis?

Radionucleotide bone scanning is more sensitive than CT for the detection of early discitis. CT, however, demonstrates to better advantage the extent of the disease and facilitates the choice of biopsy site for identification of the responsible organism. Collapse of the disc space, best seen on sagittal reformatted images, and irregular destruction of the vertebral endplates are characteristic of this disorder. Symptoms of discitis, which occur most commonly in the immediate postoperative period, include severe low back pain and the presence of localized tenderness and muscle spasm at the surgical site.

20. What is the role of electromyography (EMG) in the evaluation of radiculopathy?

In light of studies suggesting a frequency of spine CT abnormalities in 25–55% of the normal population, EMG provides neurophysiologic confirmation of the radiographic lesion. In some studies investigators find that EMG correlates better with the clinical course than myelography or CT scanning. More importantly, EMG evidence of altered innervation suggests significant nerve root compromise. The most widely accepted EMG evidence of radiculopathy is the presence of positive sharp waves and fibrillation potentials in two separate areas. EMG changes are first seen in muscles closest to the site of nerve injury, underscoring the importance of examination of the paraspinous muscles. A disadvantage of EMG is the delay in appearance of reliable abnormalities until 7–10 days after a root injury. The sequence of EMG changes begins with positive sharp waves in paraspinal muscles between days 7 and 10, then paraspinous fibrillation potentials and positive sharp waves in limb muscles between days 17 and 21.

   McGarry JD: Neurophysiologic evaluation of patients with low back pain. Semin Neurol 6:372–375, 1986.

21. What is the role of the H-reflex in an S1 radiculopathy?

The H-reflex closely mirrors variation in the ankle jerk, where a small difference in latency between the lower extremities suggests S1 root disease. The H-reflex is an evoked potential study performed by electrically stimulating the S1 root and measuring the nerve conduction velocity proximally. It complements the routine nerve conduction and EMG analysis of muscles, and is routinely performed during the same evaluation. Unlike EMG, the H-reflex may demonstrate abnormalities within 1 or 2 days following nerve root injury.

22. What is the role of EMG in differentiating spinal root, plexus, or peripheral nerve injury?

Derangement of motor, sensory, and autonomic function may be present with lesions at the level of the root, plexus, or peripheral nerve. EMG changes consistent with a lesion of the L5 root, the most common one involved in low back pain, would demonstrate altered innervation in the lumbar paraspinous muscles as well as the L5-innervated gluteus medius and extensor hallucis longus muscles. A lumbosacral plexopathy would be expected to spare the lumbar paraspinous muscles. A peroneal nerve injury could be differentiated from an L5 root or lumbosacral plexopathy by the absence of denervation in the gluteus medius.

23. What is the nonsurgical treatment for patients with acute back pain?

Patients with acute back pain who have had symptoms for less than 6 months but without a radiculopathy may reasonably expect a 90% chance of recovery. A somewhat smaller proportion, 75–85% of those with radicular features, will also recover. The first phase of treatment is aimed at immediately relieving the pain. The second is designed to maintain the patient's comfort level by self-applied programs using activity and conditioning, with minimal use of medication.

   The acute phase is managed by bed rest. Some experts also advocate manipulative therapy, emphasizing the slow application of pressure to alter spinal alignment. Bed rest is assisted by placing a board on or below the mattress, which relieves the vertical pressure on the spine and evenly supports it. Most patients quickly become comfortable and do not need narcotics, maintaining relief with aspirin or acetaminophen. Heat or ice may be applied. When comfortable, patients are ready to enter the second phase, where progressive ambulation begins and the level of activity is steadily increased. As they return to full activity, most patients can be taught proper carriage, movement patterns, and methods of lifting. Should spinal instability be suspected, a lumbosacral corset should be used to inhibit random spinal movement. Patients with acute pain and without neurologic manifestations who fail to fully recover should be reassessed by clinical, electrophysiologic, and imaging procedures.

Nachemson A: A critical look at the treatment for low back pain. Scand J Rehabil Med 11:143–147, 1979.

24. What is the nonsurgical treatment of patients with chronic pain who have failed to respond to conservative treatment?

Chronic back pain will never remit. More importantly, it will not remain at a fixed level, but rather will oscillate between recurrent exacerbations and remissions. The treatment goal is reduction of pain to a tolerable level. Some experts assert that however treated, the majority of patients, because of spontaneous stabilization of the spine, will no longer complain of severe pain after about 4 years. Assuming that the clinical assessment fails to indicate a condition requiring specific medical or surgical treatment, the elements of the treatment program for chronic pain include postural correction and avoidance of activities in which the spine may be aggravated by improper lifting techniques. Compensation for spinal segmental instability may require a lumbosacral corset, or, less often, a brace. Surgical fusion should never be undertaken for chronic spinal pain unless external immobilization has produced consistent and durable relief. Periodic movement and stretching, avoiding fixed positions at work, and adjusting the height and inclination of work surfaces may relieve most diurnal discomfort. Maintenance of the range of spinal motion can be assured by simple exercises.

25. What are the current surgical techniques for common clinical radicular syndromes?

Although an epidural injection might not ordinarily be considered a surgical procedure, it is an invasive one that has proved to be quite effective in hastening spontaneous relief of root entrapment syndromes. Microdiscectomy is the current equivalent of the traditional unilateral laminectomy for removal of a herniated disc. A smaller skin incision and lesser dissection are afforded. Lateral recess stenosis with or without disc herniation can be treated with laminectomy plus medial facetectomy. When bilateral and associated with foraminal stenosis, foraminotomy plus fusion is required.

26. What are the most common causes of the failed (surgical) back?

1. The diagnosis was wrong. Therefore, even if the surgical treatment was technically flawless, the patient must be regarded as having never been treated and requires thorough reassessment, with generation of a new treatment plan.

2. The diagnosis was correct but the treatment was technically flawed, inappropriate, or incompetent.

3. Whether or not the diagnosis was correct, something new has happened—perhaps an immediate or late consequence of treatment or an unrelated but intercurrent complication. This situation usually occurs when two or more pain-generating mechanisms coexist, such as in disc herniation, when removal of disc material improves radicular symptoms but fails to address the mechanical pain produced by the spinal instability after the herniation.

4. A complication of diagnosis or treatment has arisen: for example, development of arachnoiditis, injury to a nerve root, or disc space infection.

5. No counseling has been given. Physicians must negotiate a plan of postsurgical treatment, stressing patient participation in functional restoration, and dispelling unrealistic expectations of complete restoration to normal.

Horenstin S: Chronic low back pain and the failed low back syndrome. Neurol Clin 7:361–386, 1989.

27. What is the most common postoperative complication of spinal surgery?
Chronic arachnoiditis at the surgical site is the most common postoperative complication. Although the pathophysiology remains uncertain, its association with the use of oil-based myelographic dyes and other intrathecal agents suggests an inflammatory etiology. Diagnosis is by CT myelography, which enhances the wall of the thecal sac and clumped nerve roots.

28. What is the clinical presentation of a thoracic disc herniation?
Pain is the most common initial symptom in thoracic disc herniation, occurring in approximately 60% of cases. The pain usually occurs near the midline, unilaterally or bilaterally, and may have a characteristic radicular distribution. The second most common symptom is numbness. Motor weakness involving the lower extremities is an initial symptom in 28% of patients. Bladder involvement is a rare initial symptom but can be present in 30% of patients at the time of presentation.

29. What is the incidence, level, and pathogenesis of herniated thoracic discs?
Less than 1% of protruded discs occur in the thoracic spine. Over 75% of herniated thoracic discs develop below T8, with the highest incidence at the T11/12 level. The protrusion is usually central. The majority of patients have a degenerative process as the main causative factor, with trauma accounting for only 10–20% of protruded discs.

30. What is the differential diagnosis of thoracic pain?

Malignant or benign tumors of the spine	Thoracic compression fractures
Ankylosing spondylosis	Intraabdominal processes
Thoracoabdominal neuropathy (diabetes)	(gallbladder disease, gastric ulcer, pancreatitis)
Intercostal neuralgia	Cardiac causes
Herpes zoster	An intramedullary lesion such as a demyelinating process

31. What are the clinical features of cervical spondylitic neurologic dysfunction?
Neurologic dysfunction from cervical spondylosis can be separated into four distinct but overlapping groups.

1. The **lateral or radicular syndrome** occurs when disc material, osteophytes, or hypertrophic facets impinge on nerve roots. Pain in the neck is often lateralized and radiates into the occiput or scapula. The pain is often aggravated by neck movement, and the cervical spine is often tender to percussion. Radicular pain and paresthesia in the upper limb are frequent features of the syndrome and are sometimes precipitated or aggravated by neck movement, coughing, sneezing, or straining. Objective neurologic findings follow dermatomal patterns and include weakness, fasciculations, atrophy, loss of reflexes, and a decrease in pain or temperature sensation. In the pure lateral syndrome, long tract signs are absent.

2. The **medial or spinal syndrome** produces pure myelopathy without root symptoms or signs. Neck pain is variable, but most patients have some limitation of neck mobility. The earliest symptoms are usually stiffness and weakness of the lower extremities, which can be asymmetric. Gait ataxia and paresthesia of the feet are also common. Examination reveals spasticity with exaggerated reflexes and extensor plantar responses.

3. The **combined medial and lateral syndrome** accounts for the largest group of patients. Symptoms or signs of root disease in the upper extremities accompany long tract signs in the lower limbs.

4. A **vascular syndrome** represents a fourth group of patients with spondylosis and symptoms distinct from those already described. They characteristically have little or no pain or root symptoms. The acute or subacute onset of the myelopathy differentiates this

group from the more common spondylitic myelopathy, which is insidious in onset. This syndrome develops quickly, with some patients awakening with the deficit.

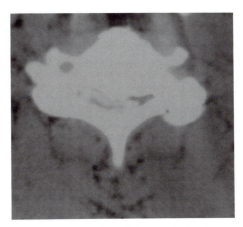

The CT scan above shows compression of the cervical spinal cord caused by severe cervical spondylosis.

Cusick JF: Neurosurgical considerations of cervical myelopathy. Semin Neurol 9:193–199, 1989.

32. What is Spurling's sign?
A patient suffering from an acute cervical disc herniation may have significantly increased neck pain on lateral neck movements, especially toward the side of the lesion (Spurling's sign). The pain is also referred within the distribution of the spinal nerve, which is compressed. On examination, the neck usually appears rigidly held and sometimes slightly flexed toward the side of the lesion.

33. What are the clinical differences between compression of the sixth and seventh cervical nerve roots?
Compression of the sixth cervical root (from either osteophytes or disc herniation at the C5/6 level) produces weakness of the deltoid and biceps muscles, a diminished biceps reflex, and diminished skin sensation in the thumb and index finger. Compression of the seventh cervical nerve root (from either osteophytes or disc herniation at the C6/7 level) produces weakness of the triceps muscle, a diminished triceps reflex, and diminished skin sensation in the index and middle finger.

34. What causes cervical spondylosis?
Cervical spondylosis includes both degenerative disc disease and degenerative joint disease. Although less common than degenerative disease of the lumbar spine, cervical spondylosis shares a similar pathogenesis. Initially, degeneration in the nucleus pulposus leads to segmental instability due to segmental narrowing. Subsequent development of degenerative joint disease in the posterior facet joints with osteophyte formation leads finally to herniation of the intervertebral disc. The segments commonly affected by such degenerative changes in the cervical spine are C5/6 and C6/7, which, like the lower lumbar segments, are particularly mobile and in the area of maximum lordosis.

35. What are the current surgical techniques recommended for cervical radiculopathy?
Cervical radiculopathy may be surgically treated with either an anterior or posterior approach. An anterior approach is recommended for medial disc herniation or when fusion is contemplated. Either approach is effective for lateral or foraminal cervical disc herniation.

36. What are the current nonsurgical techniques recommended for cervical radiculopathy?
Patients with slight to moderate disability usually do well when treated conservatively. Response to conservative management over time is also important. Bed rest and activity modification are important acutely and should be combined with anti-inflammatory agents, including a brief and quickly tapered course of low-dose corticosteroids if severe. Muscle relaxants may provide benefit to patients with secondary cervical paraspinal spasm due to the radiculopathy. Patients with more severe disability and signs of progressive myelopathy, however, often fare poorly with conservative, nonsurgical management.

BIBLIOGRAPHY

1. Adams R, Victor M. Principles of Neurology, 4th ed. New York, McGraw-Hill, 1989.
2. Kranzler LI, Penn RD, Dohrmann GJ (eds): Neurol Clin 3(2):1985.

7. MYELOPATHIES

Richard M. Armstrong, M.D.

1. What is the anatomic organization of the spinal cord?

The gray matter forms a butterfly-shaped column in the center of the cord, containing the cell bodies of many of the motor, sensory, and autonomic neurons. These neurons are grouped into various zones (Rexed's laminae), depending on their function. Surrounding the gray matter are the white matter pathways, or long tracts, which carry ascending and descending information throughout the cord.

2. What are the most important long tracts in the spinal cord? Where in the cord is each located?

Long Tracts in the Spinal Cord

TRACT	LOCATION	FUNCTION
Gracile	Medial dorsal column	Proprioception from the leg
Cuneate	Lateral dorsal column	Proprioception from the arm
Spinocerebellar	Superficial lateral column	Muscular position and tone
Pyramidal	Deep lateral column	Upper motor neuron
Lateral spinothalamic	Ventrolateral column	Pain and thermal sensation

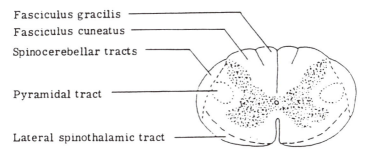

The major long tracts of the spinal cord. (From Joynt R: Clinical Neurology. Philadelphia, J.B. Lippincott, 1992, with permission.)

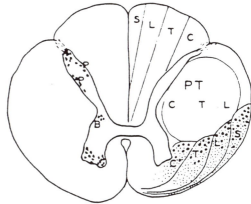

The somatotopic organization of the major long tracts of the spinal cord. The dorsal columns have lower-extremity fibers (sacral and lumbar) lying medially, while the pyramidal and spinocerebellar tracts have lower-extremity fibers lying laterally. C = cervical, T = thoracic, L = lumbar, S = sacral, PT = pyramidal tract. (From Joynt R: Clinical Neurology. Philadelphia, J.B. Lippincott, 1992, with permission.)

3. What is the pyramidal tract?

The pyramidal tract is made up of those axons arising in the posterior frontal and anterior parietal cortex that terminate in the cord after passing through the pyramid of the medulla. It helps control motor function.

4. What is pyramidal decussation?

At the level of the lower medulla, the majority (80%) of the fibers derived from one hemisphere cross the midline and innervate cells in the cord contralateral to the side of origin.

5. What results from nondecussation of the pyramids?

Nondecussation may occur in association with some anomaly of the medullary cord junction. Clinically, it may be expressed as mirror movements.

6. Where are the long tracts that regulate bladder function?

The pathways for micturition lie in the lateral columns of the cord.

7. What are the fasciculi proprii?

The fasciculi proprii, or ground bundles, are short fiber connections between segments of the cord. They help control spinal reflex patterns.

8. What is the intermediolateral cell column?

The intermediolateral cell column is composed of neurons that lie in a column in the lateral horn of the gray matter of the cord from T1 to L3 segments. These neurons give rise to sympathetic efferent nerves.

9. Where are the neurons that innervate the axial musculature located?

Axial musculature neurons are in the ventral horn of the gray matter in the cord and lie medially to those neurons innervating the limb musculature.

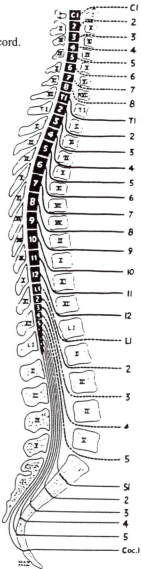

10. What are myotomes and dermatomes?

The cord is organized segmentally, with a pair of spinal nerves exiting from each of its 29 segments. Each pair supplies a specific group of muscles (the myotome) and a specific area of the skin (the dermatome).

11. What are the dermatomes at the umbilicus? At the nipple line?

The umbilicus is at T10. The nipple line is at T5.

12. What is the relationship of the cord segment and its spinal nerves to the vertebral body?

The spinal cord extends from the medullary cervical junction at the foramen magnum to the level of the body of the first lumbar vertebra. The spinal roots exit in relation to their corresponding vertebral body. The first seven cervical nerves exit above the vertebral body, and the eighth exits below C7. The remainder of the spinal roots exit below their corresponding vertebral body. This diagram of the sagittal section of the spinal cord and vertebral column shows the relationship of the nerve roots to the intervertebral foramina. (From Joynt R: Clinical Neurology. Philadelphia, J.B. Lippincott, 1992, with permission.)

13. What is the origin and distribution of the anterior spinal artery?

The anterior spinal artery lies along the median ventral plane of the cervical cord. It receives 6 to 8 major radicular branches, and other branches of the ascending cervical and vertebral arteries help it supply the cervical and upper thoracic cord. The anterior spinal artery gives rise to small central arteries that enter the ventral fissure and penetrate the cord to supply the anterior columns and ventral gray matter. Circumferential branches supply the anterolateral two thirds of the cord.

14. What is the artery of Adamkiewicz?

The artery of Adamkiewicz is a major radicular branch that arises from the aorta and enters the cord between T10 and L3. It supplies the lumbar and lower thoracic segments, anastomosing with the anterior spinal artery in the lower thoracic region, which is thus the watershed area of the cord. The diagram shows the blood supply of the spinal cord. The lumbar radicular artery is commonly called the artery of Adamkiewicz. (From Joynt R: Clinical Neurology. Philadelphia, J.B. Lippincott, 1992, with permission.)

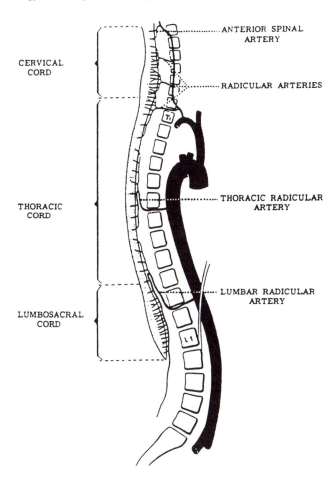

15. What is the arterial supply of the posterior third of the cord?
Paired dorsolateral arteries extend the length of the cord and supply the posterior third of the cord through circumflex and penetrating vessels.

16. What is a myelopathy?
A myelopathy is any pathologic process that affects primarily the spinal cord and causes neurologic dysfunction. The commonest causes of myelopathies are:

1. Congenital and developmental defects
   Syringomyelia
   Neural tube formation defects
2. Trauma
3. Compromise of the spinal canal
   Cervical spondylosis
   Inflammatory arthritis
   Acute disc herniation
4. Spinal neoplasms
5. Physical agents
   Decompression sickness
   Electrical injury
   Radiation
6. Toxins
   Nitrous oxide
   Triorthocresyl phosphate
7. Metabolic and nutritional disorders
   Pernicious anemia
   Chronic liver disease
8. Remote effect of cancer
9. Arachnoiditis
10. Postinfectious autoimmune disorders
    Acute transverse myelitis
    Connective tissue disease
11. Multiple sclerosis
12. Epidural infections
13. Primary infections
14. Vascular
    Epidural hematoma
    Atherosclerotic, abdominal
      aneurysm
    Malformation

17. What clinical findings suggest a myelopathy?
Myelopathies usually have a triad of clinical findings:
   1. Bilateral upper motor neuron weakness of the legs (paraparesis, paraplegia) or legs and arms (quadriparesis, quadriplegia).
   2. Bilateral impairment of sensation with a "level" that separates a region of normal sensation from a region of impaired sensation.
   3. Bowel or bladder sphincter dysfunction.

18. What is Lhermitte's sign?
Lhermitte's sign is present when the patient reports an electric shocklike sensation down the spine with neck flexion. The symptom is produced by stretching and irritation of damaged fibers in the dorsal columns of the cervical cord. It may occur in cervical spondylogenic myelopathy or with intramedullary lesions such as a demyelinating plaque.
   Goldblatt D, Levy L: The electric sign and the incandescent lamp. Semin Neurol 5:191–193, 1985.

19. What is the Brown-Sequard syndrome?
The Brown-Sequard syndrome is caused by a lateral hemisection of the spinal cord, usually at or below the cervical enlargement, that severs the pyramidal tract (which has already crossed in the medulla), the uncrossed dorsal columns, and the crossed spinothalamic tract.
   Ipsilateral and below the level of the lesion there is upper motor neuron weakness or paralysis, and loss of tactile discrimination and position and vibration sense. The tendon reflexes become hyperactive with subsequent spasticity and an extensor plantar response. Contralateral to the lesion there is loss of sense of pain and temperature to a dermatome one or two levels below the lesion.

20. What is spinal shock?
If the cord is transected suddenly by mechanical trauma, ischemia, or compression, there is an initial period when reflex activity begins to function autonomously, and hyporeflexia

with flaccidity may occur. Development of upper motor neuron signs may take several weeks. There may also be autonomic dysfunction with diffuse sweating and hypotension.

21. What are the signs of anterior spinal artery occlusion?
Anterior spinal ischemia causes bilateral impairment of pain and temperature below the lesion, accompanied by weakness and bladder dysfunction. The reflexes may be hyperactive below the level of the lesion. Dorsal column function (position and vibration) is spared.

22. What is transverse myelitis?
Transverse myelitis is an inflammatory process that is localized over several segments of the cord and functionally transects the cord. It may occur as an infectious or parainfectious illness, or as a manifestation of multiple sclerosis, vasculitis, or an autoimmune process. In a significant number of cases (40%), no specific etiology is ever identified.

Ford B, Tampieri D, Francis G: Long-term follow-up of acute partial transverse myelopathy. Neurology 42:250–252, 1992.

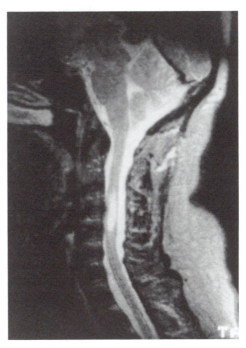

Sagittal T2-weighted MRI shows increased signal within the cervical cord caused by acute inflammatory transverse myelitis.

23. What are the clinical features of acute transverse myelitis?
The sudden onset of weakness and sensory disturbance in the legs and trunk is the usual presenting feature. Ultimately, sphincter dysfunction is common. Pain and temperature are usually affected but proprioception and vibration are often spared. The tendon jerks below the lesion may be initially depressed and then hyperactive. A sensory level indicates the level of the lesion.

24. What is the management of the patient with transverse myelitis?
Appropriate imaging studies of the cord and spinal column should be obtained to exclude a compressive lesion. Diagnostic studies (hematologic, CSF analysis) should exclude, if possible, multiple sclerosis, vasculitis, or an infectious process (zoster, HIV, HTLV-I, etc.).

Supportive nursing care and careful management of bladder and bowel function are essential. A trial of high-dose intravenous corticosteroids may be tried if infectious causes and compressive lesions have been excluded.

Helgason C, Arnason BTW: Transverse myelitis. Autoimmun Forum 6:2–11, 1992.

25. What is syringomyelia?

Syringomyelia is a longitudinal cystic cavity that develops within the substance of the cord. It may extend over a few or many segments of the cord, and may extend into the medulla (syringobulbia). The cavity is irregular and tends to intrude into the anterior horns of the gray matter and the gray matter dorsal to the central canal. The cavity wall is unremarkable, with only gliosis present.

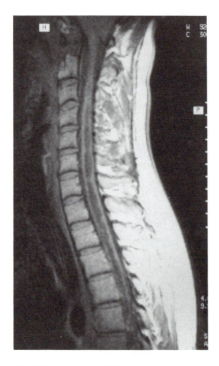

Sagittal MRI shows an extensive syrinx cavity in the cervical and thoracic spinal cord. This syrinx is associated with a developmental defect—an Arnold-Chiari malformation at the base of the skull (protrusion of the cerebellar tonsils down through the foramen magnum).

26. What are the clinical features of syringomyelia?

Classically there is a dissociated sensory loss (loss of temperature and pain with intact proprioception) and lower motor neuron weakness (flaccid paralysis, atrophy, fasciculations) that result from the cavity extension and destruction of central spinal gray matter. This most commonly occurs in the lower cervical and upper thoracic segments in a capelike distribution. Long tract signs may be evident below the level of the lesion, and sphincter abnormalities and sympathetic dysfunction (Horner's syndrome) may also develop.

27. What causes syringomyelia?

The formation of the syrinx cavity is not fully understood. Primary syringomyelia is presumed to be a developmental abnormality. It has been suggested that it is a form of dysraphism resulting from incomplete closure of the neural tube, or that it results from an intramedullary vascular anomaly that causes tissue necrosis and cavitation. Another theory proposes that it results from pulsing pressure waves transmitted from the fourth ventricle because of anomalies in the fourth ventricle foramina.

Secondary syringomyelia is recognized as a cavity formed in relation to an acquired injury, such as an intramedullary tumor, traumatic damage, or central necrosis resulting from ischemia.

28. What is the treatment for syringomyelia?

The standard therapy for progressive syringomyelia is surgical decompression and shunting of the cavity. Unfortunately, results are seldom impressive, and symptoms often continue to progress.

Logue V, Edwards MR: Syringomyelia and its surgical treatment—an analysis of 75 cases. J Neurol Neurosurg Psychiatry 44:273–278, 1981.

29. What is cervical spondylosis?

Cervical disc narrowing and osteophytic proliferation are common (>50%) in persons 40 years or older. These changes may result in cord compression if the canal diameter is small, and may also compromise the circulation to the cord. Spondylitic changes can also compress the spinal nerves that exit through the foramen.

30. What is spondylogenic myelopathy?

This myelopathy is caused by spondylitic changes compressing the cord. It occurs in middle to late age and is more common in men than women. Long tract involvement resulting from cord compromise may be associated with radicular features.

Upper motor neuron weakness (paresis, hypertonia, hyperreflexia) may appear before sensory impairment. When sensory loss does develop, dorsal columns tend to be more affected than lateral spinothalamic tracts. Bladder and bowel dysfunction is less common.

31. How is spondylogenic myelopathy best managed?

The management of spondylogenic myelopathy is controversial. In a patient with severe disease, a significantly narrowed canal, and severe neurologic compromise, surgical treatment is probably indicated to prevent further deterioration. Many patients with features of myelopathy and radicular pain are managed conservatively with a cervical collar and anti-inflammatory medication. The course tends to be chronic, in which there may be intermittent exacerbations, improvement, or long periods of stable symptomatology.

32. What are the other common causes of cord compression?

Causes of spinal cord compression are best conceptualized in terms of their anatomic location, either inside or outside the cord (medulla) and surrounding meninges (especially the dura).

1. Intramedullary and Intradural
     Primary cord neoplasms
     Syringomyelia
     Metastasis or abscess within the substance of the cord (rare)
2. Extramedullary and Intradural
     Neurofibroma and schwannoma
     Meningioma
3. Extramedullary and Extradural
     Epidural metastases from a remote primary neoplasm. The most common
         metastases that compress the cord arise from the breast, lung, GI tract,
         lymphoma/myeloma, and prostate.
     Epidural abscess
     Epidural hematoma

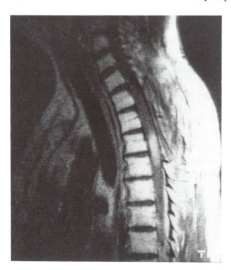

Sagittal T1-weighted MRI (*left*), after gadolinium enhancement, shows an astrocytoma arising within the thoracic spinal cord (an intramedullary, intradural lesion).

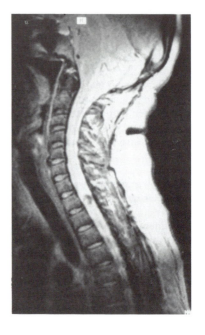

Sagittal T2-weighted MRI (*right*) shows a neurofibroma displacing the thoracic spinal cord (an extramedullary, intradural lesion).

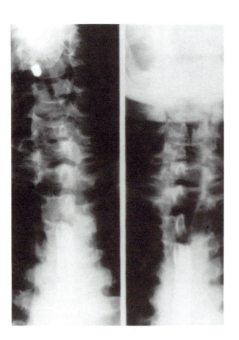

Myelogram (*left*) shows a block of the column of dye at T2 caused by spinal cord compression from metastatic prostate cancer (an extramedullary, extradural lesion).

33. What are the commonest neoplasms arising within the spinal cord?

Most primary spinal cord tumors are either astrocytomas or ependymomas.

34. What is tropical spastic paraparesis?

This disorder has been recognized clinically for many years in tropical areas and in Japan. It is characterized by a chronic course in which mild to severe leg weakness develops with increased muscle tone and extensor plantar responses. Half the patients have posterior column sensory signs and 15% have optic nerve involvement. The condition is caused by infection with a retrovirus, HTLV-I. For this reason, it is sometimes called HTLV-I associated myelopathy (HAM).

Janssen RS, Kaplan JE, Khabbaz RF, et al: HTLV-I associated myelopathy/tropical spastic paraparesis in the United States. Neurology 41:1355–1357, 1991.

35. What is subacute combined degeneration of the spinal cord?

This condition is the result of vitamin B12 deficiency. In the cord, there is demyelination and vacuolar degeneration of the posterior columns and the corticospinal tracts. Frequently there is an associated peripheral neuropathy that often presents clinically as peripheral neuropathy accompanied by accentuated tendon jerks and extensor plantar responses (because of the corticospinal tract involvement). The sensory impairment resulting from posterior column damage may be much more severe than the loss of spinothalamic modalities. Nitrous oxide exposure may produce a similar pathologic picture.

36. Does myelopathy occur as part of acquired immunodeficiency syndrome (AIDS)?

HIV infection may affect the spinal cord and produce a picture of acute or subacute myelitis. Myelopathy is found in approximately 25% of AIDS autopsies. The pathologic picture is vacuolar degeneration similar to that seen in vitamin B12 deficiency.

Petito CK, Navia BA, Cho ES, et al: Vacuolar myelopathy pathologically resembling subacute combined degeneration in patients with the acquired immunodeficiency syndrome. N Engl J Med 312:874–879, 1985.

BIBLIOGRAPHY

1. Adams RD, Victor M: Principles of Neurology, 4th ed. New York, McGraw-Hill, 1989.
2. DeMyer W. Anatomy and clinical neurology of the spinal cord. In Joynt R (ed): Clinical Neurology. Philadelphia, J.B. Lippincott, 1992.
3. Kincaid JC: Myelitis and myelopathy. In Joynt R (ed): Clinical Neurology. Philadelphia, J.B. Lippincott, 1992.

8. BRAINSTEM DISEASE

Eugene C. Lai, M.D., Ph.D.

CLINICAL ANATOMY OF BRAINSTEM

1. What is the functional importance of the brainstem?
The brainstem is a small, narrow region connecting the spinal cord with the diencephalon and cerebrum. It lies ventral to the cerebellum, which it links via the cerebellar peduncles. Its functions are critical to survival. The brainstem is densely packed with many vital structures such as long ascending and descending pathways that carry sensory and motor information to and from higher brain regions. It contains the nuclei of cranial nerves III through XII and their intramedullary fibers. It also possesses groups of neurons that are the major source of noradrenergic, dopaminergic, and serotonergic inputs to most parts of the brain. In addition, other specific nuclear groups such as the reticular formation, the olivary bodies, and the red nucleus lie with the brainstem. In short, it is a complicated but highly organized structure that controls motor and sensory activities, respiration, cardiovascular functions, and mechanisms related to sleep and consciousness. Consequently, a small lesion in the brainstem can affect contiguous structures and cause disastrous neurologic deficits for the patient.

2. What are the main divisions of the brainstem?
The brainstem can be divided into three major regions—medulla, pons and midbrain.

3. What is the function of the medulla?
The medulla (bulb) is the direct rostral extension of the spinal cord. It contains the nuclei of the lower cranial nerves (mainly IX, X, XI and XII) and the inferior olivary nucleus. The dorsal column pathways decussate in its central region to form the medial lemniscus, while the corticospinal tracts cross on the ventral side as they descend caudally. Together with the pons, the medulla also participates in vital autonomic functions such as digestion, respiration, and the regulation of heart rate and blood pressure.

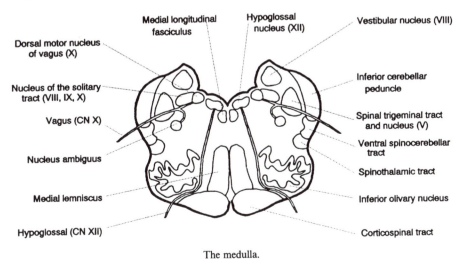

The medulla.

4. What is the function of the pons?

The pons (bridge) lies rostral to the medulla and appears as a bulge mounting from the ventral surface of the brainstem. Cranial nuclei in the pons include those for cranial nerves V, VI, VII, and VIII. There are also a large number of neurons that relay information about movement from the frontal cerebral hemispheres to the cerebellum (frontopontocerebellar pathway). Other clinically pertinent pathways in the pons are those for the control of saccadic eye movements (medial longitudinal fasciculus) and the auditory connections.

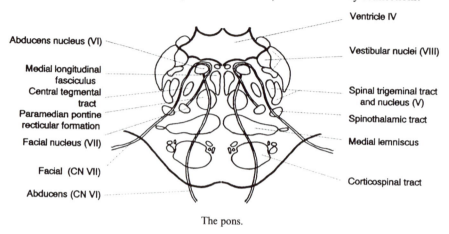

The pons.

5. What is the function of the midbrain?

The midbrain, the smallest and most rostral component of the brainstem, plays an important role in the control of eye movements and the coordination of visual and auditory reflexes. It contains the nuclei for cranial nerves III and IV. Other important structures are the red nuclei and the substantia nigra. The periaqueduct area has an important but poorly understood influence on consciousness and pain perception.

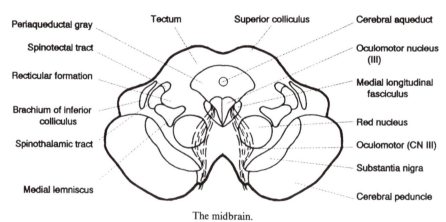

The midbrain.

6. Which cranial nerves are not found in the brainstem?

There are twelve pairs of cranial nerves that are numbered in rostral-caudal sequence. The brainstem contains the nuclei of all the cranial nerves except two, and they are the optic (II) nerve, which terminates in the thalamus, and the olfactory (I) nerve, which synapses in the olfactory bulb.

7. What are the main functions of the cranial nerves?

The cranial nerves have three main functions. Some of them provide motor or general sensory functions, whereas others mediate special senses such as vision, hearing, olfaction, and taste. The rest carry the parasympathetic innervation that controls visceral functions.

8. What are the locations and functions of the individual cranial nerves?

Location and Function of Cranial Nerves

NERVE	LOCATION OF NUCLEI	FUNCTION
Olfactory (I)	Olfactory bulb	Sensory: smell and olfactory reflex
Optic (II)	Thalamus	Sensory: vision and visual reflexes
Oculomotor (III)	Midbrain	Motor: eye movement, eyelids, pupillary constriction, accommodation of lens
Trochlear (IV)	Midbrain	Motor: eye movement (superior oblique)
Trigeminal (V)	Midbrain	Sensory: proprioception for chewing
	Pons	Sensory: from face and cornea. Motor: to masticatory muscles and tensor tympani muscle
	Medulla	Sensory: from face and mouth
Abducens (VI)	Pons	Motor: eye movement (lateral rectus)
Facial (VII)	Pons	Sensory: from skin of external ear, taste from anterior tongue. Motor: facial expression, stapedius muscle movement, salivation, and lacrimation
Vestibulocochlear (VIII)	Pons and medulla	Sensory: equilibrium and hearing
Glossopharyngeal (IX)	Medulla	Sensory: from middle ear, palate, pharynx, and posterior tongue, taste from posterior tongue. Motor: swallowing, parotid gland salivation
Vagus (X)	Medulla	Sensory: from pharynx, larynx, thorax, and abdomen, taste from epiglottis. Motor: swallowing and phonation. Autonomic: parasympathetics to thoracic and abdominal viscera
Spinal accessory (XI)	Medulla	Motor: sternocleidomastoid and upper trapezius muscles
Hypoglossal (XII)	Medulla	Motor: tongue

9. How can understanding the anatomy and function of individual cranial nerves assist in localizing brainstem lesions?

The relatively compact positioning of the cranial nerve nuclei and their intramedullary nerve fibers at specific levels, as well as their proximity to certain vertically directed fiber tracts, creates a series of anatomic patterns that provide a basis for the localization of brainstem lesions. Generally speaking, the motor nuclei of the cranial nerves are situated medially, the spinothalamic fibers run along the dorsal lateral portion, and the corticospinal fibers run along the ventral portion of the brainstem.

10. What is the approach to localizing a brainstem lesion?

As a consequence of the unique anatomic arrangements in the brainstem, a unilateral lesion within this structure often causes "crossed syndromes," in which ipsilateral dysfunction of one or more cranial nerves is accompanied by hemiplegia and/or hemisensory loss on the contralateral body. Exquisite localization of a brainstem lesion depends on signs of long-tract (corticospinal and spinothalamic pathways) dysfunction to identify the lesion in the longitudinal (or sagittal) plane, and on signs of cranial nerve dysfunction to establish its position in the cross-sectional (or axial) plane. Localization of disorders of the brainstem can be simplified by summarizing the patient's neurologic deficits to answer the following questions: Is the lesion affecting unilateral or bilateral structures of the brainstem? What is the level of the lesion? If the lesion is unilateral, is it medial or lateral in the brainstem?

11. What are the common symptoms and signs of brainstem lesions?

Common Symptoms of Brainstem Lesions

1. Double vision	4. Incoordination	7. Hoarseness
2. Vertigo	5. Gait imbalance	8. Difficulties with swallow-
3. Nausea	6. Numbness of the face	ing and speaking

Common Signs of Brainstem Lesions

1. Multiple cranial nerve dysfunctions	8. Dysphonia
2. Gaze palsies	9. Tongue deviation or atrophy
3. Nystagmus	10. Paresis or dysesthesia of the face with contralateral motor or sensory deficits in the body (crossed symptoms)
4. Sympathetic dysfunction (Horner's syndrome)	
5. Hearing loss	11. Unilateral hemiparesis with ataxia
6. Dysphagia	12. Significant bilateral brainstem lesions produce altered mental status or coma.
7. Dysarthria	

12. What is the approach to localizing an isolated cranial nerve deficit?
An isolated cranial nerve defect, especially that of VI and VII, is most often due to a peripheral and not a brainstem lesion.

13. How do the presentations of an intra-axial lesion of the brainstem differ from those of an extra-axial one?
A lesion that directly affects the tissues of the brainstem is called intra-axial or intramedullary. It usually presents with simultaneous cranial nerve and long-tract symptoms and signs. A lesion outside the brainstem is called extra-axial. It affects the brainstem by initially compressing and interfering with the functions of individual cranial nerves. Later, as it enlarges, neighboring structures within the brainstem may then be affected, causing additional long-tract signs.

14. What is the differential diagnosis for a brainstem lesion?

Differential Diagnosis for a Brainstem Lesion

INTRA-AXIAL LESIONS		EXTRA-AXIAL LESIONS	
Neoplasm	Vascular malformation	Acoustic neuroma	Aneurysms
Ischemia/infarct	Demyelinating disease	Meningioma	Epidermoid
Hemorrhage	Inflammatory lesion	Chordoma	Arachnoid cyst

15. What is the radiographic examination of choice for brainstem lesions?
Magnetic resonance imaging (MRI) is the examination of choice for suspected brainstem lesions. It provides a highly sensitive and noninvasive method of evaluating the posterior

fossa, unhampered by skull base artifact. Enhancement with gadolinium may be useful to characterize breakdown of the blood-brain barrier. MR angiography may also be helpful to investigate further the major branches of the vertebrobasilar system in brainstem ischemia or infarction.

16. What is the practical approach to characterizing intra-axial brainstem lesions by MRI?

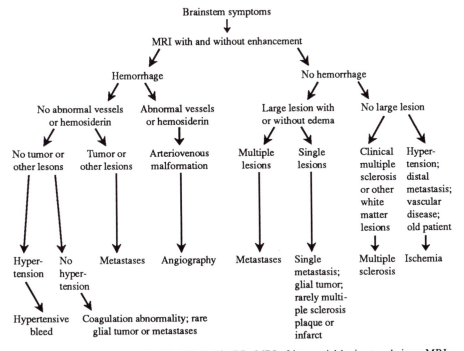

Adapted from Gaskill MF, Wiot JG, Lukin RR: MRI of intra-axial brain stem lesions. MRI Decis 3:2–11, 1989.

BRAINSTEM VASCULAR DISEASES

17. What is the vascular supply of the brainstem?

The blood supply of the brainstem is derived from the vertebrobasilar system of the posterior circulation. (Reproduced with permission from Baker AB, Joynt RJ: Clinical Neurology, Vol 3, ch. 40, Philadelphia, J.B. Lippincott, 1988.)

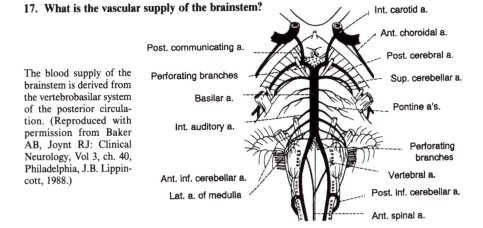

The paired **vertebral arteries** arise from the subclavian artery on each side and join at the pontomedullary junction to form the **basilar artery**. The main branches of the vertebral artery are the **anterior spinal**, the **posterior spinal**, and the **posterior inferior cerebellar** (PICA) arteries. Branches of the basilar artery include the **anterior inferior cerebellar** (AICA), the **internal auditory**, and the **superior cerebellar arteries**. The basilar artery then terminates by dividing into the two posterior cerebral arteries at the midbrain level.

18. What is the vascular supply of the medulla?
The medulla is supplied by the vertebral arteries and their branches. Its blood supply may be further subdivided into two groups, the **paramedian bulbar** and the **lateral bulbar arteries**. The paramedian bulbar arteries are penetrating branches, mainly from the vertebral artery, that supply the midline structures of the medulla. At the lower medulla, branches from the anterior spinal artery also contribute to this paramedian zone. The lateral portion of the medulla is supplied by the lateral bulbar branches of the vertebral artery or the posterior inferior cerebellar artery.

19. What is the vascular supply of the pons?
The basilar artery is the principal supplier of the pons. It gives off three types of branches. The **paramedian arteries** supply the medial basal pons, including the pontine nuclei, the corticospinal fibers, and the medial lemniscus. The **short circumferential arteries** supply the lateral aspect of the pons and the middle and superior cerebellar peduncles. The **long circumferential arteries** together with branches from the anterior inferior cerebellar and superior cerebellar arteries supply the pontine tegmentum and the dorsolateral quadrant of the pons.

20. What is the vascular supply of the midbrain?
Arteries supplying the midbrain include branches of the superior cerebellar artery, the posterior cerebral artery, the posterior communicating artery, and the anterior choroidal artery. Branches of these arteries, like those of the pons, can be grouped into **paramedian arteries**, which supply the midline structures, and the **long and short circumferential arteries**, which supply the dorsal and lateral midbrain.

Because the blood supply to the brainstem at each level is divided into several territories (usually medial and lateral), occlusion of specific arteries manifests clinical features that reflect their vascular distribution.

21. What is the medial medullary syndrome?
The **medial medullary (Dejerine's) syndrome** is caused by occlusion of the anterior spinal artery or its parent vertebral artery, resulting in the following signs:
    1. Ipsilateral paresis of the tongue (damage to cranial nerve XII), which deviates toward the lesion
    2. Contralateral hemiplegia (damage to the corticospinal tract) with sparing of the face
    3. Contralateral loss of position and vibratory sensation (damage to the medial lemniscus)

22. What is the consequence of occlusion of a dominant anterior spinal artery?
The central medullary area may be supplied by a single dominant anterior spinal artery. Occlusion of this vessel then leads to bilateral infarction of the medial medulla, resulting in quadriplegia (with face sparing), complete paralysis of the tongue, and complete loss of position and vibratory sensation. The patient will be mute although fully conscious.

23. What is the lateral medullary syndrome?
The **lateral medullary (Wallenberg's) syndrome** is often due to vertebral artery or posterior inferior cerebellar artery occlusion. Vertebral artery dissection can also be a cause.

Damage to the dorsolateral medulla and the inferior cerebellar peduncle results in the following signs:

1. Ipsilateral loss of pain and temperature sensation of the face (damage to the descending spinal tract and nucleus of cranial nerve V)

2. Ipsilateral paralysis of palate, pharynx, and vocal cord (damage to nuclei or fibers of IX and X) with dysphagia and dysarthria

3. Ipsilateral Horner's syndrome (damage to descending sympathetic fibers)

4. Ipsilateral ataxia and dysmetria (damage to inferior cerebellar peduncle and cerebellum)

5. Contralateral loss of pain and temperature on the body (damage to the spinothalamic tract)

6. Vertigo, nausea, vomiting, and nystagmus (damage to the vestibular nuclei)

7. Other signs and symptoms may include hiccups, diplopia, or unilateral posterior headache

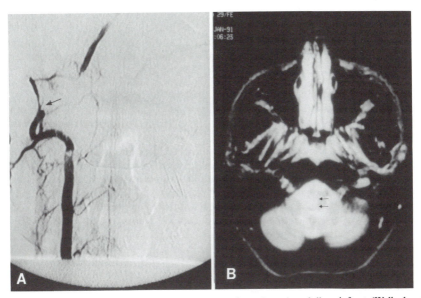

Dissection of the right vertebral artery (*A*, arrow) causing a lateral medullary infarct (Wallenberg's syndrome), seen as an area of increased signal on a T2-weighted MRI of the brainstem (*B*).

24. What is the ventral pontine syndrome?

The **ventral pontine (Millard-Gubler) syndrome** is caused by paramedian infarction of the pons and results in the following signs:

1. Ipsilateral paresis of the lateral rectus (damage to cranial nerve VI) with diplopia

2. Ipsilateral paresis of the upper and lower face (damage to cranial nerve VII)

3. Contralateral hemiplegia (damage to the corticospinal tract) with sparing of the face

25. What is the lower dorsal pontine syndrome?

The **lower dorsal pontine (Foville's) syndrome** is caused by lesions in the dorsal tegmentum of the lower pons, resulting in the following signs:

1. Ipsilateral paresis of the whole face (damage to the nucleus and fibers of VII)

2. Ipsilateral horizontal gaze palsy (damage to paramedian pontine reticular formation and/or VI nucleus)

3. Contralateral hemiplegia (damage to corticospinal tract) with sparing of the face

26. What is the upper dorsal pontine syndrome?

The **upper dorsal pontine (Raymond-Cestan) syndrome** is caused by obstruction of the long circumferential branches of the basilar artery and results in:

1. Ipsilateral ataxia and coarse intention tremor (damage to the superior and middle cerebellar peduncles)

2. Ipsilateral paralysis of muscles of mastication and sensory loss in face (damage to sensory and motor nuclei and tracts of V)

3. Contralateral loss of all sensory modalities in the body (damage to medial lemniscus and spinothalamic tract)

4. Contralateral hemiparesis of the face and body (damage to corticospinal tract) may occur with ventral extension of the lesion.

5. Horizontal gaze palsy may occur, as in the lower dorsal pontine syndrome.

27. What is the ventral midbrain syndrome?

The **ventral midbrain (Weber's) syndrome** is caused by occlusion of median and paramedian perforating branches and may result in:

1. Ipsilateral oculomotor paresis, ptosis, and dilated pupil (damage to fascicle of cranial nerve III, including parasympathetic fibers)

2. Contralateral hemiplegia, including the lower face (damage to corticospinal and corticobulbar tracts)

28. What is the dorsal midbrain syndrome?

The **dorsal midbrain (Benedikt's) syndrome** results from a lesion in the midbrain tegmentum caused by occlusion of paramedian branches of the basilar or posterior cerebral arteries, or both. Its signs are:

1. Ipsilateral oculomotor paresis, ptosis, and dilated pupil (damage to fascicle of cranial nerve III, including parasympathetic fibers as in Weber's syndrome)

2. Contralateral involuntary movements, such as intention tremor, ataxia, and chorea (damage to the red nucleus)

3. Contralateral hemiparesis may be present if the lesion extends ventrally.

4. Contralateral hemianesthesia may be present if the lesion extends laterally, affecting the spinothalamic tract and the medial lemniscus.

29. What is the dorsolateral midbrain syndrome?

The **dorsolateral midbrain syndrome** is caused by infarction of the circumferential arteries and results in:

1. Ipsilateral Horner's syndrome (damage to the sympathetic tract)

2. Ipsilateral severe tremor that may be present at rest and grossly worsened by attempted movement (damage to superior cerebellar peduncle prior to crossing to the opposite red nucleus). Tremor and ataxia can be present bilaterally if both the superior cerebellar peduncle and red nucleus are affected.

3. Contralateral loss of all sensory modalities (damage to the spinothalamic tract and the medial lemniscus that now ascend together).

30. What are the symptoms of brainstem transient ischemic attacks?

Transient circulatory insufficiency in the vertebrobasilar distribution causes brief episodes of brainstem dysfunction characterized by a more patchy and variable presentation. The symptoms of the recurrent attacks may be identical or they may vary in detail. In basilar artery disease, each side of the body may be affected alternately. All the structures in the same ischemic distribution may be affected simultaneously, or symptoms of brainstem dysfunction may spread from one region to another. The symptoms may then end abruptly or fade gradually. They are often premonitory symptoms of impending brainstem strokes that may result in devastating consequences for the patient.

Transient brainstem ischemic attacks affecting the medulla occur particularly often. Vertigo, dysarthria, dysphagia, and tingling around the mouth suggest dysfunction in this region. At pontine levels, vertigo, imbalance, hearing abnormalities, tingling, numbness, or weakness of the limbs and diplopia are frequent symptoms. Midbrain ischemia may cause diplopia, ataxia, sudden loss of consciousness, and weakness of limbs. Symptoms of brainstem ischemia are usually multiple, and isolated findings (such as vertigo or diplopia) are more often caused by peripheral lesions affecting individual cranial nerves.

Ausman JI, Shrontz CE, Pearce JE, et al: Vertebrobasilar insufficiency: A review. Arch Neurol 42:803–808, 1985.

31. What are the commonest causes of brainstem transient ischemic attacks?

Causes of transient brainstem ischemia include atherosclerotic stenosis of vessels in the vertebrobasilar system, embolization from the heart or ulcerated plaques, recurrent hypotension, vertebral steal syndrome, and cervical spondylosis compromising the vertebral circulation. Transient brainstem ischemic episodes may also occur in the prodromal phase of migraine (especially in basilar migraine in which the entire attack may be dominated by a prolonged brainstem ischemic event).

32. What is the "top of the basilar" syndrome?

Occlusion of the rostral basilar artery, usually embolic, often results in the "top of the basilar" syndrome caused by infarction of the midbrain, thalamus, and portions of the temporal and occipital lobes. This syndrome should be suspected in a patient with sudden onset of unresponsiveness, confusion, amnesia, abnormal eye movement, and visual defect. The neurologic signs may be variable and the most common ones are:

1. **Impairments of ocular movements**—unilateral or bilateral vertical (upgaze, downgaze, or complete) gaze palsy, skew deviation, hyperconvergence or convergence spasms causing pseudo-VI-nerve palsy, convergence-retraction nystagmus, and retraction of the upper eyelids.

2. **Abnormalities in pupils**—small with incomplete light reactivity (diencephalic dysfunction), large or mid-position and fixed (midbrain dysfunction), ectopic pupils (corectopia), oval pupils.

3. **Alterations of consciousness and behavior**—stupor, somnolence, apathy, lack of attention, memory deficits, agitated delirium.

4. **Defects in vision**—homonymous hemiopsia, cortical blindness, Balint's syndrome (impaired visual form discrimination and color dysnomia), and abnormal color vision.

5. **Motor weakness, sensory deficits, and reflex abnormalities** are usually variable and subtle, and due to the involvement of long tracts at the infarcted region.

This syndrome may be reversible in patients who are younger and do not have significant risks for cerebrovascular disease.

Caplan LR: "Top of the basilar" syndrome. Neurology 30:72–79, 1980.
Mehler MF: The rostral basilar artery syndrome: Diagnosis, etiology, prognosis. Neurology 39:9–15, 1989.

33. What is the locked-in syndrome?

This syndrome occurs in patients with bilateral ventral pontine lesions. Its etiology is most frequently pontine infarction. Other common causes include pontine hemorrhage, trauma, central pontine myelinolysis, tumor, and encephalitis. The patient is quadriplegic due to bilateral damage of the corticospinal tracts in the ventral pons. He or she is unable to speak and incapable of facial movement because of involvement of the corticobulbar tracts. Horizontal eye movements are also limited by the bilateral involvement of the nuclei and fibers of cranial nerve VI. Consciousness is preserved because the reticular formation is not damaged. The patient has intact vertical eye movements and blinking because the supranuclear ocular motor pathways that run dorsally are spared. The patient is able to communicate by movement of the eyelids, although otherwise completely immobile. Sometimes an incomplete state of this syndrome may occur when the patient retains some horizontal gaze and facial movement. The locked-in syndrome must be distinguished from the persistent neurovegetative state (such as coma vigil or akinetic mutism), in which the patient appears awake but does not react to environmental stimuli and is unable to communicate in any form (thought to be due to a lesion in the rostral midbrain, in the basal-medial frontal region, or in the limbic lobes).

Patterson JR, Grabois M: Locked-in syndrome: A review of 139 cases. Stroke 17:758–764, 1986.

34. What are the common causes of brainstem hemorrhage?

Pontine hemorrhage is usually caused by uncontrolled systemic hypertension, resulting in a sudden loss of consciousness, quadriparesis, and pinpoint pupils. Progressive central herniation from supratentorial mass lesions can compress the brainstem and cause hemorrhage in the midline of the midbrain (Duret hemorrhage), producing coma and bilateral large and fixed pupils. Diencephalic bleeding, such as thalamic hemorrhage, can dissect into the cerebral peduncles and midbrain, producing acute severe headache, hemiparesis, and III nerve palsy. Small petechial hemorrhages occur in the brainstem of patients with head injuries, blood dyscrasias, or hemorrhagic disorders. Ruptured aneurysms or arteriovenous malformations of the vertebrobasilar system may result in subarachnoid hemorrhage that injures the brainstem.

OTHER BRAINSTEM SYNDROMES

35. What is Parinaud's syndrome?

The Parinaud syndrome is also known as the dorsal midbrain or collicular syndrome. The lesion is in the rostral dorsal midbrain, damaging the superior colliculi and pretectal structures. The patient with this condition reports difficulty looking up and blurring of distant vision. The common tetrad of findings are:

1. Paralysis of upgaze and accommodation, but sparing of other eye movements
2. Normal to large pupils with light-near dissociation (loss of pupillary reflex to light with preservation of pupilloconstriction in response to convergence)
3. Eyelid retraction
4. Convergence-retraction nystagmus (eyes make convergent and retracting oscillations following an upward saccade)

This disorder may result from tumors of the pineal gland, stroke, hemorrhage, trauma, hydrocephalus, or multiple sclerosis. The upgaze palsy in this syndrome can be mimicked by progressive supranuclear palsy, thyroid ophthalmopathy, myasthenia gravis, Guillain-Barré syndrome, or congenital upgaze limitation.

Vogel R: Parinaud's syndrome and other related pretectal syndromes. Ophthalmic Semin 1:287–370, 1976.

36. What is internuclear ophthalmoplegia?

Internuclear ophthalmoplegia (INO) is a disorder of horizontal ocular movement due to a lesion in the brainstem (usually in the pons, and specifically along the medial longitudinal fasciculus between the VI and III nuclei). Horizontal gaze requires the coordinated activity of the lateral rectus muscle of the abducting eye (innervated by the VI nerve) and the medial rectus muscle of the adducting eye (innervated by the III nerve). This integrated function is regulated by the paramedian pontine reticular formation (or pontine gaze center). This structure receives inputs from the contralateral occipital and frontal eyefields, and sends fibers to the ipsilateral abducens (VI) nucleus and the contralateral oculomotor (III) nucleus. Fibers from the pontine gaze center run rostrally together with vestibular and other fibers to make up the medial longitudinal fasciculus (MLF).

The cause is commonly multiple sclerosis in young adults, especially when the syndrome is bilateral. In the older population, the syndrome is often unilateral and caused by occlusion of the basilar artery or its paramedian branches. Occasionally INO can be caused by lupus erythematosus and drug (e.g., barbiturates, phenytoin, or amitriptyline) overdose. Pseudo-INO occurs rarely as a feature of myasthenia gravis, Wernicke's encephalopathy, and the Guillain-Barré syndrome.

Many patients with INO have no symptoms, but some have diplopia or blurred vision. On lateral gaze, the signs of this syndrome include:

1. Impaired or paralyzed adduction of the eye ipsilateral to the lesion. The deficit can range from complete medial rectus paralysis to slight slowing of an adducting saccade.

2. Horizontal nystagmus of the abducting eye contralateral to the lesion.

3. Bilateral INO results in defective adduction to the right and left, and nystagmus of the abducting eye on both directions of gaze.

4. Convergence is usually preserved. Skew deviation and vertical gaze nystagmus are sometimes present.

Carlow TJ, Bicknell JM: Abnormal ocular motility with brainstem and cerebellar disorders. Int Ophthalmol Clin 18:37–56, 1978.

37. What is the "one-and-a-half" syndrome?

This syndrome is also a disorder of horizontal ocular movement, characterized by a lateral gaze palsy when looking toward the side of the lesion, together with INO on looking in the other direction. The location of the lesion is the paramedian pontine reticular formation or VI nerve nucleus. Median longitudinal fasciculus (MLF) fibers crossing from the contralateral VI nucleus are also involved, causing INO. The common causes of this syndrome are similar to those of INO, such as multiple sclerosis and stroke. Hemorrhage or tumor in the lower pons is also in the differential diagnosis. Pseudo-one-and-a-half syndromes may occur with myasthenia gravis, Wernicke's encephalopathy, or the Guillain-Barré syndrome. The clinical signs of this syndrome are:

1. Horizontal gaze palsy when looking toward the side of the lesion ("one").

2. INO when looking away from the side of the lesion ("half"). This paralyzes adduction and causes nystagmus on abduction. As a result, the ipsilateral eye has no horizontal movement, and the only lateral ocular movement that remains is abduction and nystagmus of the contralateral eye.

3. Associated signs include skew deviation, gaze-invoked nystagmus on vertical gaze, and exotropia of the eye contralateral to the lesion.

4. Vertical ocular movements and convergence are usually intact.

Wall M, Wray SH: The one-and-a-half syndrome: A unilateral disorder of the pontine tegmentum: A study of 20 cases and review of the literature. Neurology 33:971–980, 1983.

38. What is bulbar palsy?

The "bulb" is the medulla, and the term bulbar palsy refers to a syndrome of lower motor neuron paralysis, affecting muscles innervated by cranial nerves (mainly IX to XII) that have their nuclei closely approximated in the lower brainstem. Muscles of the face, palate, pharynx, larynx, sternocleidomastoid, upper trapezius, and tongue are usually affected. Patients may present clinically with dysarthria, dysphagia, hoarseness, nasal voice, palatal deviation, diminished gag reflex, or weakness of the sternocleidomastoid, upper trapezius, or tongue. Atrophy and fasciculations may be evident. Bulbar palsy may result from a variety of conditions involving the motor nuclei of the lower brainstem or their intramedullary fibers, the corresponding peripheral nerves, the myoneural junction, or the musculature. Etiologies of intra-axial lesions include brainstem infarct, syringobulbia, glioma, poliomyelitis, encephalitis, and motor neuron disease (amyotrophic lateral sclerosis or progressive bulbar palsy). Extra-axial causes are neoplasms (meningioma or neurofibroma), chronic meningitis, aneurysms, neck trauma, and congenital abnormalities (Chiari malformation or basilar impression). Myasthenia gravis, the Guillain-Barré syndrome, myositis, and diphtheria are other conditions that can also present with similar signs and symptoms.

39. What is pseudobulbar palsy?

Pseudobulbar palsy is a syndrome of upper motor neuron paralysis that affects the corticobulbar system above the brainstem bilaterally. Although it presents with most of the signs and symptoms of bulbar palsy, the causative lesion is not in the brainstem. This condition causes dysphagia, dysarthria, and paresis of the tongue (without atrophy or fasciculations). In contrast to bulbar palsy, the reflex movements of the soft palate and pharynx are frequently hyperactive. The jaw jerk is brisk. Frontal signs (grasp, snout, suck, and glabellar reflex) may be present. Emotional incontinence with exaggerated crying (or less often, laughing) also occurs commonly and may be due to disruption of frontal efferents subserving emotional expression. Multiple lacunar infarcts or chronic ischemia in the hemispheres affecting bilateral corticobulbar fibers usually causes this syndrome. Other causes are amyotrophic lateral sclerosis and multiple sclerosis. In amyotrophic lateral sclerosis, there is often a combination of upper and lower motor neuron disease, resulting in coexisting bulbar and pseudobulbar palsies (wasting and fasciculations of the tongue associated with brisk jaw jerk).

OTHER BRAINSTEM DISEASES

40. What is a brainstem glioma?

Brainstem glioma is the most frequent neoplasm affecting the brainstem. It occurs mostly in children and adolescents and is often associated with neurofibromatosis. The tumor arises in the region of the VI nerve nucleus and gradually enlarges to involve the VI and VII nerves and adjacent vestibular structures. Vestibular, cerebellar, and lower cranial nerve symptoms may be present and slowly progressive over a period of months or years before the diagnosis is made because motor and sensory symptoms in the body are usually absent.

41. What other neoplasms affect the brainstem?

Ependymomas occur in the fourth ventricle and can cause obstruction, resulting in intermittent noncommunicating hydrocephalus accompanied by headache and protracted vomiting from involvement of the chemoreceptor trigger zone on the floor of the fourth ventricle. **Metastatic lesions** of the brainstem may arise from malignant melanoma or from neoplasms of the lung and breast, but are relatively rare.

42. What are the common metabolic causes of brainstem dysfunction?

Extraocular movements and cerebellar pathways are vulnerable to damage by metabolic insults because they are highly metabolically active. These dysfunctions are usually acute and reversible. The common presentations are ataxia, vertigo, nausea, vomiting, dysarthria, nystagmus, and gaze palsies such as INO. Common causes are alcohol intoxication and overdose of sedative drugs (e.g., barbiturates) and anticonvulsants (e.g., phenytoin).

43. How does thiamine deficiency affect the brainstem?

Wernicke's encephalopathy is a complication of alcoholism and malnutrition resulting in thiamine deficiency. It usually presents with characteristic mental changes of gross confusion, ataxia, extraocular movement abnormalities, and other signs of brainstem dysfunction. The brainstem signs can be readily reversed by parenteral thiamine therapy, but the confusional state may resolve more slowly.

44. How does demyelinating disease affect the brainstem?
Multiple sclerosis often results in demyelination of the fast-conducting, heavily myelinated nerve fibers traveling along the brainstem. These include the cerebellar-vestibular pathways, the medial longitudinal fasciculus, and the pyramidal pathways. Bilateral INO is almost pathognomonic of multiple sclerosis. Another hallmark of brainstem multiple sclerosis is the combination of bilateral cerebellar and pyramidal signs producing ataxia and pathologically brisk reflexes.

45. What is central pontine myelinolysis?
Central pontine myelinolysis is another demyelinating disease that affects the brainstem white matter, mostly in the central pons and occasionally the cerebral hemispheres. It occurs primarily in patients suffering from malnutrition or alcoholism complicated by hyponatremia. Rapid correction of the hyponatremia has been implicated as a cause of the demyelination. This disorder develops as a subacute progressive quadriparesis with lower cranial nerve involvement. It is usually fatal, but survival with recovered neurologic function is possible. It can be prevented by correcting the electrolyte disturbance gradually, rather than rapidly.

Gocht A, Colmant HJ: Central pontine and extrapontine myelinolysis: A report of 58 cases. Clin Neuropathol 6:262–270, 1987.

VERTIGO

46. What is vertigo?
Vertigo is a false sense of movement, either of oneself or of the environment. The feeling may involve the whole body or be limited to the head. It should be distinguished from dizziness or giddiness resulting from near syncope, postural hypotension, hyperventilation, multiple sensory deficits, ataxia, or other etiologies. The spinning or swirling sensations of vertigo are related to disturbances of the vestibular system.

47. What are the common causes of vertigo?
The causes of vertigo are central (due to a brainstem lesion) or peripheral (due to an inner ear or vestibular nerve lesion). Central vertigo is almost always accompanied by other signs of brainstem dysfunction, such as double vision, weakness or numbness of the face, dysarthria, dysphagia, etc. Peripheral vertigo is usually accompanied by tinnitus or hearing loss but no other neurologic abnormalities.

Common Causes of Vertigo

CENTRAL	PERIPHERAL
Brainstem stroke or transient ischemic attack	Vestibular neuronitis
Multiple sclerosis	Benign positional vertigo
Neoplasms	Meniere's disease
Syringobulbia	Local trauma or posttraumatic
Arnold-Chiari deformity	Physiologic (e.g., motion sickness)
Basilar migraine	Drugs/toxins (e.g., antibiotics, diuretics, antineoplastics, or anticonvulsants)
Cerebellar hemorrhage	Posterior fossa tumors/masses (e.g., acoustic neuroma)

48. What are the signs and symptoms that can help distinguish central from peripheral vertigo?

Central vs. Peripheral Vertigo

SIGNS AND SYMPTOMS	CENTRAL VERTIGO	PERIPHERAL VERTIGO
Nystagmus	Often vertical or rotatory; nystagmus may change with direction of gaze; increases when looking toward side of lesion	Mostly horizontal or sometimes rotatory; unidirectional and conjugate; nystagmus increases when looking away from side of lesion
Latency of onset and duration of nystagmus	No latency after head motion; persistent and lasts >60 sec	Latency after head motion; fatigable and lasts <60 sec
Caloric test	May be normal	Abnormal on side of lesion
Brainstem or cranial nerve signs	Often present	Absent
Hearing loss, tinnitus	Absent	Often present
Nausea and vomiting	Usually absent	Usually present
Vertigo	Usually mild	Severe, often rotational
Falling	Often falls toward the side of the lesion	Often falls to side opposite the nystagmus
Visual fixation or eye closing	No change or increase of symptoms	Inhibits nystagmus and vertigo

CONSCIOUSNESS

49. What are the functions of the reticular formation in the brainstem?
The reticular formation is composed of a network of diffuse aggregations of neurons distributed throughout the central parts of the medulla, pons, and midbrain. It fills the spaces between cranial nerve nuclei and olivary bodies, and it intermixes between ascending and descending fiber tracts. Its neurons receive afferent information from the spinal cord, cranial nerve nuclei, cerebellum, and cerebrum, and they send efferent impulses to the same structures. Their widespread connections give them extensive influence over many neuronal activities. The main functions of the reticular formation are:

    1. Activation of the brain for behavioral arousal and for different levels of awareness

    2. Modulation of segmental stretch reflexes and muscle tone for control of motor function

    3. Coordination of autonomic functions, such as control of breathing and cardiovascular activities

    4. Modulation of the perception of pain

50. How do you examine for brainstem dysfunction in a comatose patient?
When examining a comatose patient, one should be aware of the signs and symptoms that indicate the coma is due to brainstem (reticular formation) dysfunction. This is especially true of impending brainstem failure from increased intracranial pressure causing herniation down into the posterior fossa. This dysfunction travels in a rostral-caudal direction, ending in death with medullary involvement. Emergency management to reduce the intracranial pressure should be implemented immediately to try to reverse this life-threatening situation. The following observations are used to monitor the patient's status in this condition:

- Mental status
- Breathing pattern
- Pupillary size and light response
- Spontaneous eye movement or deviation
- Oculocephalic relfex on head turning (doll's eye movement)

- Oculovestibular test of gaze response to ice-water calorics
- Motor response to supraorbital nerve pressure (noxious stimulus)
- Presence of other brainstem reflexes (corneal, gag, and ciliospinal)

51. How does the clinical examination localize the level of brainstem dysfunction in a comatose patient?

Localization of Level of Brainstem Dysfunction

SIGNS AND SYMPTOMS	SUBCORTICAL	MIDBRAIN	PONS	MEDULLA
Consciousness	Lethargy or stupor	Coma	Coma	Coma
Breathing	Cheyne-Stokes	Central hyperventilation	Apneustic or cluster	Atactic
Pupils	Small and reactive	Mid-position and fixed (III nucleus); unilateral dilated and fixed (III nerve); large and fixed (pretectal)	Pinpoint	Mid-position and fixed, often irregular in shape
Oculocephalic and oculovestibular responses	Present	Absent or abnormal	Absent or abnormal	Absent
Motor response to stimulation	Decortication	Decerebration	Decerebration or no response	No response

52. How do you test for irreversible loss of brainstem function?
Brain death is a clinical diagnosis of irreversible cessation of all cerebral and brainstem function. Complete loss of brainstem function begins with apneic coma. On examination, all brainstem reflexes (corneal, pupillary, gag, ciliospinal) are absent. The pupils are mid-position or large and fixed. Oculocephalic and oculovestibular reflexes are both absent. Muscle tone is flaccid and there is no spontaneous facial movement and no motor response to noxious stimuli. This condition should be present for 6–24 hours in adults. Metabolic causes (hypothermia, hypotension) and drug effects (neuromuscular blockers, sedative drugs) of brainstem dysfunction need to be ruled out.

53. What is the apnea test?
The apnea test is an essential test for the cessation of brainstem function. It stimulates the respiratory centers in the brainstem by inducing hypercarbia. The President's Commission on Brain Death recommends ventilation of the patient with 100% oxygen for 10–30 minutes (depending on the severity of any underlying lung injury) followed by disconnection from the respirator and administration of 100% oxygen through a catheter in the trachea or via T-piece at a flow rate of 6 L/min. Absence of spontaneous respiratory effort with a $PaCO_2$ of above 60 mm Hg confirms clinical apnea. Arterial blood gas should be checked before and after the withdrawal of ventilation. Sometimes the test cannot be completed because of

ventricular arrhythmias or hypotension. In that situation, the diagnosis of irreversible brainstem dysfunction is made by clinical judgment.

Report of the Medical Consultants on the Diagnosis of Death to the President's Commission for the Study of Ethical Problems in Medicine and Biomedical and Behavioral Research: Guidelines for the determination of death. JAMA 246:2184–2186, 1981.

BIBLIOGRAPHY

1. Adams RD, Victor M: Principles of Neurology, 4th ed. New York, McGraw-Hill, 1989.
2. Baker AB, Joynt RJ: Clinical Neurology. Philadelphia, J.B. Lippincott, 1988.
3. Bradley WG, Daroff RB, Fenichel GM, Marsden CD: Neurology in Clinical Practice. Boston, Butterworth-Heinemann, 1991.
4. Brazis PW, Masdeu JC, Biller J: Localization in Clinical Neurology, 2nd ed. Boston, Little, Brown, 1990.
5. Duus P: Topical Diagnosis in Neurology, 2nd ed. New York, Thieme, 1989.
6. Johnson RT: Current Therapy in Neurologic Disease–3. Philadelphia, B.C. Decker, 1990.
7. Kandel ER, Schwartz JH, Jessell TM: Principles of Neural Science, 3rd ed. New York, Elsevier, 1991.
8. Leigh RJ, Zee DS: The Neurology of Eye Movements, 2nd ed. Philadelphia, F.A. Davis, 1991.
9. Plum F, Posner JB: The Diagnosis of Stupor and Coma, 3rd ed. Philadelphia, F.A. Davis, 1982.
10. Rosenberg RN: Comprehensive Neurology. Raven Press, New York, 1991.
11. Rowland LP: Merrit's Textbook of Neurology, 8th ed. Philadelphia, Lea & Febiger, 1989.
12. Swash M, Oxbury J: Clinical Neurology, Edinburgh, Churchill Livingstone, 1991.

9. CEREBELLAR DISEASE

Eugene C. Lai, M.D., Ph.D.

1. What is the functional importance of the cerebellum?

The cerebellum coordinates movement and maintains equilibrium and muscle tone through a complex regulatory and feedback system. It receives somatosensory input from the spinal cord, motor information from the cerebral cortex, and input about balance from the vestibular organs of the inner ears. It integrates all this information and aids in organizing the range, velocity, direction, and force of muscular contractions to produce steady volitional movements and posture. It accomplishes this by constantly screening its sensory inputs and modulating its motor outputs. The cerebellum also plays an important role in the coordination of the planning of limb movements. In addition, it participates in learning motor tasks, as its function can be modified by experience.

Damage to the cerebellum alone does not impair sensory perception or muscle strength. Rather, it disrupts coordination of limb and eye movements, impairs balance, and decreases muscle tone.

2. What is the basic anatomy of the cerebellum?

The cerebellum can be divided into three major lobes by transverse fissures. The primary fissure, located on the upper surface of the cerebellum, divides the cerebellum into an **anterior lobe** and a **posterior lobe**. The posterolateral fissure on the underside of the cerebellum separates the large posterior lobe from the small **flocculonodular lobe**. The cerebellar cortex consists of three layers based on its microscopic anatomy: the molecular cell layer, the Purkinje cell layer, and the granule cell layer. Three pairs of deep nuclei are present within the cerebellum. From medial to lateral these are the fastigial, interposed (may be separated into globose and emboliform), and dentate nuclei. A more functionally useful method of describing the cerebellum is based on its longitudinal zonal patterns and their different connections. There is a midline zone, known as the **vermis**, that separates the two cerebellar hemispheres on each side. Each hemisphere in turn is composed of an **intermediate zone** and a **lateral zone**. These three zones, together with the flocculonodular lobe, represent the major functional subdivisions of the cerebellum by virtue of their distinct input and output pathways.

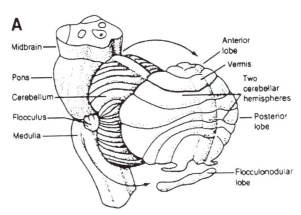

A

Midbrain

Pons

Cerebellum

Flocculus

Medulla

Anterior lobe

Vermis

Two cerebellar hemispheres

Posterior lobe

Flocculonodular lobe

The cerebellum is divided into anatomically distinct lobes. *A*, The cerebellum is unfolded to reveal the lobes normally hidden from view. *(Continued on next page.)*

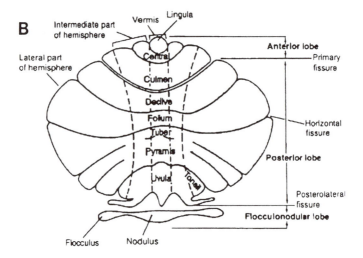

B, The main body of the cerebellum is divided by the primary fissure into anterior and posterior lobes. The posterolateral fissure separates the flocculonodular lobe. Shallower fissures divide the anterior and posterior lobes into nine lobules. The cerebellum has three functional regions: the central vermis and the lateral and intermediate zones in each hemisphere. (Reproduced with permission from Ghez C: The cerebellum. In Kandel ER, et al (eds): Principles of Neural Science. New York, Elsevier, 1991.)

3. What are the connections and functions of the major divisions of the cerebellum?

Connections and Functions of Major Divisions of the Cerebellum

FUNCTIONAL DIVISION	MAJOR INPUT	MAJOR OUTPUT	FUNCTION
Flocculonodular lobe (vestibulocerebellum)	Vestibular nuclei, labyrinth, visual system	Vestibular nuclei, medial and lateral vestibular tracts	Equilibrium (axial), eye movements, vestibular reflexes
Vermis (spinocerebellum)	Vestibular, visual, and auditory systems, face, proximal body parts	Vestibular nucleus, reticular formation, contralateral motor cortex, and medial descending system via the **fastigial** nucleus	Axial and proximal muscle control and execution, progressive movement
Intermediate zone (spinocerebellum)	Spinal cord (distal body parts)	Contralateral red nucleus, motor cortex, and lateral descending system via the **interposed** nucleus	Distal muscle control and execution, progressive movement
Lateral zone (cerebrocerebellum)	Contralateral cerebral cortex via pontine nuclei	Contralateral red nucleus, thalamus, motor and premotor cortex via **dentate** nucleus	Motor planning initiation and timing

4. What are the principal afferent and efferent pathways of the cerebellum?

The afferent and efferent pathways to and from the cerebellum course through three pairs of tracts (cerebellar peduncles) that connect the cerebellum to the brainstem:

1. The **inferior cerebellar peduncle** (restiform body) consists of mainly afferent fibers. A single efferent tract, the fastigiobulbar tract, goes to the vestibular nucleus from the flocculonodular lobe. Afferent fibers enter the inferior cerebellar peduncle from at least five sources, including (1) the vestibulocerebellar tract, (2) the olivocerebellar tract, (3) the dorsal spinocerebellar tract, (4) the cuneocerebellar tract, and (5) the reticulocerebellar tract.

2. The **middle cerebellar peduncle** (brachium pontis) consists almost entirely of crossed afferent fibers from the pontine nuclei that transmit impulses from the cerebral cortex to the intermediate and lateral zones of the cerebellum (corticopontocerebellar tract).

3. The **superior cerebellar peduncle** (brachium conjunctivum) consists principally of efferent projections from the cerebellum. Rubral, thalamic, and reticular projections arise from the dentate and interposed nuclei. The fastigiobulbar tracts run with this peduncle for a short distance before it enters the inferior cerebellar peduncle. Afferent fibers include the ventral spinocerebellar tract and the trigeminocerebellar and tectocerebellar projections.

5. What are the blood supplies to the cerebellum?

The vertebral and basilar arteries give off three paired branches to the cerebellum: the superior, the anterior inferior, and the posterior inferior cerebellar arteries, which are interconnected by anastomoses. The superior cerebellar artery runs over the superior surface of the cerebellum, while the other arteries supply the inferior surface.

The **superior cerebellar artery** arises from the rostral part of the basilar artery and supplies the lateral midbrain and pontine tegmentum, superior cerebellar peduncle, upper segment of middle cerebellar peduncle, dentate nucleus, rostral vermis, and the superior portion of the rostral cerebellar hemisphere.

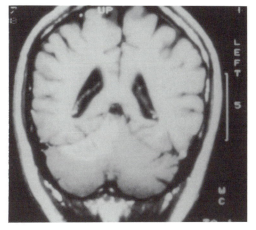

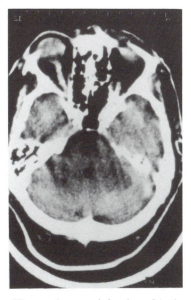

T-1 weighted MRI shows a hemorrhagic infarction of the right superior cerebellar artery territory.

The **anterior inferior cerebellar artery** arises from the caudal basilar artery and supplies the smallest territory of all the cerebellar arteries. It provides supply to the lateral pontomedullary tegmentum, lower segment of the middle cerebellar peduncle, flocculus and adjacent inferior surface of the cerebellar hemispheres. Penetrating branches supply part of the dentate nucleus and nearby white matter.

CT scan shows an infarction of both interior inferior cerebellar arteries.

The **posterior inferior cerebellar artery** derives from the vertebral artery and supplies the lateral medullary tegmentum, inferior cerebellar peduncle, and the caudal portions of the cerebellar nuclei, inferior vermis, and inferior cerebellar hemisphere, including the tonsils.

6. What are the main clinical features of cerebellar diseases?

Cerebellar diseases comprise a disturbance of equilibrium, muscle tone, and execution of movement. The following findings can be present: hypotonia, ataxia, dysmetria, dysdiadochokinesia, nystagmus, rebound phenomenon, postural instability, scanning speech, and intention tremor. These findings vary in severity depending on whether the lesion is acute or chronic, bilateral or unilateral, hemispheric or midline. The common findings of cerebellar dysfunction can be remembered by the mnemonic **HANDS Tremor:**

H	=	Hypotonia (loss of muscle tone)
A	=	Asynergy (lack of coordination)
N	=	Nystagmus (ocular oscillation)
D	=	Dysarthria (speech abnormalities)
S	=	Station and gait (imbalance, gait ataxia)
Tremor		Tremor (coarse intention tremor)

7. What are the clinical tests for cerebellar dysfunction?

Tests for Cerebellar Dysfunction

ABNORMALITY	METHODS OF EXAMINATION
Hypotonia	Passive movement of extremities to check muscle tone; pendular patellar reflexes; rebound phenomenon; inspect for rag doll (flaccid) posture
Asynergy	Finger-nose-finger, heel-to-shin, and rapid-alternating supernation-pronation tests to evaluate rate, range, force, and accuracy of voluntary movement
Nystagmus	Ocular oscillations through the fields of gaze
Dysarthria	Abnormalities in articulation and prosody (scanning or explosive speech, altered accent)
Stance and gait	Broad-based stance and gait, difficulty with tandem walk, and postural instability
Tremor	Limb tremor at rest, with sustained posture, and during action

Because most of the tests for cerebellar functions require the cooperation and volitional movement of the patient, clinical features of cerebellar dysfunction cannot be elicited from a paralyzed or comatose patient.

8. How do you differentiate cerebellar and sensory ataxia?

The cerebellum can coordinate and equilibrate movement only if it receives the proper proprioceptive information. Therefore, if the proprioceptive system is defective, the patient has imbalance and ataxia. The proprioceptive defect can be compensated by visual guidance, and so the patient with sensory loss will exhibit worsening of movement with his eyes closed.

Cerebellar vs. Sensory Ataxia

CLINICAL FINDING	CEREBELLAR ATAXIA	SENSORY ATAXIA
Hypotonia	Present	Present
Asynergy, dysmetria	Present	Absent
Nystagmus	Present	Absent
Dysarthria	Present	Absent
Tremor	Present	Absent
Loss of vibration and position sense	Absent	Present
Areflexia	Absent	Present
Dystaxia much worse with eyes closed (Romberg test)	Absent	Present

9. What are the general principles in localizing a cerebellar lesion?

Specific cerebellar regions possess distinct functions. There is also a topical representation of individual body parts in the cerebellum. Thus, signs of cerebellar dysfunction may have localizing significance. Some general principles include:

- Lesions of the rostral midline impair coordination involving stance and gait.
- Lesions of the caudal midline impair axial truncal posture and equilibrium.
- Lateral lesions impair the limbs ipsilateral to the cerebellar lesion.
- Lesions of the cerebellar hemisphere ultimately impair movement on the ipsilateral side of the body because of a doublecrossing of the pathways. The ascending cerebello-cortical fibers cross in the midbrain and project to the contralateral cortex, and then the descending corticospinal fibers cross back in the medulla to project to the contralateral body.
- Lesions of the afferent or efferent pathways to the cerebellum may cause signs similar to lesions of the cerebellum itself.
- Lesions of the superior cerebellar peduncle and the deep nuclei usually produce the most severe disturbance of cerebellar dysfunction.

10. What are the major cerebellar syndromes?

There are four major cerebellar syndromes: the rostral vermis syndrome, the caudal vermis syndrome, the hemispheric syndrome, and the pancerebellar syndrome. They are distinguished by their presentations and the anatomical regions affected. Recognition of these syndromes may help narrow the differential diagnosis of the cerebellar lesions.

Cerebellar Syndromes

CLINICAL SYNDROMES	REGION(S) INVOLVED	DISTRIBU-TION OF DEFICITS	COMMON CAUSES	HYPO-TONIA	INCOORDINATION OF:			NYSTAGMUS	DYS-ARTHRIA
					Arms	Legs	Gait & Trunk		
Cerebellar hemisphere syndrome	Unilateral intermediate and lateral zones	Ipsilateral head and body	Infarct, neoplasm, abscess, demyelination	+	+	+	+	+ (bidirectional, coarser, slower on gaze to side of lesion; faster, finer on gaze to other side)	+
Rostral vermis syndrome	Anterior and superior vermis	Gait and trunk	Alcoholism, thiamine deficiency	+ −	+	+	+	−	−

Table continued on next page.

Cerebellar Syndromes (Continued)

| CLINICAL SYNDROMES | REGION(S) INVOLVED | DISTRIBU- TION OF DEFICITS | COMMON CAUSES | HYPO- TONIA | INCOORDINATION OF: | | | | |
					Arms	Legs	Gait & Trunk	NYSTAGMUS	DYS- ARTHRIA
Caudal vermis syndrome	Flocculo- nodular and posterior vermis	Axial disequi- librium	Midline neoplasm	+ −	−	+ −	+	+ (variable)	−
Pancerebellar syndrome	All regions	Bilateral signs of cerebellar dysfunction	Toxic/ metabolic, infectious/ postinfectious, paraneoplastic, degenerative disorders	+	+	+	+	+ (variable type)	+

11. What are the common acquired diseases of the cerebellum?
Acquired cerebellar diseases frequently present as acute ataxia with or without other cerebellar signs. They are often treatable if recognized early. Therefore, one should be astute with the differential diagnosis of acute ataxia so that the disorder can be identified and management plans initiated as early as possible. Cerebellar diseases have a broad differential diagnosis. Initially, they may be divided by their etiology into acquired or inherited disorders. Some common acquired cerebellar diseases are as follows:

1. **Vascular diseases**
   Infarction (mostly thrombotic, sometimes embolic)
   Hemorrhage (from hypertension, vascular malformation, or tumor)
   Transient ischemic attacks
   Basilar migraine (usually in children)
   Vascular malformation
   Systemic vasculitides (systemic lupus erythematosus)

2. **Neoplasms**
   Primitive neuroectodermal tumor (PNET or medulloblastoma; in children)
   Astrocytoma (often cystic; midline in children and hemispheric in adults)
   Hemangioblastoma (may be associated with von Hippel–Landau disease)
   Metastatic tumor (may be multiple)

3. **Infections**
   Acute cerebellar ataxia of childhood (possible viral etiology)
   Tuberculosis or tuberculoma
   Cysticercosis
   Bacterial infection and abscess (through direct extension of mastoid infection)
   Chronic panencephalitis of congenital rubella infection
   Viral encephalitis (involving cerebellum or brainstem)

4. **Inflammatory or autoimmune disorders**
   Multiple sclerosis
   Acute postinfectious cerebellitis
   Postinfectious disseminated encephalomyelitis
   Miller-Fisher variant of acute inflammatory polyneuropathy

5. **Paraneoplastic syndromes**
   Paraneoplastic cerebellar degeneration (commonly associated with lung, ovarian, or breast carcinomas)
   Opsoclonus-myoclonus (secondary to neuroblastoma)

6. **Metabolic disorders**
   Hypothyroidism
   Hyperthermia
   Hypoxia
   Deficiencies of thiamine (in alcoholics), niacin (pellagra), vitamin E,
   essential amino acids, and zinc

7. **Drugs and toxins**
   Anticonvulsant: phenytoin, carbamazepine, barbiturates
   Chemotherapeutic agents: 5-fluorouracil, cytosine arabinoside
   Heavy metals: thallium, lead, organic mercury
   Alcohol (may be indirectly due to malnutrition)
   Toluene

8. **Developmental abnormalities**
   Chiari malformations
   Dandy-Walker syndrome
   Cerebellar aplasia
   Basilar impression

9. **Trauma**
   Postconcussion
   Hematoma or contusion

12. What are some of the major inherited cerebellar diseases?
The classification of inherited cerebellar diseases is confusing and nonuniform. These diseases usually cause progressive degeneration and atrophy of the cerebellum. They are also known as hereditary ataxias because their common major neurologic sign is ataxia, or clumsiness and incoordination of movement. These diseases can be classified according to their time of onset, inheritance pattern, known or unknown etiology, clinical features, etc. Only some of the more common ones will be listed here.

1. **Friedreich's ataxia**
   This autosomal recessive disorder is listed separately because it is relatively
   common, with a prevalence of about 1 in 100,000.

2. **Syndromes associated with defective DNA repair** (autosomal recessive)
   Ataxia telangiectasia (low IgA and IgE levels)
   Xeroderma pigmentosum

3. **Mitochondrial encephalopathies**
   Leigh's disease
   Kearns-Sayre syndrome

4. **Syndromes of known metabolic etiology**
   Abetalipoproteinemia or hypobetalipoproteinemia (deficient apolipoprotein B)
   Wilson's disease (low or absent copper ceruloplasmin)
   Refsum's disease (deficient phytanic acid hydroxylase)
   Aminoacidurias (Hartnup disease)
   Disorders of pyruvate and lactate metabolism (metabolic acidosis)
   Urea cycle enzyme defects (hyperammonemia)
   Biotinase deficiency (metabolic acidosis)
   Hexosaminidase deficiency
   Leukodystrophies (metachromatic, Krabbe's)
   Ceroid lipofuscinosis
   Niemann-Pick disease

5. **Syndromes of unknown etiology**
    Autosomal dominant diseases:
      Olivopontocerebellar atrophy (ataxia, ophthalmoplegia, optic atrophy)
      Spinocerebellar ataxia (ataxia, dysarthria, sensory loss)
      Machado-Joseph disease (variable cerebellar, extrapyramidal,
        and pyramidal involvement)
    Autosomal recessive diseases:
      Ramsay-Hunt syndrome (ataxia and myoclonus)
      Behr's syndrome (ataxia, optic atrophy, mental retardation)
    X-linked spinocerebellar ataxia (rare)

   Harding AE: The Hereditary Ataxias and Related Disorders. Edinburgh, Churchill Livingstone, 1984.

13. What are the clinical features of Friedreich's ataxia?

Freidreich's ataxia is an autosomal recessive disease affecting the cerebellum, spinal cord, peripheral nerve, and heart. Carbohydrate metabolism is also altered. It has an early onset, before age 20, and a rapidly progressive course. The initial presentation is frequently gait ataxia, but arm ataxia may also be significant. Scoliosis and dysarthria are common in these patients. Loss of all tendon reflexes, loss of vibration and position sense, and extensor plantar responses are typical. Other associated features include muscle weakness and atrophy, hypertrophic cardiomyopathy, pes cavus, abnormal ocular motility, diabetes, and deafness. Most patients are confined to a wheelchair by early adulthood. The etiology of Friedreich's ataxia is unknown, but recently the genetic defect has been localized to chromosome 9. There is presently no effective treatment for this disease. Symptomatic treatment of scoliosis by orthopedic intervention, and cardiac abnormalities by appropriate medication, may prolong survival.

   Stumf DA: The inherited ataxias. Pediatr Neurol 1:129, 1985.

14. What is the difference in the diagnosis of posterior fossa neoplasms in children versus adults?

Posterior fossa neoplasms account for approximately 50% of the total number of neoplasms in the pediatric population. The four major types are cerebellar astrocytoma, medulloblastoma (primitive neuroectodermal tumor), ependymoma of the fourth ventricle, and brainstem glioma. In adults, posterior fossa neoplasms are much rarer. They consist of mainly hemangioblastoma, metastatic tumor, acoustic neuroma (schwannoma), and meningioma.

   Albright L: Posterior fossa tumors. Neurosurg Clin North Am 3:881–891, 1992.

15. What are the presentations of cerebellar infarction or hemorrhage? What are the management concerns?

The presentation of cerebellar infarction and hemorrhage may be indistinguishable. Abrupt onset of headache, vomiting, vertigo, and ataxia, especially in a hypertensive patient, should be considered a neurologic emergency, and a vascular etiology should be ruled out. A high index of suspicion can lead to the proper diagnosis with CT or MRI scanning. Expanding hematoma or edema may rapidly lead to brainstem compression and cerebellar herniation accompanied by signs including hemiparesis, pontine gaze abnormalities, depressed consciousness, irregular breathing, or coma. Prompt surgical evacuation of the hematoma or removal of necrotic cerebellar tissue may be life-saving in this situation.

   Amarenco P: The spectrum of cerebellar infarctions. Neurology 41:973–979, 1991.
   van der Hoop HG, Vermeulen M, van Gijn J: Cerebellar hemorrhage: Diagnosis and treatment. Surg Neurol 29:6–10, 1988.

16. What are the clinical features and causes of the cerebellopontine angle syndrome?

Lesions at the space between the cerebellum and the pons often present themselves by compressing and interfering with the functions of the cranial nerves that are in close proximity at the location, namely cranial nerves V, VII, and VIII. Involvement of cranial nerve V is often detected by depression or absence of the ipsilateral corneal reflex. Later, other sensory and motor functions may be affected, as manifested by numbness of the face and weakness of the mastication muscles. Involvement of cranial nerve VII may produce facial myokymia (involuntary contraction of the facial musculature) or a lower motor neuron paralysis of the ipsilateral face. Hearing loss, tinnitus, and vertigo are features of damage to cranial nerve VIII. As the lesion enlarges, distortion of the brainstem may occur, producing bilateral long-tract signs or obstruction of the aqueduct to cause hydrocephalus and symptoms of increased intracranial pressure. Compression of the cerebellar hemisphere adjacent to the cerebellopontine angle presents with ipsilateral limb ataxia and intention tremor, or nystagmus.

17. What is an acoustic neuroma?

The acoustic neuroma (or schwannoma) is the most common extra-axial lesion that causes the cerebellopontine angle syndrome. It originates from schwann cells in the sheath of cranial nerve VIII, close to the attachment of the nerve to the brainstem. It can be distinguished from other lesions of the cerebellopontine angle by the fact that it involves cranial nerve VIII early; the functions of cranial nerve VII are usually resistant to this tumor and are not affected until much later. The early involvement of cranial nerve VII is sufficient cause to consider the possibility of other lesions, such as meningioma, epidermoidoma, craniopharyngioma, glomus jugulare tumor, and aneurysm of the basilar artery. Intra-axial masses of the brainstem and cerebellum can also cause the syndrome if they are sufficiently large and extend into the cerebellopontine space.

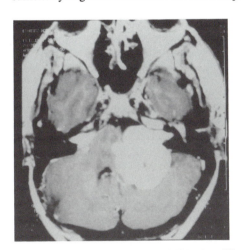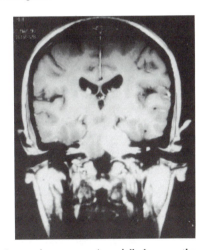

Gadolinium-enhanced T1-weighted MRIs show bilateral acoustic neuromas (especially large on the left) in a patient with neurofibromatosis.

18. What are the clinical features of the cerebellar herniation syndromes?

Mass lesions in the cerebellum, particularly neoplasms and hematomas, often initially present as nonspecific symptoms such as headache. As the lesions enlarge, the increased pressure causes the cerebellum to herniate in one of two directions, downward or upward.

Downward herniation of the cerebellum is most common. Increased pressure in the posterior fossa pushes the cerebellar tonsils downward through the foramen magnum to compress the medulla. It is characterized by progressive vomiting, stiff neck, skew deviation of the eyes, coma, ataxic breathing, apnea, and death. There are no pupillary changes until the patient is terminal. This condition is fatal if not anticipated and prevented early.

Upward herniation occurs when the cerebellar mass pushes the cerebellum and upper brainstem through the tentorial opening. The clinical features are caused by progressive compression of the pons and midbrain. The patient is usually obtunded or comatose with small pupils (reactive at first) or anisocoria. There is abnormal oculocephalic and oculo-vestibular responses. Hemiparesis may progress to quadriparesis and decorticate posturing. Abnormal breathing (central hyperventilation or apneustic breathing) can be observed.

19. What is the treatment for cerebellar herniation?

Osmotic agents and hyperventilation may provide temporary relief, but definitive treatment for cerebellar herniations consists of surgical decompression and removal of the mass if possible.

20. What is paraneoplastic cerebellar degeneration?

Paraneoplastic cerebellar degeneration (PCD) is the most common remote effect of neoplasm affecting the brain. It is associated with lung (especially small cell), ovarian and breast neoplasms, and Hodgkin's disease. Cerebellar signs usually begin with gait ataxia, developing over a few weeks to months. The symptoms may progress rapidly to severe and symmetric truncal and limb ataxia with dysarthria and nystagmus. Vertigo is also common. Often, neurologic symptoms precede the detection of neoplasms. Thus, when an adult develops a rapidly progressing and symmetrical cerebellar syndrome, PCD should be promptly considered. Pathologically, there is a severe loss of Purkinje cells, affecting all parts of the cerebellum. Neuroimaging studies are typically normal early, but later show signs of progressive cerebellar atrophy. Cerebellar symptoms may improve in some patients when the causative neoplasms are removed, but they are not improved by plasmapheresis.

21. What is the cause of paraneoplastic cerebellar degeneration?

An autoimmune process may be the cause of this syndrome, and antibodies to cerebellar Purkinje cells are observed in patients' sera and spinal fluid. The two main antibodies may be used as markers for patients with PCD. The Yo antibodies (or anti-Purkinje cell cytoplasmic antibodies) are found in gynecologic cancer patients with PCD, whereas the Hu antibodies (antineuronal nuclear antibodies) are present in some patients with small-cell lung cancer with PCD. The pathogenic basis of these antibodies is still uncertain.

Posner JB: Paraneoplastic syndromes. Neurol Clin 9:919–936, 1991.

BIBLIOGRAPHY

1. Adams RD, Victor M: Principles of Neurology, 4th ed. New York, McGraw-Hill, 1989.
2. Baker AB, Joynt RJ: Clinical Neurology. Philadelphia, J.B. Lippincott, 1988.
3. Bradley WG, Daroff RB, Fenichel GM, Marsden CD: Neurology in Clinical Practice. Boston, Butterworth-Heinemann, 1991.
4. Brazis PW, Masdeu JC, Biller J: Localization in Clinical Neurology, 2nd ed. Boston, Little, Brown, 1990.
5. Duus P: Topical Diagnosis in Neurology, 2nd ed. New York, Thieme, 1989.
6. Gilman S, Bloedel JR, Lechtenberg R: Disorders of the Cerebellum. Philadelphia, F.A. Davis, 1981.
7. Johnson RT: Current Therapy in Neurologic Disease-3. Philadelphia, B.C. Decker, 1990.
8. Kandel ER, Schwartz JH, Jessell TM: Principles of Neural Science, 3rd ed. New York, Elsevier, 1991.
9. Rosenberg RN: Comprehensive Neurology. New York, Raven Press, 1991.
10. Rowland LP: Merrit's Textbook of Neurology, 8th ed. Philadelphia, Lea & Febiger, 1989.
11. Swash M, Oxbury J: Clinical Neurology. Edinburgh, Churchill Livingstone, 1991.

10. BASAL GANGLIA AND MOVEMENT DISORDERS

Francisco Cardoso, M.D., and Joseph Jankovic, M.D.

ANATOMY AND PHYSIOLOGY

1. What are the components of the basal ganglia?

The basal ganglia are a group of nuclei situated in the deep part of the cerebrum and upper part of the brainstem. In addition to the striatum, encompassing the caudate and putamen, and the pallidum, composed of the internal (medial) and external (lateral) parts of globus pallidus (GP), the subthalamic nucleus (STN) and the substantia nigra (SN), with pars compacta (SNc) and reticulata (SNr), are also components of the basal ganglia. These interrelated structures are primarily responsible for control of motor functions.

Alexander GE, Crutcher MD: Functional architecture of basal ganglia circuits: Neural substrates of parallel processing. Trends Neurosci 13:266, 1990.

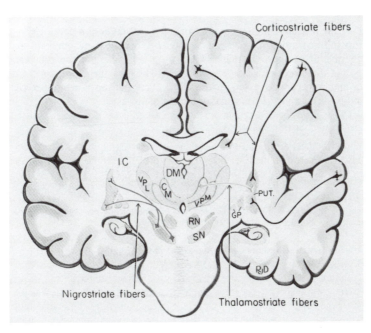

The basal ganglia and thalamus. PUT = putamen, GP = globus pallidus, SN = substantia nigra, RN = red nucleus, IC = internal capsule, VPL = ventral posterior lateral nucleus; VPM = ventral posterior medial nucleus, CM = centromedian nucleus, DM = dorsomedian nucleus.

2. How are the basal ganglia organized?

There are three levels of organization within the basal ganglia. The first level consists of the two major striatal outputs: (1) the indirect pathway to the external segment of the GP (GPe) and (2) the direct pathway to the SNr and internal segment of the GP (GPi). The second level of organization consists of pathways from the cerebral cortex (sublaminae of layer V) to the patch and matrix compartments of the striatum (which are organized in a mosaic pattern). The third level of organization is related to the topography of cortical projections to other regions of the striatum.

Gerfen CR: The neostriatal mosaic: Multiple levels of compartmental organization. Trends Neurosci 15:133, 1992.

3. How can the matrix and patch compartments of the striatum be distinguished?

These two subpopulations of striatal medium spiny neurons have distinct neurochemical properties as well as distinct afferents and efferents. Neurochemically, the patches are enriched in μ opiate receptors and display weak acetylcholinesterase staining. The limbic-related allocortex projects predominantly to the patches. The output from the patches is directed at cholinergic neurons mainly situated in the ventral GP and dopaminergic neurons in the SNc. On the other hand, the neurons of the matrix mainly receive fibers from the neocortical areas such as sensorimotor cortex that project chiefly to the GABAergic neurons of the SNr and GPe.

In summary, the patches are more related to limbic and nonspecific functions and the matrix is involved with more specific, sensorimotor tasks. However, these distinctions are not absolute because there are transitional areas that display overlap of the above-mentioned features.

Nieoullion A, Kerkerian-Le Goff L: Cellular interactions in the striatum involving neuronal systems using "classical" neurotransmitters: Possible functional implications. Mov Disord 7:311, 1992.

4. What are the neurotransmitters of the two major striatal output pathways?

The majority of the neurons in the striatum are GABAergic medium spiny cells that project to the GPe and SNr. Approximately 50% of these cells also contain substance P and dynorphin, and these project to the SNr and GPi. The other half of the neurons express enkephalin and project their axons to the GPe. These pathways are respectively called striatonigral or direct and striatopallidal or indirect pathways.

Gerfen CR, et al: D1 and D2 dopamine receptor-regulated gene expression of striatonigral and striatopallidal neurons. Science 250:1429, 1990.

5. What is the role of the STN in the neurophsyiology of the basal ganglia?

The STN receives inhibitory input from the striatopallidal pathway. The SNr is the main target of the output of the STN. The likely neurotransmitter of the STN projection neurons is glutamate, an excitatory amino acid.

Bergman H, Wichman T, DeLong MR: Reversal of experimental parkinsonism by lesion of the subthalamic nucleus. Science 249:1436, 1990.

6. What is the source of the major output of the basal ganglia?

The GABAergic neurons of the SNr and the GPi, which may be considered as a single neuronal complex, innervate the mediodorsal and ventral tier thalamic nuclei (which provide feedback to the frontal cortex), the intralaminar thalamic nuclei (which provide feedback to the striatum), the superior colliculus (important in the control of the ocular movements), and the pedunculopontine nucleus (seemingly involved in the maintenance of posture).

7. What is the neurotransmitter of the nigrostriatal system?

The nigrostriatal system is composed of the dopaminergic neurons in the SNc which project to the medium spiny neurons of the striatum.

8. How many types of dopamine receptors have been identified?

There are five dopamine receptors, D1–D5, that have now been pharmacologically charac-terized and cloned. The activation of D1 and D5 receptors increases the intracellular level of cAMP, and these receptors have been mapped, respectively, to chromosomes 5 and 4. The D1 receptor is localized chiefly in the caudate, putamen, nucleus accumbens, and olfactory tubercle, whereas the D5 receptor is predominantly expressed in the hippocampus and hypothalamus. The D2 and D4 receptors have been linked to chromosome 11, and the gene for the D3 receptor has been identified on chromosome 3. The D2 receptor, expressed in two isoforms (D2S and D2L), decreases the intracellular level of cAMP and has the same distribution as the D1 receptor. The D3 receptor, apparently also acting by decreasing the cAMP level, has been identified in the olfactory tubercle, hypothalamus, and nucleus accumbens. A similar mechanism of action has been proposed for the D4 receptor, found in the frontal cortex, medulla, and midbrain.

The functional significance of this multitude of receptors is not clearly understood. The role of the D1 and D2 receptors in the motor systems has been studied more extensively; activation of the D1 receptors appears to be important in mediating dystonic movements, whereas activation of the D2 receptors may result in chorea. A specific blocker for the D4 receptor, clozapine, is an effective antipsychotic agent that does not induce or exacerbate movement disorders.

Factor SA, Brown D: Clozapine prevents recurrence of psychosis in Parkinson's disease. Mov Disord 7:125, 1992.

Sibley DR, Monsma FJ: Molecular biology of dopamine receptors. Trends Pharmacol Sci 13:61, 1992.

9. How are the D1 and D2 dopamine receptors expressed in the striatum?

The D1 dopamine receptor is predominantly expressed on the striatonigral neurons, while the D2 receptors are primarily found on the striatopallidal neurons. Evidence suggests that in the striatum the D1 and D2 receptors have, respectively, an excitatory and inhibitory action.

Engber TM, et al: Chronic levodopa treatment alters basal and dopamine agonist-stimulated cerebral glucose utilization. J Neurosci 10:3889, 1990.

PARKINSONISM

10. What are the neurophysiologic changes in the basal ganglia in Parkinson's disease (PD)?

Neuronal loss in the SNc with consequent dopamine depeletion in the striatum is the neurochemical-pathological hallmark of PD. This dopaminergic deafferentation produces an imbalance in the striatal activity, with hypoactivity of the striatonigral pathway and hyperactivity of striatopallidal pathways. This results in decreased inhibition (disinhibition) of the STN and increased activity of the SNr neurons, causing increased inhibition of the thalamic ventral tier nuclei. As these nuclei are responsible for the activation of the cortical areas involved in the generation of movements, the final effect of the dopamine deficiency is poverty or slowness of movements (hypokinesia). In fact, monkeys with parkinsonism induced by 1-methyl-4-phenyl-1,2,3,6-tetrahydropyridine (MPTP) had their akinesia reversed by subthalamotomy.

Albin RL, et al: The functional anatomy of basal ganglia disorders. Trends Neurosci 12:366, 1989.

Bergman H, et al: Reversal of experimental parkinsonism by lesions of the subthalamic nucleus. Science 249:1436, 1990.

11. What are the cardinal symptoms and signs of parkinsonism?

Tremor at rest is one of the most typical signs of parkinsonism. It is characterized by an oscillatory pronation-supination at a 3–5 Hz frequency. In addition to the hands, where it assumes an appearance of pill rolling, this type of tremor is commonly observed in the facial musculature (lips and chin) and legs. Head tremor, however, is rare in parkinsonism and its presence should suggest the diagnosis of essential tremor (ET).

The term **bradykinesia** is used to describe slowness of movements that often causes difficulties for patients in getting dressed, feeding, and maintaining personal hygiene. Bradykinesia is evident when a person performs rapid alternating movements such as pronation and supination of the forearms.

Rigidity, often associated with the cogwheel phenomenon, is another hallmark of parkinsonism. Impairment of the postural reflexes is responsible for the falls that are frequently experienced by parkinsonian patients. Parkinsonian gait often reflects a combination of bradykinesia, rigidity, and postural instability.

In addition to the above-mentioned features, there are other important symptoms and signs in parkinsonism. Approximately 50% of patients who have PD experience pain, which may be their presenting symptom. Micrography, or small-sized handwriting, is another frequent and precocious sign of PD. The coexistence of rigidity and bradykinesia in the facial musculature accounts for decreased blinking rate and facial expression (hypomimia or mask facies). Seborrhea, weight loss, and various signs of autonomic dysfunction are also often found in PD patients. Involvement of the upper and lower GI tract in PD is evidenced respectively by dysphagia and constipation.

The chronology of appearance as well as the pattern of combination of these clinical features depend on the cause of the parkinsonism. For example, in progressive supranuclear palsy (PSP), postural reflex impairment occurs early in the course of the disease, whereas prominent rest tremor at onset suggests the diagnosis of PD.

12. What are the most common causes of parkinsonism?

In a highly selected population, such as that attending a Movement Disorders Clinic, PD is responsible for 77.7% of the cause of parkinsonism. The other most most frequent causes are parkinsonism-plus syndrome (12.2%), secondary parkinsonism (8.2%), and heredodegenerative parkinsonism (0.6%).

Jankovic J: Parkinsonism-plus syndrome. Mov Disord 4(Suppl 1):S95, 1989.

Causes of Parkinsonism

  I. Idiopathic Parkinsonism
      Parkinson's disease (PD)
        Sporadic form
        Familial form

 II. Secondary Parkinsonism
      Drug-induced
        Dopamine receptor blockers (neuroleptics, including antiemetics
          such as metoclopramide)
        Dopamine depleters (reserpine, tetrabenazine)
        Calcium channel blockers (flunarizine, cinnarizine, diltiazem)
        Lithium
        Methyldopa
      Hemiatrophy-hemiparkinsonism
      Hydrocephalus
        Normal pressure hydrocephalus
        Noncommunicating hydrocephalus
      Hypoxia
      Infectious
        AIDS
        Creutzfeldt-Jakob disease
        Fungus
        Intracytoplasmic hyaline inclusion disease
        Postencephalitic parkinsonism
        Subacute sclerosing panencephalitis
      Metabolic
        Acquired hepatocerebral degeneration (chronic liver insufficiency)
        Hypocalcemic parkinsonism
      Paraneoplastic parkinsonism
      Syringomesencephalia

Table continued on next page

Causes of Parkinsonism (Continued)

II. Secondary Parkinsonism *(Cont.)*
  Toxin
    Carbon disulfide
    Carbon monoxide
    Cyanide
    Disulfiram
    Ethanol
    Manganese
    Methanol
    1-Methyl-4-phenyl-1,2,3,6-tetrahydropyridine (MPTP)
  Trauma
  Tumor
  Vascular
    Multi-infarct
    Binswanger's disease
    Lower body parkinsonism

III. Parkinsonism-plus Syndromes
  Alzheimer's disease-parkinsonism
  Cortical basal ganglionic degeneration (CBGD)
  Diffuse Lewy-body disease
  Multiple system atrophy (MSA)
    Shy-Drager syndrome
    Sporadic olivopontocerebellar atrophy (OPCA)
    Striatonigral degeneration
  Parkinsonism-dementia-amyotrophic lateral sclerosis
  Progressive pallidal atrophy
  Progressive supranuclear palsy (PSP)

IV. Heredodegenerative Diseases
  Ceroid-lipofuscinosis
  Gerstmann-Strausler-Scheinker disease
  Familial OPCA
  Hallervorden-Spatz disease
  Huntington's disease
  Levodopa-responsiveness (fluctuating) dystonia
  Machado-Joseph disease (Azorean heredoataxia)
  Mitochondrial cytopathies with striatal necrosis
  Neuroacanthocytosis
  Thalamic dementia syndrome
  Wilson's disease
  X-linked dystonia-parkinsonism

13. What causes PD?

Although PD was first described in 1817, its cause is still unknown. The recognition that MPTP can produce in humans and nonhuman primates a parkinsonian syndrome very similar to PD led to the hypothesis that an MPTP-like substance present in the environment could cause PD. This theory was strengthened by the finding that subjects living in rural areas and exposed to pesticides that are structurally related to MPTP, such as paraquat, had a relatively high risk for developing PD. MPTP exerts its neurotoxic action by inhibiting complex I of the respiratory chain of the innner mitochondrial membrane. This group of enzymes has been reported to be impaired in patients with PD. Despite these striking similarities, there are definite differences between MPTP-induced parkinsonism (MPTP-P) and PD. Rest tremor is less frequently found in humans with MPTP-P and is virtually absent in monkeys exposed to MPTP. PD is a progressive disease, but there is no evidence of progression of MPTP-P. Typical Lewy bodies (LB) found in the brains of patients with PD have not been demonstrated in MPTP-P.

One theory on the cause of PD is that afflicted persons have a defective antioxidant system, leading to an increased formation of highly reactive and toxic free oxygen radicals (oxidative stress). Indeed, the findings of increased nigral basal lipid peroxidation, reduced glutathione levels, increased total iron, and decreased ferritin in the SN suggest that there is increased generation of free radicals. Despite all this evidence, the precise role of oxidative mechanisms in the pathogenesis of PD remains to be established.

A growing body of evidence supports the notion that genetic factors play an important role in the etiology of PD. Families with otherwise typical PD with an autosomal dominant transmission have been described, as have monozygotic twins concordant for the disease. The possibility of involvement of maternal transmission has been raised by several reports of mutations of mitochondrial DNA in the SN. Other areas of the brain of persons with PD, such as the striatum, and the SN of persons with multiple system atrophy (MSA), do not display this abnormality.

The etiology of PD is still speculative but there may be a combination of environmental factors associated with a genetic predisposition.

Johnson WG, et al: Twin studies and the genetics of Parkinson's disease: A reappraisal. Mov Disord 5:187, 1990.

Dexter DT, et al: Alterations in the levels of iron, ferritin and other trace metals in Parkinson's disease and other neurodegenerative diseases affecting the basal ganglia. Brain 114:1953, 1991.

Jenner P, Schapira AHV, Marsden CD: New insights into the cause of Parkinson's disease. Neurology 42:2241, 1992.

14. What are the clinical and pathologic hallmarks of PD?

Patients with PD may have several combinations of parkinsonian symptoms. Typically, the onset is insidious in the sixth decade of life, and the symptoms usually begin unilaterally or predominate on one side of the body. It is possible to recognize two clinical types of PD: a **tremor-dominant** form and a **postural instability and gait difficulty** form.

Pathologically, there is loss of dopaminergic neurons in the SNc, and the surviving neurons contain LB. Although to a lesser degree than the SNc, other pigmented nuclei of the brainstem, such as locus ceruleus and tegmental ventral area, are also involved by a similar process. A recent clinicopathologic study showed that the presence of a resting tremor is more likely to be associated with LB at autopsy.

Jankovic J, et al: Variable expression of Parkinson's disease: A base-line analysis of the DATATOP cohort. Neurology 40:1529, 1990.

Rajput AH, et al: Mode of onset and prognosis in Parkinson's disease. Neurology 42(Suppl 3): 419, 1992.

15. How specific is the clinical diagnosis of PD?

Two recent clinicopathologic studies (Rajput et al, 1991; Hughes et al, 1992a) addressed this question. In both series, 24% of the patients with the clinical diagnosis of PD were found to have other diagnosis at necropsy. These studies show that patients with typical symptomatology may have variable pathologic findings and, conversely, typical pathologic findings can be expressed by very dissimilar signs. Findings of asymmetric onset, no evidence for other causes of parkinsonism, and no atypical features of PD increased the specificity of the clinical diagnosis in the London series to 92%, but 32% of the PD cases did not satisfy these criteria, indicating that these criteria have a low sensitivity.

Rajput AH, et al: Accuracy of clinical diagnosis in parkinsonism: A prospective study. Can J Neurol Sci 18:275, 1991.

Hughes AJ, et al: Diagnosis of idiopathic Parkinson's disease: A clinico-pathological study of 100 cases. J Neurol Neurosurg Psychiatry 55:181, 1992a.

Hughes AJ, et al: What features improve the accuracy of clinical diagnosis in Parkinson's disease: A clinicopathologic study. Neurology 42:1142, 1992b.

16. Are there tests that support an antemortem diagnosis of PD?
Currently, there is no biologic marker that would allow an in vivo diagnosis of PD. However, some tests may be helpful in supporting the diagnosis of PD. The values of homovanillic acid, a metabolite of dopamine, in the cerebrospinal fluid (CSF) are usually low, but computerized tomography (CT) scans and magnetic resonance imaging (MRI) of the head are usually normal.

Positron emission tomography (PET) scanning with 18F-fluorodopa, a radioactive isomer of levodopa, provides an index of the nigrostriatal integrity. In PD there is reduction of 18F-fluorodopa uptake, particulary in the putamen. Dopamine D2 receptor ligands, such as raclopride and spiperone, can be imaged with PET to demonstrate increased density of these receptors in PD patients not exposed to dopaminergic drugs. This receptor up-regulation probably reflects denervation hypersensitivity secondary to the loss of nigrostriatal axons. Despite its usefulness, PET scanning is a cumbersome and expensive method of assessing the integrity of striatal dopaminergic terminals. It is not a practical diagnostic test for PD.

Single photon emission tomography (SPECT) may be more practical and less expensive than PET, but its spatial resolution is limited. Preliminary studies using IBZM, a ligand of D2 receptors, and iodine-123 labeled RTI-55 to image presynaptic dopamine uptake sites have suggested that eventually SPECT may be used to aid the early diagnosis of PD. The presynaptic dopamine uptake sites are impaired in early PD as a result of the loss of dopaminergic terminals, and therefore the RTI SPECT could be helpful in the early detection of PD.

Sawle GV, et al: The identification of presymptomatic parkinsonism: Clinical and {[18]F} dopa positron emission tomography studies in an Irish kindred. Ann Neurol 32:609, 1992.

Brooks DJ, et al: Striatal D2 receptor status in patients with Parkinson's disease, striatonigral degeneration, and progressive supranuclear palsy, measured with 11C-raclopride and positron emission tomography. Ann Neurol 31:184, 1992.

Schwarz J, et al: 123I-iodobenzamide-SPECT predicts dopaminergic responsiveness in patients with de novo parkinsonism. Neurology 42:556, 1992.

Shaya EK, et al: In vivo imaging of dopamine reuptake sites in the primate brain using single photon emission computed tomography (SPECT) and iodine-123 labeled RTI-55. Synapse 10:169, 1992.

17. What is the rationale for using deprenyl in PD?
Deprenyl is an inhibitor of the enzyme monoamine oxidase B (MAOB). The conversion of MPTP to MPP+, which is the active substance that produces parkinsonism, is catalyzed by MAOB. In nonhuman primates it was shown that inhibitors of MAOB prevent the formation of MPP+ and so prevent the development of MPTP-P. If PD is caused by an MPTP-like substance, then antioxidant therapy may be a rational protective treatment. Three double-blind studies assessed the role of deprenyl in the treatment of PD and showed that MAOB inhibitors delayed the need for levodopa. However, the interpretation of this result is still disputed, and some authors argue that instead of changing the rate of neurodegeneration, deprenyl exerts a minimal symptomatic effect. Because deprenyl may indeed provide a protective effect and is well tolerated by most patients, it is recommended during the early therapy of PD. The patients are usually started on one 5-mg tablet after breakfast in the first week and one tablet after break-fast and lunch thereafter. The most common untoward effects of the 10-mg dose are headache and nausea. Dosages higher than 10 mg/day should be avoided because both MAOA and B may be inhibited. This may be associated, then, with cardiovascular side effects.

Juncos JL, et al: Does selegiline have a subclinical therapeutic effect on Parkinson' disease? Neurology 42(Suppl 3):357, 1992.

Parkinson Study Group: Effects of tocopherol and deprenyl on the progression of disability in early Parkinson's disease. N Engl J Med 328:176, 1993.

18. What is the role of anticholinergic drugs and amantadine in the treatment of PD?

In the early stages of the disease, combined with deprenyl, these medications may be used as the primary treatment of PD. With the progression of the disease, patients require the addition of levodopa. Even in this cricumstance, some patients still benefit from using anticholinergics and amantadine. Tremor is occasionally resistant to dopaminergic therapy and this symptom may be better controlled with the use of levodopa in association with these ancillary medications. In contrast to the anticholinergics, amantadine, a drug that has mild anticholinergic effects and increases the release of dopamine, also improves rigidity and bradykinesia.

The anticholinergic medications must be used cautiously because, in addition to causing dryness of the mouth and bladder retention, they may produce disorientation, confusion, and memory loss, particularly in the elderly. Amantadine in some patients may also cause cognitive side effects as well as livedo reticularis, ankle swelling, and worsening of congestive heart failure.

Jankovic J, Marsden CD: Therapeutic strategies in Parkinson's disease. In Jankovic J, Tolosa E (eds): Parkinson's Disease and Movement Disorders, 2nd ed. Baltimore, Williams & Wilkins, 1993.

19. When should levodopa therapy be started in the treatment of PD?

The mainstay in the treatment of PD is the replacement of dopamine. This therapy was introduced in the 1960s. Instead of using dopamine, which does not cross the blood-brain barrier, the current approach combines levodopa and carbidopa. The first is transformed into dopamine and the latter is a peripheral inhibitor of the enzyme dopa decarboxylase. The inhibition of this enzyme in the periphery, but not in the brain, decreases substantially the required dosage of levodopa and the occurrence of GI side effects (nausea and vomiting). In Europe and other countries, benseraside is available as an inhibitor of dopa decarboyxlase.

The controversy about the best timing for introducing levodopa is not yet settled. One argument for early use is that levodopa is the most effective treatment for PD; therefore there is no reason to deprive the patients of its benefits. The proponents of early levodopa therapy also argue that the occurrence of central side effects of levodopa (e.g., dyskinesias and clinical fluctuations) are related to progression of the disease and not to the duration or cumulative dosage of levodopa. Conversely, those who prefer postponing the use of levodopa argue that levodopa is neurotoxic, and that it directly contributes to the development of complications such as the wearing-off effect and dyskinesia.

A rational strategy is to start levodopa when the parkinsonian symptoms begin to impair activities of daily living or interfere with social and occupational functioning. The usual starting dose is in a form of Sinemet CR (50/200), half a tablet twice a day, increased by half a tablet every 3 days until a satisfactory improvement is noted. Other formulations of Sinemet include Sinemet 10/100, 25/100, and 25/250.

Hefti F, et al: Long-term administration of levodopa does not damage dopaminergic neurons in the mouse. Neurology 31:1194, 1981.

Markham CH, et al: Long-term follow-up of early dopa treatment in Parkinson's disease. Ann Neurol 19:365, 1986.

Fahn S, Bressman SB: Should levodopa therapy for parkinsonism be started early or late? Evidence against early treatment. Can J Neurol Sci 11:2000, 1984.

Cedarbaum JM, et al: "Early" initiation of levodopa treatment does not promote the development of motor response fluctuations, dyskinesias, or dementia in Parkinson's disease. Neurology 41:622, 1991.

Mena MA, et al: Neurotoxicity of levodopa on catecholamine-rich neurons. Mov Disord 7:23, 1992.

Nutt JG, et al: Effect of long-term therapy on the pharmacodynamics of levodopa: Relation to on-off effect. Arch Neurol 49:1123, 1992.

20. What are the most common peripheral side effects of levodopa therapy? How are they managed?

Nausea and vomiting are common occurrences in the beginning of the use of levodopa. Most patients overcome this difficulty by taking the medication after meals. In some patients extra amounts of carbidopa (typically, one 25-mg tablet together with each dose of Sinemet) may be necessary. A small proportion of patients will have nausea and vomiting despite these measures. Treatment of the GI side effects should not include dopamine blockers, such as metoclopramide, because they may cause worsening of PD. Diphenidol and cyclizine are useful alternatives.

The most common cardiovascular undesired effect is orthostatic hypotension. The management of this complication involves the adding of salt to the diet, wearing elastic stockings, and using medications such as fluodrocortisone and indomethacin.

Parkes DJ: Domperidone and Parkinson's disease. Clin Neuropharmacol 6:517, 1986.

Jankovic J, et al: Neurogenic orthostatic hypotension: A double-blind placebo controlled study with midodrine. Am J Med (in press).

21. What are the clinical fluctuations recognized in PD?

Although the most dramatic fluctuations in patients with PD are related to levodopa therapy, some who have not been previously treated with dopaminergic drugs exhibit fluctuations in the severity of symptoms and signs. Fluctuations are not exclusively motor phenomena. It is well recognized that the mood and autonomic functions also fluctuate. For example, some patients display depression when they are "off," and euphoria when they are "on." Fatigue and stress usually make these more prominent. The most dramatic example of spontaneous fluctuations is paradoxical dyskinesia: when under extreme stress, patients completely immobilized by their parkinsonism are suddenly able to get up and run.

Levodopa-induced fluctuations are the most important motor fluctuations because of their potential to cause significant disability. The most common type of clinical fluctuation is the shortening of the response to levodopa (wearing-off phenomenon), as a consequence of which antiparkinsonian benefits ("on" period) are lost after 2–3 hours (or even less) and the parkinsonian symptoms re-emerge ("off" period). Occasionally, the action of levodopa ends suddenly, the so-called on-off effect. Motor fluctuations are probably caused by a loss of dopaminergic terminals in the striatum, with consequent impairment of the brain's ability to buffer the shifts in levodopa availability. Among the most challenging problems in the treatment of PD are the motor blocks, or freezing. They consist of sudden episodes of inability to move the legs, usually triggered by being in crowded places and walking through narrow passages. Attempts at overcoming these episodes by moving the upper part of the body are common causes of falls in these patients. This symptom is probably not related to dopaminergic changes. Therefore, use of levodopa or dopamine agonists is usually ineffective. Although desipramine may benefit a few patients, the most effective treatment consists of using sensory, especially visual, cues to guide the motor planning. An inverted L-shaped cane has been shown to be helpful to many patients, who can overcome their freezings by stepping over the handle of the cane.

Jankovic J, et al: Comparison of Sinemet CR-4 and standard Sinemet: Double-blind and long-term open trial in parkinsonian patients with fluctuations. Mov Disord 4:303, 1989.

Menza MA, et al: Mood changes and "on-off" phenomena in Parkinson's disease. Mov Disord 5:148, 1990.

Dietz MA, et al: Evaluation of a modified inverted walking stick as a treatment for parkinsonian freezing episodes. Mov Disord 5:243, 1990.

Cedarbaum JM, Olanow CW: Dopamine sulfate in ventricular cerebrospinal fluid and motor function in Parkinson's disease. Neurology 41:1567, 1991.

Vaamonde J, et al: Subcutaneous lisuride infusion in Parkinson's disease: Response to chronic administration in 34 patients. Brain 114:601, 1991.

Sage JI, Mark MH: Nighttime levodopa infusions to treat motor fluctuations in advanced Parkinson's disease: Preliminary observations. Ann Neurol 30:616, 1991.

Clinical Fluctuations in Parkinson's Disease

FLUCTUATION	MANAGEMENT
End-of-dose deterioration ("wearing off")	Increase frequency of levodopa doses Sinemet CR Dopamine agonists Deprenyl Amantadine Infusions of levodopa or dopamine agonists
Delayed onset of response	Give before meals Reduce protein Antacids Infusions of levodopa or dopamine agonists
Drug-resistant "offs"	Increase levodopa dose and frequency Give before meals Infusions of levodopa or dopamine agonists
Random oscillation ("on-off")	Dopamine agonists Deprenyl Infusions of levodopa or dopamine agonists Levodopa withdrawal
Freezing*	Increase dose Dopamine agonists Desipramine Inverted L-shaped cane

* May not be related to levodopa therapy.

22. How can the continuous-release form of Sinemet (Sinemet CR) be useful to the management of fluctuations in PD?

The controlled-release preparation of carbidopa/levodopa, Sinemet CR (50/200 mg tablets), represents a useful alternative to the standard Sinemet (10/100, 25/100, 25/250) for the treatment of these patients. The transition from the regular to the controlled preparation of Sinemet has to be carefully planned. Because of lower bioavailability of the CR preparation, the authors usually increase the daily dosage of levodopa by 30%; many patients require a 50% increase in the final dose of of Sinemet CR compared with the baseline dosage of the standard Sinemet. A potential problem of the CR preparation is the long latency. When present, this difficulty is usually overcome by adding one-half or one tablet of the Sinemet 25/100 to the first morning dose of the Sinemet CR. Unfortunately, many patients have a coexistence of clinical fluctuations and peak-dose dyskinesias. The latter side effect tends to deteriorate with the increased dopaminergic stimulation provided by the Sinemet CR.

23. What are the most common types of levodopa-induced dyskinesias (LID)? How are they treated?

After 3 years of treatment with levodopa, approximately 50% of the patients with PD display some degree of involuntary movements related to this drug. Phenomenologically, LID may be classified into three main categories: (1) **"peak dose" dyskinesias** (improvement–dyskinesia–improvement or I–D–I) coincide with the time of maximum clinical improvement and usually consist of choreatic movements. (2) **Diphasic dyskinesias** (dyskinesia–improvement–dyskinesia or D–I–D) occur at the onset and/or at the end of the "on" period, and usually consist of dystonia and repetitive stereotypic movements of the legs. Some patients display a combination of these two types and have dyskinesia the entire "on" period (square wave dyskinesias). (3) **"Off" dyskinesias**, typically painful dystonias, coincide with the period of decreased mobility. The most common example is early morning dystonia. Dopaminergic stimulation increases "on" dyskinesias and decreases the other two types. Conversely, antidopaminergic drugs improve all forms of LID, although they worsen the PD. Dystonia induced by levodopa may improve significantly with the use of baclofen, an agonist of gamma-aminobutyric acid receptors.

Nutt JG: Levodopa-induced dyskinesia: Review, observations, and speculations. Neurology 40:340, 1990.

Luquin MR, et al: Levodopa-induced dyskinesias in Parkinson's disease: Clinical and pharmacological classification. Mov Disord 7:117, 1992.

Jankovic J: Natural course and limitations of levodopa therapy. Neurology 42(international symposium):14, 1992.

Levodopa-Induced Dyskinesias

PATTERN	PHENOMENOLOGY	MANAGEMENT
Peak-dose (I-D-I)	Chorea	Reduce each dose of levodopa Add dopamine agonists
	Dystonia	Reduce each dose of levodopa Clonazepam Baclofen Anticholinergics
	Pharyngeal dystonia	Reduce each dose of levodopa Add anticholinergics
	Respiratory dyskinesia	Reduce each dose of levodopa Add dopamine agonists
	Myoclonus	Clonazepam Valproate Methysergide
	Akathisia*	Anxiolytics Propranolol Opioids
Diphasic (D-I-D)	Dystonia	Increase each dose of levodopa Baclofen Sinemet CR
	Stereotypies	Increase each dose of levodopa Baclofen
Off dyskinesia	Dystonia	Baclofen Dopamine agonists Anticholinergics Sinemet CR Tricyclics Lithium Botulinum toxin
	Akathisia*	Anxiolytics Propranolol Opioids
Striatal posture*	Dystonia	Increase levodopa Anticholinergics Thalamotomy Botulinum toxin

I-D-I = improvement-dyskinesia-improvement
D-I-D = dyskinesia-improvement-dyskinesia
* May be unrelated to levodopa therapy.

24. What is the role of dopamine agonists in the treatment of PD?

Dopamine agonists directly stimulate dopamine receptors, and, in contrast to levodopa, do not require enzymatic transformation into metabolites. Because dopamine agonists bypass the presynaptic elements of the nigrostriatal system, they have some advantages in relation to levodopa. Dyskinesias and clinical fluctuations, for example, are less frequently caused by these drugs and they usually have a levodopa-sparing effect. The most established use of these medications is as an adjunct to levodopa, especially in patients with clinical fluctuations and dyskinesias. There is evidence that early introduction of dopamine agonists decreases the possibility of development of complications of long-term levodopa therapy by maintaining the doses of levodopa at low levels.

25. Name the dopamine agonists available to treat PD. What are their most common side effects?

Bromocriptine and pergolide are the two dopamine agonists commercially available in the U.S. Both are ergot derivatives, but bromocriptine stimulates dopamine D2 receptors and inhibits D1 receptors, whereas pergolide stimulates both D1 and D2 receptors. Although they display fewer side effects than levodopa, peak-dose dyskinesias may be exacerbated by these medications, and other dopaminergic undesired effects such as nausea, vomiting, anorexia, malaise, orthostatic hypotension, confusion, and hallucinations may also occur. Additionally, vasospasm with acroparesthesias and angina, exacerbation of peptic ulcer disease, and erythromelalgia (a painful reddish discoloration of the skin) are other side effects reported with these drugs. Bromocriptine has been found to rarely cause retroperitoneal fibrosis. The difference in the mechanism of action between these two drugs suggests that pergolide has more efficacy than bromocriptine. However, this has not been confirmed in clinical trials, although bromocriptine seems to be less tolerated than pergolide.

Jankovic J: Long-term study of pergolide in Parkinson's disease. Neurology 35:296, 1985.
Jankovic J, Marsden CD: Therapeutic strategies in Parkinson's disease. In Jankovic J, Tolosa E (eds): Parkinson's Disease and Movement Disorders, 2nd ed. Baltimore, Williams & Wilkins, 1993.

26. What is the role of surgery in the treatment of PD?

Thalamotomy is the most established neurosurgical procedure used in the treatment of PD. This procedure consists of lesioning some thalamic nuclei, especially ventral inferior medial nucleus, involved in the generation of parkinsonian tremor. This treatment is reserved for patients with predominantly unilateral parkinsonism who fail to respond to conservative therapy. In approximately 80% of the PD patients who undergo this procedure, there is improvement of the tremor without significant side effects. Bilateral surgery is not recommended, however, because of the complication of dysarthria.

The recognition that in PD there is hyperactivity of the subthalamic nucleus led to a successful treatment of MPTP-P in monkeys by subthalamotomy. Some human patients, inadvertently treated with subthalamotomy instead of thalamotomy, noted improvement not only in their tremor, but also in their bradykinesia. Further studies are needed before subthalamotomy can be recommended in the treatment of parkinsonian symptoms.

Lateral pallidotomy has been reported to provide improvement not only in contralateral tremor, but also bradykinesia. The long-term efficacy of this technique in the treatment of PD, however, also remains to be established.

Sellal F, et al: Contralateral disappearance of parkinsonian signs after subthalamic hematoma. Neurology 42:255, 1992.

27. What is the role of transplant surgery in the treatment of PD?

Interest in the transplantation of adrenal medulla into the basal ganglia was sparked by the hypothesis that the adrenal chromaffin cells will produce dopamine when implanted into parkinsonian striatum. After initial encouraging reports, this procedure has been virtually abandoned in the U.S. because of its modest benefits and high risk of morbidity.

Several ongoing studies are testing the possibility of transplanting human fetal dopamine neurons extracted from the mesencephalic tegmentum into the putamen. The rationale is that the embryonic cells will proliferate, establish connections, and produce dopamine in the striatum. Some studies have shown a modest clinical improvement. Because of ethical and legal issues involved, the development of this procedure in the treatment of PD has been slow, and it is unlikely that it will ever be adopted as a routine treatment.

Goetz CG, et al: United Parkinson Foundation Neurotransplantation Registry on Adrenal Medullary Transplants: Presurgical, and 1- and 2-year follow-up. Neurology 41:1719, 1991.

Lindvall O, et al: Transplantation of fetal dopamine neurons in Parkinson's disease: One-year clinical and neurophysiological observations in two patients with putaminal implants. Ann Neurol 31:155, 1992.

Freed CR, et al: Survival of implanted fetal dopamine cells and neurologic improvement 12 to 46 months after transplantation for Parkinson's disease. N Engl J Med 327:1549, 1992.

Spencer DD, et al: Unilateral transplantation of human fetal mesencephalic tissue into the caudate nucleus of patients with Parkinson's disease. N Engl J Med 327:1541, 1992.

28. Is there any relationship between Alzheimer's disease (AD) and PD?

Currently available data do not support a common etiology. However, approximately 20% of patients with PD have troublesome dementia. AD accounts for an unknown proportion of these cases. Unlike AD, the pattern of dementia in PD is characterized by lack of cortical signs, such as aphasia and apraxia, and the presence of forgetfulness, bradyphrenia, and depression. This suggests that different mechanisms are responsible for cognitive dysfunction in both diseases, and pathologic studies support this distinction. PD is characterized by relative sparing of the cortex and by neuronal loss in the SN and other subcortical structures, such as the locus ceruleus. LB are found in the remaining cells. On the other hand, cerebral cortex is the area primarily involved in AD, where neurofibrillary tangles and deposits of amyloid are the most important lesions. However, a recent study shows that over 50% of patients with AD will display parkinsonism and myoclonus during the course of the disease.

Chen JY, et al: Cumulative risks of developing extrapyramidal signs, psychosis, or myoclonus in the course of Alzheimer's disease. Arch Neurol 48:1141, 1991.

German DC, et al: Disease-specific patterns of locus coeruleus cell loss. Ann Neurol 32:667,1992.

29. What are the main clinical features of progressive supranuclear palsy (PSP)?

PSP is the second most common cause of idiopathic parkinsonism. Typically, the onset is in the seventh decade, with no family history. Patients have ophthalmoparesis of downgaze, parkinsonism, pseudobulbar palsy, and fontal lobe signs. Eyelid abnormalities are common in this condition. One of the examples is eyelid freezing: patients have difficulty either opening or closing the eyes owing to inhibition of, respectively, levator palpebrae and orbicularis oculi muscles. The presence of dementia in PSP is controversial. The prevalence of dystonia in patients with pathologically-proven PSP is about 13%.

30. What is the cause of PSP?

The cause is unknown. Radiologic and pathologic evidence shows that a multi-infarct state can cause a picture identical to PSP. Idiopathic PSP is pathologically character-ized by marked neuronal cell loss in subcortical structures, such as nucleus basalis of Meynert, the pallidum, subthalamic nucleus, substantia nigra, locus ceruleus, and superior colliculi. Other pathologic features include neurofibrillary tangles, granulovacuolar degeneration, and gliosis. Atrophy, generalized or focal (midbrain or cerebellum), is the most common neuroradiologic finding in idiopathic PSP. However, up to 25% of the patients with a diagnosis of PSP do not have any abnormality on CT and/or MRI of the brain.

Dubinsky RM, Jankovic J: Progressive supranuclear palsy and a multi-infarct state. Neurology 37:570, 1987.

Jankovic J, et al: Progressive supranuclear palsy: Motor, neurobehavioral, and neuro-ophthalmic findings. In Streifler MB, et al (eds): Advances in Neurology, Vol 53: Anatomy, Pathology, and Therapy. New York, Raven Press, 1990, p 293.

Rivest J, Quinn N, Marsden CD: Dystonia in Parkinson's disease, multiple system atrophy, and progressive supranuclear palsy. Neurology 40:1571, 1990.

31. How can PSP be distinguished from PD?

The most distinctive feature of PSP is supranuclear downgaze palsy, which is not found in PD, the most common misdiagnosis of PSP. The differentiation is particularly difficult when the chracteristic supranuclear ophthalmoparesis is not evident, as may be the case in the early stages of the disease. Some patients never develop this finding, but at autopsy are found to have PSP. The difficulty in establishing the diagnosis of PSP is suggested by an average delay in making the diagnosis of 3.6 years after the onset of symptoms.

Maher ER, Lees AJ: The clinical features and natural history of the Steele-Richardson-Olszewski syndrome (progressive supranuclear palsy). Neurology 36:1005, 1986.

Golbe LI, et al: Prevalence and natural history of progressive supranuclear palsy. Neurology 38:1031, 1988.

Cardoso F, Jankovic J: Progressive supranuclear palsy. In Calne DB (ed): Neurodegenerative Diseases. Philadelphia, W.B. Saunders, 1993.

Differential Diagnosis of PD and PSP

CLINICAL FEATURES	PSP	PD
Age at onset (decade)	7th	6th
Initial symptoms	Postural and gait disorder	Tremor and bradykinesia
Family history	−	±
Multi-infarct state	±	−
Dementia	± (visual/motor)	±
Downgaze ophthalmoparesis	+	−
Lid abnormalities	+	±
Pseudobulbar palsy	+	±
Gait	Wide, stiff, unsteady	Slow, shuffling, narrow, festinating
Rigidity	Axial (neck)	Generalized
Facial expression	Astonished, worried	Hypomimia
Tremor at rest	−	+
Dystonia	+	±
Cortico-bulbar-spinal signs	±	−
Symmetry of findings	+	−
Weight loss	−	+
Improvement with DA drugs	−	+
Levodopa-induced dyskinesias	−	+

+ = yes or present; − = no or absent; PSP = progressive supranuclear palsy; PD = Parkinson's disease; and DA = dopamine.

32. What is the treatment of PSP?

Levodopa and dopamine agonists are most frequently used in the treatment of PSP. However, even when using high doses, these drugs usually provide only a transient and slight improvement of parkinsonian symptoms. The loss of dopamine receptors in the striatum and the presence of extensive lesions involving other neurotransmitters, such as acetylcholine, probably account for the failure of pharmacologic therapy. No effective drug currently provides any sustained relief in patients with PSP. With the progression of the disease, patients usually become bedridden and unable to swallow or talk. Gastrostomy is necessary in these advanced stages. Death, usually related to respiratory complications, occurs after a mean disease duration of 7–8 years.

Golbe LI, Davis PH: Progressive supranuclear palsy. In Jankovic J, Tolosa E (eds): Parkinson's Disease and Movement Disorders, 2nd ed. Baltimore, Williams & Wilkins, 1993.

33. What are the most important characteristics of vascular parkinsonism?

Multiple vascular lesions in the basal ganglia may be associated with parkinsonism. Tremor at rest is not a common finding, and bradykinesia and rigidity tend to be more significant in the legs. In some patients the findings are virtually limited to the lower extremities, hence the designation "lower body parkinsonism." Unlike in PD, in vascular parkinsonism the gait is characterized by a broad base. In some patients there is stepwise progression. Associated findings, such as dementia, spasticity, weakness, and Babinski signs, are commonly observed. Neuroradiologic studies, especially MRI, show a multi-infarct state. The response to dopaminergic therapy is usually poor.

Fitzgerald PM, Jankovic J: Lower body parkinsonism: Evidence for vascular etiology. Mov Disord 4:249, 1989.

34. Is it possible clinically to distinguish drug-induced parkinsonism from PD?

Drugs are one of the most common causes of parkinsonism in the general population. Drugs that block postsynaptic dopamine receptors and/or deplete presynaptic dopamine may cause parkinsonism. Some of these medications are listed in the table on p. 130–131. Clinical studies indicate that patients with drug-induced parkinsonism are indistinguishable from those with PD. Discontinuation of the offending drug is enough to promote remission of the syndrome in the majority of cases, although sometimes the parkinsonism persists. These patients may have subclinical PD and may require dopaminergic therapy.

Hardie RJ, Lees AJ: Neuroleptic-induced Parkinson's syndrome: Clinical features and results of treatment with levodopa. J Neurol Neurosurg Psychiatry 51:850, 1988.

35. What is multiple-system atrophy (MSA)?

MSA is a neuropathologic term that encompasses Shy-Drager syndrome (SDS), sporadic forms of olivopontocerebellar atrophy (OPCA), and striatonigral degeneration (SND). The first is characterized by parkinsonism, occasionally responsive to dopaminergic therapy, associated with dysautonomia. Although cerebellar findings dominate the picture of OPCA, mild parkinsonism and pyramidal signs are also usually recognized. Patients with SND typically have parkinsonism and pyramidal signs with laryngeal stridor, although in some cases they are indistinguishable from patients with PD. There is controversy whether MSA should be subdivided into SDS, OPCA, and SND. Although usually clinically distinct at onset, with progression there is a substantial overlap in symptoms. These syndromes have a common pathologic substratum consisting of cell loss and gliosis in the striatum, substantia nigra, locus ceruleus, inferior olive, pontine nuclei, dorsal vagal nuclei, cerebellar Purkinje cells, and intermediolateral cell columns of the spinal cord. Glial cytoplasmic inclusions, especially in oligodendrocytes, are claimed to be relatively specific for MSA.

36. What is the treatment of MSA?

Dopaminergic drugs are the mainstay of treatment. Despite the use of high doses of levodopa, no significant improvement is usually observed. The loss of cells in the striatum and widespread lesions of other neurotransmitters probably account for the failure of treatment.

Stacy M, Jankovic J: Differential diagnosis of Parkinson's disease and parkinsonism plus syndromes. Neurol Clin 10:341, 1992.

Papp M, Lantos P: Accumulation of tubular structures in oligodendroglial and neuronal cells as the basic alteration in multiple system atrophy. J Neurol Sci 107:172, 1992.

Hughes AJ, et al: The dopaminergic response in multiple system atrophy. J Neurol Neurosurg Psychiatry 55:1009, 1992.

Doody RS, Jankovic J: The alien hand and related signs. J Neurol Neurosurg Psychiatry 55:806, 1992.

37. What is cortical basal ganglionic degeneration (CBGD)?

Patients with CBGD display a combination of cortical (pyramidal signs, myoclonus, and apraxia) and subcortical findings (rigidity and dystonia) as well as a distinctive alien limb sign. CBGD is virtually the only disease that can cause this constellation of symptoms and signs. Until the late stages of the disease, patients with CBGD do not experience cognitive decline or dysautonomia. Convergence disturbances and oculomotor apraxia are common neuro-ophthalmic signs. The neuropathologic hallmarks are swollen achromatic neurons, neuronal loss and gliosis in the cerebral cortex, SN, lateral nuclei of the thalamus, striatum, locus ceruleus, and Purkinje layer of the cerebellum. The etiology is entirely obscure. No familial forms have been reported. The disease progresses relentlessly until death, usually within 10 years after onset. No treatment is available.

Riley DE, et al: Cortical-basal ganglionic degeneration. Neurology 40:1203, 1990.

TREMORS

38. What is essential tremor (ET)?

ET is a neurologic disease characterized by action tremor of the hands in the absence of any identifiable causes, such as drugs or toxins. There is general agreement that other types of tremor, such as isolated head and voice tremor, are also expressions of ET. It is estimated that at least 5 million Americans are affected by ET. Characterized by action-postural tremor of the hands and arms, ET may be asymmetric at onset and may have a kinetic component. Patients with a severe form of ET may display tremor at rest. The postural component is observed upon the maintenance of postures, such as holding the arms outstretched in front of the body. The kinetic component, often more severe than the postural component, is apparent during the performance of some tasks, such as handwriting or the finger-to-nose maneuver. Although sometimes labeled as "benign," ET may be a source of marked disability and embarrassment. ET is presumably transmitted by an autosomal dominant gene with variable expression. However, in about 35% of patients with ET, there is no family history. Supportive criteria for diagnosis of ET include improvement with alcohol, propranolol, and primidone. Findings of a survey of 350 patients with ET seen at the Baylor College of Medicine Parkinson's Disease Center and Movement Disorders Clinic are summarized in the table below.

Essential Tremor: Clinical Correlates

VARIABLE	RESULT	N
Gender	179 M/171 F	350
Age at evaluation (yr)	58.4 ± 16.4	350
Duration of symptom (yr)	18.7 ± 17.5	326
Family history		350
First-degree relative(s)	219 (62.5%)	
Other relatives	25 (7.1%)	

Table continued on next page

Essential Tremor: Clinical Correlates (Continued)

VARIABLE	RESULT	N
Anatomical distribution		350
Hands	314 (89.7%)	
Head	143 (40.8%)	
Voice	62 (17.4%)	
Leg	48 (13.7%)	
Jaw	25 (7.1%)	
Face	8 (2.9%)	
Trunk	6 (1.7%)	
Tongue	5 (1.4%)	
Orthostatic	2 (0.6%)	
Associated disorders		350
Dystonia	165 (47.1%)	
Cervical dystonia	94 (26.8%)	
Writer's cramp	48 (13.7%)	
Blepharospasm	26 (7.4%)	
Laryngeal dystonia	14 (4.0%)	
Others	21 (6.0%)	
Parkinsonism	72 (20.2%)	
Myoclonus	8 (2.2%)	
Improvement with drugs		
Alcohol	96 (66.7%)	144
Propranolol	22 (68.0%)	32
Primidone	8 (72.1%)	13

From Lou JS, Jankovic J: Essential tremor: Clinical correlates in 350 patients. Neurology 41:234, 1991, with permission.

39. How can enhanced physiologic tremor be differentiated from ET?

Physiologic tremor is a rhythmic oscillation with a frequency of 8–12 Hz determined largely by the mechanical properties of the oscillating limb. Under several circumstances (listed in the table below) this tremor can be enhanced and will appear identical to ET. Enhanced physiologic tremor is the most common cause of postural tremor. Unlike ET, however, its frequency can be reduced by mass loading.

Elble RJ, Koller WC: The measurement and quantification of tremor. In Tremor. Baltimore, The John Hopkins University Press, 1990, p 10.

Causes of Enhanced Physiologic Tremor

Stress-induced	Drugs
Anxiety	Beta agonists
Emotion	Theophylline, terbutaline,
Exercise	epinephrine, etc.
Fatigue	Cyclosporine
Fever	Dopaminergic drugs
Endocrine	Levodopa, dopamine agonists
Adrenocorticosteroids	Methylxanthines
Hypoglycemia	Coffee, tea
Pheochromocytoma	Psychiatric drugs
Thyrotoxicosis	Lithium, neuroleptics, tricyclics
Toxins	Stimulants
As, Bi, Br, ethanol	Amphetamines, cocaine
withdrawal, Hg, Pb	Valproic acid

40. What physiopathologic mechanisms underlie ET?

Only 14 patients with ET have had thorough pathologic examination, and no specific abnormality has been found. It has been suggested that the postural tremor of ET arises from spontaneous firing of the inferior olivary nucleus, which drives the cerebellum and its outflow pathways via the thalamus to the cerebral cortex and then to the spinal cord. This is supported by the finding that the metabolism of glucose in the inferior olive increases significantly when patients with ET perform finger-to-nose tests, and that the postural tremor of ET is associated with markedly increased blood flow to both cerebellar hemispheres. Clinical data also support a cerebellar role in the pathogenesis of ET: over 50% of ET patients have difficulty performing tandem gait, which is considered an indicator of cerebellar function, and hemispheric cerebellar stroke can abolish ipsilateral ET.

Dubinsky R, Hallet M: Glucose hypermetabolism of the inferior olive in patients with essential tremor. Ann Neurol 22:118, 1987.

Dupuis MJM, et al: Homolateral disappearance of essential tremor after cerebellar stroke. Mov Disord 4:183, 1989.

Colebatch JG, et al: Preliminary report: Activation of the cerebellum in essential tremor. Lancet 2:1028, 1990.

Rajput AH, et al: Clinicopathological observations in essential tremor: Report of six cases. Neurology 41:1422, 1991.

41. Is there an association between ET and PD?

According to different sources, the prevalence of ET in patients with PD ranges from 3–8.5%. There is lack of agreement as to the prevalence of PD in ET (4.5–21.8%). The relatively high frequency of familial tremor (15–23%) among patients with PD supports the existence of an etiologic link between PD and ET. Further epidemiologic and genetic studies are needed before the controversy about the relationship between PD and ET can be resolved.

Jankovic J: Essential tremor and other movement disorders. In Findley LJ, Koller W (eds): Handbook of Tremor Disorders. New York, Marcel Dekker, 1993.

42. What is the relationship between ET and dystonia?

Although tremor is frequently found in patients with dystonia, it is not always clear whether the oscillatory movement is a form of dystonia, hence a dystonic tremor, or whether it represents coexistent ET. Postural hand tremor, phenomenologically identical to ET, may precede or be the initial manifestation of dystonia. The lack of demographic and other differences between patients with ET and ET-dystonia supports the notion that ET is a single disease entity whose clinical spectrum often includes dystonia. Some investigators argue, however, that the postural tremor seen in patients with dystonia has different clinical characteristics, such as an irregularity and a broader range of frequencies, asymmetry of contractions, and the presence of associated myoclonus which distinguish this tremor from ET.

Rivest J, Marsden CD: Trunk and head tremor as isolated manifestations of dystonia. Mov Disord 5:60, 1990.

Jankovic J, et al: Cervical dystonia: Clinical findings and associated movement disorders. Neurology 41:1088, 1991.

Jedynak CP, Bonnet AM, Agid Y: Tremor and idiopathic dystonia. Mov Disord 6:230, 1991.

43. What is orthostatic tremor? How is it treated?

Orthostatic tremor (OT) is a relatively rare but frequently misdiagnosed disorder. It is more common in women, and the onset is typically in the sixth decade. It consists of a rapid (13–14 Hz) tremor of the legs triggered by standing. Postural tremor of the hands and a family history of ET are frequent features, suggesting that OT is a variant of ET. Clonazepam is the treatment of choice, and other less effective options are propranolol, primidone, and phenobarbital.

FitzGerald PM, Jankovic J: Orthostatic tremor: An association with essential tremor. Mov Disord 6:60, 1991.

44. What other tremors are variants of ET?

Besides OT, other types of tremor are considered to be variants of ET. However, some authors argue that the pharmacologic differences between these tremors and ET support the notion that they represent distinct entities. There is evidence, for example, that some isolated site-specific (head tremor) and task-specific tremors, such as primary handwriting tremor, actually represent forms of dystonic tremor. This controversy will not be settled until a biologic marker for ET and for dystonia is available.

Rosenbaum F, Jankovic J: Task-specific focal dystonia and tremor: Categorization of occupational movement disorders. Neurology 38:522, 1988.

Rivest J, Marsden CD: Trunk and head tremor as isolated manifestations of dystonia. Mov Disord 5:60, 1990.

Elble RJ, et al: Primary writing tremor: A form of focal dystonia? Mov Disord 5:118, 1990.

Variants of Essential Tremor

VARIANT	TREATMENT
Chin tremor	Propranolol, primidone
Facial tremor	Clonazepam, propranolol, primidone
Head tremor	Clonazepam, primidone, propranolol, trihexyphenidyl
Orthostatic tremor	Clonazepam, propranolol, primidone, phenobarbital
Shuddering attacks (childhood)	Propranolol
Task-specific tremor (writing)	Propranolol, primidone, trihexyphenidyl, botulinum toxin
Tongue tremor	Propranolol, primidone
Truncal tremor	Clonazepam, propranolol, primidone
Voice tremor	Propranolol, ethanol, botulinum toxin

45. What is the treatment of ET?

Propranolol is the most effective medication for ET, although other beta blockers also have an antitremor activity. Daily doses of up to 360 mg may be necessary to control tremor. Fatigability, depression, bradycardia, hypotension, weight gain, and sexual impotence are potential side effects of propranolol and, to a lesser degree, of the other beta blockers. Contraindications for their use include COPD, asthma, congestive heart failure, and insulin-dependent diabetes mellitus.

Primidone, an anticonvulsant medication, has also been shown to be effective for the treatment of ET in both open and controlled studies. This drug should be started at very low doses (25 mg QHS) to avoid the occasional, acute, idiosyncratic toxic reaction characterized by severe nausea, vomiting, sedation, confusion, and ataxia. The daily dosage may be increased to 300 mg. If the patient does not improve on this dosage, further increments are usually useless. Fewer side effects occur with the long-term use of primidone than with propranolol.

Less effective but occasionally useful medications are lorazepam, clonazepam, alprazolam, and diazepam. Alcohol, although effective in approximately two-thirds of patients with ET, is not recommended as a treatment because of the possibility of addiction, although ET does not appear to increase the risk of alcoholism.

Pilot trials have demonstrated that **botulinum toxin** injected into the affected musculature is a useful alternative in the treatment of patients with ET that is unresponsive to other measures. As a last resort in clinically intractable ET, contralateral thalamotomy is efficient and well tolerated. More recently, chronic high-frequency thalamic stimulation has been reported to completely suppress disabling ET. Unlike thalamotomy, this procedure can be performed bilaterally.

Hubble JP, et al: Essential tremor. Clin Neuropharmacol 12:453, 1989.

Banabid AL, et al: Long-term suppression of tremor by chronic stimulation of the ventral intermediate thalamic nucleus. Lancet 1:403, 1991.

Jankovic J, Schwartz K: Botulinum toxin treatment of tremors. Neurology 41:1185, 1991.

46. What are the characteristics and most common causes of kinetic tremor?

Kinetic tremors occur after lesions of the cerebellar outflow pathways. This tremor has a 3–4 Hz frequency and is typically observed on the finger-to-nose test. When caused by cerebellar lesions, titubation (anterior/posterior oscillation of the trunk and head) and postural tremor of the hands are often seen in addition to the kinetic tremor. Patients with lesions in the midbrain, involving the superior cerebellar peduncle and the nigrostriatal system, also display tremor at rest (midbrain tremor).

Multiple sclerosis, trauma, stroke, Wilson's disease, phenytoin intoxication, acute alcoholic intoxication, cerebellar parenchymatous alcoholic degeneration, and tumor are the most important causes of kinetic tremor.

The treatment of kinetic tremors remains unsatisfactory. Drugs useful in the treatment of ET, such as propranolol and primidone, are ineffective in the treatment of kinetic tremors. Isoniazid, carbamazepine, and glutethimide may control this type of tremor in some patients. Attaching weights to the wrist may be also only modestly helpful. Injections of botulinum toxin or thalamotomy may benefit some selected patients.

47. What is neuropathic tremor?

There are reports of tremor associated with several neuropathies. Approximately 40% of the patients with hereditary motor and sensory neuropathy (Charcot-Marie-Tooth disease) display action tremor. There is no relationship between tremor and severity of the neuropathy. The features of this tremor (age at onset, anatomic distribution, response to alcohol, and family history of tremor) overlap with ET, suggesting an association between the two conditions. Patients with chronic relapsing and dysgammaglobulinemic neuropathies have also been reported to display tremor. One study showed that, like ET, the tremor in patients with chronic relapsing radiculoneuropathies is associated with activation of both cerebellar hemispheres.

Brooks DJ, et al: A comparison of the abnormal patterns of cerebral activation associated with essential and neuropathic tremor. Neurology 42(Suppl 3):423, 1992.

48. What is the relationship between tremor and peripheral trauma?

The occurrence of tremor and other movement disorders, especially dystonia and myoclonus, after peripheral trauma is well established. Typically, the peripherally-induced tremors have rest and action components. Some patients develop a typical picture of parkinsonism, with rest tremor, bradykinesia, hypomimia, and response to levodopa. The physiopathology of this movement disorder is unknown. Although in only less than half of patients conventional neurophysiologic studies do show abnormalities of the peripheral nerves, it is reasonable to speculate that damage to the peripheral nervous system causes sustained changes in the central nervous system, which accounts for the movement disorders. The common association with reflex sympathetic dystrophy suggests that dysautonomia plays a role in the generation of these posttraumatic movement disorders. In about 60% of the patients there are predisposing factors such as personal and family history of ET and exposure to neuroleptics.

The treatment of this condition is difficult. Anticholinergic agents and antitremor medications, such as propranolol and primidone, are usually ineffective. Clonazepam may provide moderate relief in some patients. Some authors have successfully used injections of botulinum toxin into the affected musculature to control posttraumatic movement disorders. Thalamotomy is another consideration in patients when conservative treatment fails.

Jankovic J, Van Der Linden C: Dystonia and tremor induced by peripheral trauma: Predisposing factors. J Neurol Neurosurg Psychiatry 51:1512, 1988.

Deuschl G, et al: Tremor in reflex sympathetic dystrophy. Arch Neurol 48:1247, 1991.

DYSTONIA

49. What is torsion dystonia?

Torsion dystonia is a neurologic condition characterized by sustained contractions of both agonist and antagonist muscles, frequently causing twisting and repetitive movements or abnormal postures. As there is no biochemical, pathologic, or radiologic marker for dystonia, the diagnosis is based on the recognition of clinical features. A characteristic feature of dystonia, which helps differentiate it from other hyperkinetic movement disorders, is that dystonic movements are repetitive and patterned. For reasons that are poorly understood, patients with dystonia have the ability to suppress or decrease the involuntary movements by gently touching the affected area (sensory trick or *geste antagonistique*). Stress and fatigue make dystonia worse and sleep and relaxation improve it.

Jankovic J, Fahn S: Dystonic disorders. In Jankovic J, Tolosa E (eds): Parkinson's Disease and Movement Disorders, 2nd ed. Baltimore, Williams & Wilkins, 1993.

Classification of Dystonia

I. Etiology		
	Idiopathic	
	Familial	
	Sporadic	
	Symptomatic	
II. Age at onset		
	Childhood-onset:	0–12 years
	Adolescent onset:	13–20 years
	Adult-onset:	>20 years
III. Distribution		
	Focal:	a single body part
	Segmental:	one or more contiguous body parts
	Multifocal:	two or more noncontiguous body parts
	Generalized:	segmental crural dystonia and dystonia in at least one additional body part
	Hemidystonia:	one-half of the body

50. What features suggest the diagnosis of secondary dystonia?

Secondary forms of dystonia, which account for 25% of the cases of dystonia, are suspected when there is history of head trauma, peripheral trauma, encephalitis, toxin exposure, drug exposure, perinatal anoxia, kernicterus, and seizures. Abnormal findings such as dementia, ocular motility abnormalities, ataxia, spasticity, weakness, or amyotrophy are often present in patients with secondary dystonia. Furthermore, onset of dystonia at rest instead of with action, early onset of speech involvement, hemidystonia, and abnormal laboratory tests and brain imaging suggest the diagnosis of secondary dystonia. The list of causes of secondary dystonia is long, but it is important to try to identify those that are potentially treatable, especially Wilson's disease and tardive dystonia.

Pettigrew LC, Jankovic J: Hemidystonia: A report of 22 patients and a review of the literature. J Neurol Neurosurg Psychiatry 48:650, 1985.

Causes of Secondary Dystonia

I. Metabolic disorders	III. Miscellaneous
Aminoacid disorders	Arteriovenous malformation
Glutaric aciduria	Atlantoaxial dislocation or
Hartnup's disease	subluxation
Homocystinuria	Brain tumor
Methylmalonic acidemia	Cerebellar ectopia and syringomyelia
Tyrosinosis	Central pontine myelinolysis
Lipid disorders	Cerebrovascular or ischemic injury
Ceroid lipofuscinosis	Drugs
GM1-gangliosidosis	Anticonvulsants
GM2-gangliosidosis	Antipsychotics
Metachromatic leukodystrophy	Bromocriptine
Miscellaneous metabolic disorders	Ergot
Leber's disease	Fenfluramine
Leigh's disease	Levodopa
Lesch-Nyhan syndrome	Metoclopramide
Mitochondrial encephalopathies	Head trauma
Triosephosphate isomerase	Infection
deficiency	Acute infectious torticollis
Vitamin E deficiency	AIDS
	Creutzfeldt-Jakob disease
II. Neurodegenerative disorders	Encephalitis lethargica
Ataxia telangiectasia	Reye syndrome
Azorean heredoataxia	Subacute sclerosing
(Machado-Joseph disease)	panencephalitis
Familial basal ganglia	Syphilis
calcifications	Tuberculosis
Hallervorden-Spatz disease	Paraneoplastic brainstem encephalitis
Huntington's disease	Perinatal cerebral injury and
Infantile bilateral striatal necrosis	kernicterus
Intraneuronal inclusion disease	Peripheral trauma
Multiple sclerosis	Plagiocephaly
Neuroacanthocytosis	Psychogenic dystonia
Parkinson's disease	Toxins
Progressive pallidal degeneration	CO
Progressive supranuclear palsy	CS_2
Rett syndrome	Methane
Wilson's disease	Wasp sting

51. What are the most common types of idiopathic dystonia?

The classic idiopathic dystonia, much more common among Ashkenazi Jews, is transmitted by an autosomal dominant gene whose expression is extremely variable. Phenocopies (sporadic cases) account for at least 20% of the cases of idiopathic dystonia. At the onset, the dystonic movements occur during the performance of voluntary movements (action dystonia). Occasionally, dystonia is triggered by specific actions, such as playing a particular musical instrument or handwriting (task-specific dystonia). With progression of the disease, the movements are brought about by less specific actions of the affected body part. With further deterioration, actions in other areas activate the dystonia (for example, torticollis worsened by handwriting). The latter phenomenon is called overflow. Dystonia at rest, with abnormal postures, is usually indicative of severe forms of idiopathic dystonia. Idiopathic dystonia starting in childhood usually has a focal onset in the feet and tends to generalize (see figure on next page), whereas most focal dystonias of adults remain restricted to the part of the body initially involved. Because axial involvement is prominent in childhood-onset forms of dystonia, this diagnosis should be entertained in children and teenagers with kyphoscoliosis.

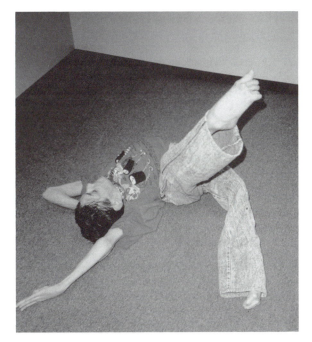

Patient with childhood-onset generalized dystonia.

Dystonia with diurnal fluctuations or dopa-responsive dystonia (Segawa variant) is responsible for less than 10% of the cases of childhood-onset dystonia. Autosomal dominant transmission is identified in about 70% of the cases. The most characteristic feature of this group of patients is significant response to small doses of levodopa.

Myoclonic dystonia is a less common form of hereditary idiopathic dystonia; it is also transmitted in an autosomal dominant fashion. Besides dystonia, these patients also exhibit shocklike, brief jerks (myoclonus), and respond dramatically to ethanol.

Paroxysmal dystonia encompasses a heterogeneous and relatively rare group of conditions. Although psychogenic dystonia accounts for some of these cases, the majority are thought to be of neurologic origin, possibly representing a form of subcortical epilepsy, arising from the basal ganglia. The organic forms, sporadic or autosomal dominant, can be categorized as either kinesiogenic or nonkinesiogenic. In the kinesiogenic variety, the attacks are precipitated by sudden movements, lasting less than 5 minutes and recurring up to 100 times a day. Anticonvulsants, such as carbamazepine and phenytoin, are usually effective in preventing the episodes. In the nonkinesiogenic paroxysmal dystonia the attacks are less frequent (3/day), last longer (minutes-hour), and are often triggered by alcohol, coffee, and fatigue. Clonazepam is partially effective in most patients. There are also secondary paroxysmal dystonias, caused by strokes, multiple sclerosis, and trauma to the peripheral and central nervous system.

Lance JW: Familial paroxysmal dystonic choreoathetosis and its differentiation from related syndromes. Ann Neurol 2:285, 1977.

Nygaard TG, et al: Dopa-responsive dystonia: Long-term treatment response and prognosis. Neurology 41:174, 1991.

52. Where is the gene for classic dystonia located?

Molecular genetic techniques link the dystonia gene to the long arm of chromosome 9 (9q32–34 region). Although there is evidence that adult-onset forms of focal dystonia are also related to the same gene, this awaits confirmation.

Ozelius L, et al: Human gene for torsion dystonia located on chromosome 9q32–34. Neuron 2:1427, 1989.

Kramer PL, et al: Dystonia gene in Ashkenazi population located on chromosome 9q32–34. Ann Neurol 27:114, 1990.

Waddy HM, et al: A genetic study of idiopathic focal dystonias. Ann Neurol 29:320, 1991.

53. What is spasmodic dysphonia (SD)?

SD is a form of focal dystonia involving the vocal cords. Laryngoscopy usually reveals adduction of the vocal cords during vocalization. It was not until the late 1970s that the concept of SD as a psychiatric condition was abandoned and the disorder became clearly recognized as a neurologic entity. Except for the voice abnormalities, these patients are usually asymptomatic. However, occasionally SD occurs in the context of craniocervical dystonia. Besides the most common adductor SD, a few patients display a breathy and whispery voice associated with abduction of the vocal cords. Unlike adductor SD, abductor SD may be intermittent and is often psychogenic. Botulinum toxin injections into the vocal cord is the treatment of choice for the adductor form of SD. Abductor SD does not improve with botulinum toxin as well as does the adductor form.

Rosenfield DB, et al: Neurologic aspects of spasmodic dysphonia. J Otolaryngol 19:231, 1990.

54. What is the most common form of focal dystonia?

The cervical region is the area most frequently affected by dystonia. Among 1,000 patients with dystonia seen at the Baylor College of Medicine Parkinson's Disease Center and Movement Disorders Clinic, 76% have cervical dystonia, alone (33% patients) or associated with involvement of other areas. It is slightly more common in women (61%). Depending on the muscle involved, different types of postures are observed.

The majority of patients with cervical dystonia have a combination of abnormal postures, such as torticollis, laterocollis, and anterocollis. Pain is a feature in about 70% of patients with neck dystonia, whereas tremor, either dystonic or essential-type, is observed in 60% of affected individuals.

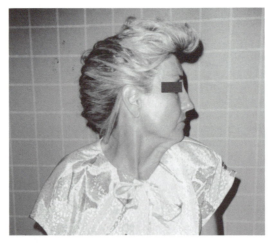

Patient with cervical dystonia manifested chiefly by torticollis to the left and marked contraction and hypertrophy of the right sternocleidomastoid muscle.

55. What are the other forms of focal dystonia?

Blepharospasm, either isolated (11%) or combined with oromandibular dystonia (23%), is the second most common form of focal dystonia. It is defined as an involuntary, bilateral eye closure produced by dystonic contractions of the orbicularis oculi muscles. Blepharospasm is three times more common in women than men. The onset is usually gradual and often, before the onset of sustained eyelid closure. Patients experience excessive blinking triggered by bright light, wind, and stress. With progression, most patients develop dystonia involving other facial muscles, as well as the masticatory and cervical musculature. Sensory tricks that help to keep the eyes open include pulling on the upper eyelids, talking, and yawning. Up to 15% of patients with blepharospasm become legally blind because of inability to keep their eyes open.

Dystonic writer's cramp is a form of task-specific dystonia associated with handwriting. Although able to use their hands when performing daily chores, after a few seconds or minutes of writing these patients develop dystonic, usually painful, spasms of the forearm musculature, which prevents them from writing further. With the progression of the disease, the dystonia becomes less task-specific, occurs during other activities, and may spread to involve more proximal muscles. Approximately 50% of patients develop similar symptoms contralaterally. Other task-specific dystonias occur among musicians (piano player's cramp, guitar player's cramp) and others whose recreational or occupational activities require fine motor coordination. The actual prevalence of these task-specific dystonias is unknown because only a few patients seek medical attention.

Jankovic J, Orman J: Blepharospasm: Demographic and clinical survey of 250 patients. Ann Ophthalmol 16:371, 1984.

Jankovic J, et al: Cervical dystonia: Clinical findings and associated movement disorders. Neurology 41:1088, 1991.

Marsden CD, Sheehy MP: Writer's cramp. Trends Neurosci 13:148, 1990.

56. What are the most effective medications for the treatment of generalized or segmental dystonias?

Levodopa, effective in about 10% of children with dystonia, should be tried in all childhood-onset dystonias. If there is no significant improvement in 2 months, levodopa is replaced by anticholinergics. The initial dose of trihexyphenidyl (Artane) is 2 mg BID. High doses, sometimes up to 100 mg a day, may be necessary. The benefits may not be appreciated for 3-4 months after initiation of therapy. Moderate to dramatic improvement is observed in up to 70% of patients, but the efficacy may decrease with chronic use. The usefulness of these medications, especially in adults, is limited by the occurrence of peripheral (dry mouth and blurred vision) and central (forgetfulness, confusion, hallucinations) side effects. Other drugs to be tried are baclofen, carbamazepine, benzodiazepines, and antidopaminergics. Extreme caution should be used when using dopamine receptor blocking drugs because of their potential to cause tardive dyskinesia.

Levodopa (in children) and anticholinergics (in adults) are the first options among the systemic drugs. Clonazepam is occasionally very effective in blepharospasm, whereas baclofen may be particularly useful in cranial dystonia. Systemic treatment of focal dystonias is disappointing, however. If oral medications are ineffective, local injections of botulinum toxin should be considered in patients with focal dystonia. Injections of botulinum toxin into the affected musculature is now considered the first choice of treatment for these forms of dystonia.

Burke RE, et al: Torsion dystonia: A double-blind prospective, trial of high-dosage trihexyphenidyl. Neurology 36:160, 1986.

Jankovic J, Orman J: Tetrabenazine treatment in dystonia, chorea, tics, and other dyskinesias. Neurology 38:391, 1988.

Jankovic J, Fahn S: Dystonic syndromes. In Jankovic J, Tolosa E (eds): Parkinson's Disease and Movement Disorders, 2nd ed. Baltimore, Williams & Wilkins, 1993.

57. What is the role of botulinum toxin in the treatment of dystonia?

Botulinum toxin, one of the most lethal biologic toxins, is produced by the bacteria *Clostridium botulinum*. It acts at the neuromuscular junction, where it binds to the presynaptic cholinergic terminal and inhibits the release of acetylcholine. This functional denervation causes weakness and atrophy. After a 3–4 month period, sprouting and regrowth of the nerve terminals occur. A small percentage of patients develop antibodies against botulinum toxin type A (the type conventionally used) after repeated injections, and the injections become ineffective. Under these circumstances it may be necessary to use another immunologic type of toxin (e.g., botulinum toxin type F) to obtain clinically effective chemodenervation.

Botulinum toxin has been found to be effective in 95% of patients with blepharospasm, 90% of patients with spasmodic dysphonia, 85% of patients with cervical dystonia, and a majority of patients with oromandibular and hand dystonia. Patients with generalized dystonia displaying prominent disability in a single region may benefit from botulinum toxin applied to the involved area. The complications of botulinum toxin treatment are limited to local weakness, with different consequences depending on the area. For example, patients with blepharospasm may have ptosis, whereas dysphagia is a potential complication of the treatment of cervical dystonia. Most complications, however, resolve spontaneously after 2–4 weeks.

58. What other conditions can be treated with botulinum toxin?

Conditions other than dystonia have also been successfully treated with botulinum toxin. Strabismus was the first disease to be treated with botulinum toxin. Ninety percent of patients with hemifacial spasm, a form of segmental myoclonus, improve with injections of the toxin. Over 50% of patients with tremor of the hand and/or head improve with botulinum toxin. There are reports describing efficacy of this treatment in patients with a variety of disorders associated with abnormal or inappropriate muscle contractions.

Jankovic J, et al: Botulinum toxin treatment of cranial-cervical dystonia, spasmodic dysphonia, other focal dystonias, and hemifacial spasm. J Neurol Neurosurg Psychiatry 53:633, 1990.

Jankovic J, Schwartz K: Botulinum toxin treatment of tremors. Neurology 41:1185, 1991.

Jankovic J, Brin M: Therapeutic uses of botulinum toxin. N Engl J Med 324:1186, 1991.

Jankovic J, Schwartz KS: Clinical correlates of response to botulinum toxin injections. Arch Neurol 48:1253, 1991.

TIC DISORDERS

59. What are tics?

Tics are relatively brief, sudden, rapid, and intermittent movements (motor tics) or sounds (vocal tics). They may be repetitive and stereotypic. Tics are usually abrupt in onset and fast ("clonic tics"), but they may be slow and sustained ("dystonic tics"). Simple tics are caused by contractions of only one group of muscles, causing a brief, jerklike movement or single, meaningless sound. Motor tics may also be complex, consisting of coordinated sequenced movements, resembling normal motor acts which are inappropriately intense and timed. Complex vocal tics include linguistically meaningful verbalizations. Tics, especially if dystonic, are associated with premonitory feelings that are relieved by performing the tics. Unlike other hyperkinetic dyskinesias, tics may be temporarily suppressed, leading some investigators to suggest that in many patients they are purposefully, albeit irresistibly, performed. (See table at top of following page.)

60. What are the most common causes of tic disorders?

Tourette's syndrome and related disorders are the most important and common causes of tics. However, these dyskinesias may occur in the context of other hereditary disorders as well as following acquired diseases. (See table at bottom of following page.)

Stone L, Jankovic J: Dystonic tics in patients with Tourette's syndrome. Mov Disord 6:248, 1991.

Jankovic J: Diagnosis and classification of tics and Tourette syndrome. In Chase T, et al (eds): Tourette syndrome. Advances in Neurology, Vol 58. New York, Raven Press, 1992, pp 7–12.

Phenomenologic Classification of Tics

I. Motor Tics

Simple tics	Complex tics
Clonic tics	Copropraxia (obscene gestures)
Blinking	Echopraxia (imitating gestures)
Head jerking	Head shaking
Nose twitching	Hitting
Dystonic tics	Jumping
Abdominal tensing	Kicking
Blepharospasm	Throwing
Bruxism	Touching
Oculogyric movements	
Shoulder rotation	
Sustained mouth opening	
Torticollis	

II. Vocal Tics

Simple tics	Complex tics
Blowing	Coprolalia (shouting of obscenities)
Coughing	Echolalia (repetition of someone
Grunting	else's phrases)
Screaming	Palilalia (repetition of one's own
Sneezing	utterances or phrases)
Squeaking	
Sucking	
Throat clearing	

Etiologic Classification of Tics

I. Physiologic tics	Secondary, Drugs *(Continued)*
Mannerisms	Levodopa
Gestures	Stimulants
	Amphetamine
II. Pathologic Tics	Cocaine
Primary	Methylphenidate
Transient tic disorder	Pemoline
Chronic tic disorder	Head trauma
Chronic motor tic disorder	Infections
Chronic phonic tic disorder	Creutzfeldt-Jakob disease
Tourette's syndrome	Encephalitis
Torsion dystonia	Postencephalitic parkinsonism
Huntington's disease	Sydenham's chorea
Neuroacanthocytosis	Mental retardation
Secondary ("Tourettism")	Autism
Chromosomal abnormalities	Pervasive developmental
Down syndrome	disorders
Fragile X syndrome	Rett's syndrome
XYY syndrome	Rubella syndrome
XXX + 9p mosaicism	Static encephalopathy
Drugs	Others
Anticonvulsants	Carbon monoxide poisoning
Dopamine receptor blocking	Schizophrenia
drugs	Stroke

61. What features are necessary to make the diagnosis of Tourette's syndrome (TS)?
According to the currently established diagnostic criteria, TS can be diagnosed only in the presence of all the following features: onset before age 21, multiple motor tics, one or more vocal tics, a fluctuating course, and presence of tics for more than 1 year. If the tics last less than 1 year, they are categorized as transient tic disorder (TTD). TTD is estimated to occur in 5 to 24% of school children; there is no accurate way to predict whether TTD will evolve into TS. Chronic motor tic disorder (CMTD) or chronic phonic tic disorder (CPTD) have the same criteria as TS, but the patients only display either motor or phonic (vocal) tics.

TS, defined by the motor manifestations, is three times more frequent in males, but when obsessive compulsive disorder is included the male preponderance becomes much less significant. The onset is around age 7 for facial tics, with gradual progression in a rostro-caudal fashion. The diagnosis is often delayed because there is a tendency to misinterpret or not recognize the tics or behavioral problems as abnormal. Behavioral problems usually precede the onset of tics by 2–3 years.

Singer HS, Walkup JT: Tourette syndrome and other tic disorders: Diagnosis, pathophysiology, and treatment. Medicine 70:15, 1991.

Jankovic J: Tourette's syndrome. In Appel SH (ed): Current Neurology, Vol. 13. Chicago, Year Book, 1993.

62. What is the clinical spectrum of tic disorders and TS?
A growing body of evidence supports the notion that these primary tic disorders represent a clinical spectrum, ranging from the mild TTD to TS. Several studies show that TTD, CMTD, CPTD, and TS are transmitted as inherited traits in the same families, suggesting that they might represent an expression of the same genetic defect. One problem with the current criteria of TS is that they do not take into account the extensive range of psychopathology and academic problems that are frequently present in this disease. For example, obsessive compulsive disorder (OCD) is encountered in at least 50% of the patients and is related to the same gene responsible for the expression of tics. Attention-deficit hyperactivity disorder (ADHD) is also quite frequent (50–60%) among TS patients, but the genetic association between the two conditions is less well understood. Other behavioral disturbances frequently observed in TS are aggressiveness, anxiety, conduct disorders, depression, learning difficulties, panic attacks, and sleep abnormalities.

63. How is TS genetically transmitted?
TS displays a sex-influenced, autosomal dominant mode of inheritance with variable expressivity as TS, CMTD, or OCD. A male offspring who inherits the TS gene has a 100% chance of expressing the gene as TS, CMTD, or OCD; a 99% chance of having either TS or CMTD; and a 45% possibility of having TS alone. A female offspring inheriting the same gene has a 71% chance of phenotypically having TS, CMTD, or OCD; a 56% chance of having either TS or CMTD; and a 17% likelihood of TS alone. Other investigators, however, suggest that the inheritance in TS is semirecessive semidominant; patients with mild to moderate forms are heterozygous, whereas more severe forms represent a homozygous state.

Price RA, et al: A twin study of Tourette syndrome. Arch Gen Psychiatry 42:815, 1985.

Pauls DL, Leckman JF: The inheritance of Gilles de la Tourette's syndrome and associated behaviors: Evidence for autosomal dominant transmission. N Engl J Med 315:993, 1986.

Comings DE, Comings BG: Alternative hypotheses on the inheritance of Tourette's syndrome. In Chase T, Friedhoff A, Cohen DJ (eds): Touretttte's Syndrome. New York, Raven Press, Adv Neurol, Vol. 58, 1992, p 189.

64. How is TS treated?
Tics require treatment when they are socially embarrassing, painful (dystonic tics quite often cause pain), and severe enough to interfere with the patient's functioning. Their management relies on the use of dopamine blockers such as fluphenazine, which is more

effective and associated with less sedation than other antidopaminergic drugs. Typically, a daily dose of 3–6 mg is sufficient to provide adequate relief. These drugs should be used cautiously because of the potential of causing tardive dyskinesia.

The behavioral problems present in TS usually cause more disabilities than tics cause. Clonidine is considered the first option in the management of ADHD. A significant number of patients have drowsiness in the beginning of the treatment. Once they are stabilized on this medication, they are switched to a clonidine patch. Deprenyl, a specific inhibitor of the enzyme monoamine oxidase type B, whose metabolites share some properties with amphetamines, was recently shown in an open study to represent an effective alternative in the treatment of ADHD, without causing tics. Clomipramine is the first option to treat OCD, but imipramine, fluoxetine, and sertraline may also be useful. Carbamazepine and lithium are also sometime used in patients with impulse control problems.

Mesulam M-M, Petersen RC: Treatment of Gilles de la Tourette's syndrome: Eight-year practice-based experience in a predominantly adult population. Neurology 37:1828, 1987.

Guidelines for the Treatment of Tourette's Syndrome

Feature '	Treatment
Tics	1. Fluphenazine 2. Pimozide 3. Haloperidol 4. Trifluoperazine 5. Molindone 6. Tetrabenazine 7. Botox
ADHD	1. Clonidine 2. Deprenyl 3. Methylphenidate 4. Dextroamphetamine
OCD	1. Clomipramine 2. Fluoxetine 3. Imipramine 4. Sertraline
Low impulse control	1. Carbamazepine 2. Lithium

ADHD = attention deficit hyperactivity disorder; OCD = obsessive conpulsive disorder.

CHOREA

65. What is Huntington's disease (HD)?

HD is clinically characterized by the presence of a triad composed of chorea, cognitive decline, and a positive family history. Chorea consists of involuntary, continuous, abrupt, rapid, brief, unsustained, irregular movements that flow randomly from one body part to another. Patients can partially and temporarily suppress the chorea and frequently incorporate them into semipurposeful activities (parakinesia). Affected patients have a peculiar, irregular gait. Besides chorea, other motor symptoms include dysarthria, dysphagia, postural instability, ataxia, myoclonus, and dystonia. The tone is decreased and the deep reflexes are often hung up and pendular.

All patients eventually develop dementia, mainly characterized by loss of recent memory and impairment of judgment, concentration, and acquisition. Neurobehavioral disturbances occasionally precede the motor symptoms and consist of personality changes, apathy, social withdrawal, agitation, impulsiveness, depression, mania, paranoia, delusions, hostility, hallucinations, and psychosis.

In virtually all cases there is a family history of a similar condition transmitted in an autosomal dominant fashion. Caudate and putamen atrophy on neuroimaging studies is another feature supportive of the diagnosis of HD.

66. What is the Westphal variant?

In 10% of cases of HD, the onset is before age 20 (Westphal variant). The disease is then characterized by the combination of progressive parkinsonism, dementia, ataxia, and seizures.

67. What are other common causes of chorea?

It is probable that **levodopa-induced chorea** in parkinsonism is the most common cause of chorea. Usually, there is no difficulty in this diagnosis once the history is available.

The combination of chorea and psychiatric symptoms can be found in **Wilson's disease**. In these patients, however, the diagnosis is easily made by finding a Kayser-Fleischer ring, low plasma ceruloplasmin, and evidence of hepatic dysfunction.

Sydenham's chorea is a form of autoimmune chorea, preceded by a group A streptococcus infection. Rarely encountered in the U.S., this condition is one of the most common causes of chorea in underdeveloped areas. **Systemic lupus erythematosus** and **primary antiphospholipid antibody syndrome** are other causes of autoimmune chorea.

Senile chorea is a condition in which chorea is the only feature and no family history of HD is present.

Neuroacanthocytosis is a rare sporadic or hereditary condition, with reported cases having autosomal recessive and dominant transmission. In addition to chorea, these patients have amyotrophy, areflexia, mutilatory oromandibular dystonia, vocal tics, and seizures. MRI of the head usually displays caudate atrophy. The findings of high plasma creatine phosphokinase, denervation on electromyography, and over 10% of acanthocytes on blood smears confirm the diagnosis.

Burnett L, Jankovic J: Chorea and ballism. Curr Opin Neurol Neurosurg 5:308, 1992.

Penney KB, et al: Huntington's disease in Venezuela: Seven years of follow-up on symptomatic and asymptomatic individuals. Mov Disord 5:93, 1990.

Hardi RJ, et al: Neuroacanthocytosis: A clinical, haematological and pathological study of 19 cases. Brain 114:13, 1991.

68. Is it possible to make a diagnosis of HD in asymptomatic individuals?

A marker for the HD gene has been identified near the tip of the short arm of chromosome 4. More recently, the gene of HD was also identified. These findings allow genetic testing of at-risk individuals before the onset of symptoms. However, until effective treatment is available for HD, many ethical and legal dilemmas associated with genetic testing remain to be solved.

Although neurobehavioral symptoms may precede motor disturbances, neuropsychologic tests do not differentiate between presymptomatic persons who are positive for the HD marker from those who are negative. Caudate atrophy correlates well with the degree of cognitive impairment in early HD, although putaminal atrophy on MRI is a more accurate predictor of the neurologic examination. Hypometabolism in the striatum as demonstrated by positron emission tomography and 18F-2-fluoro-2-deoxyglucose precedes caudate atrophy, but neither one allows presymptomatic diagnosis of HD.

Wexler NS, et al: Molecular approaches to hereditary diseases of the nervous system: Huntington's disease as a paradigm. Ann Rev Neurosci 14:503, 1991.

Harris GJ, et al: Putamen volume reduction on magnetic resonance imaging exceeds caudate changes in mild Huntington's disease. Ann Neurol 31:69, 1992.

Wiggins S, et al: The psychological consequences of predictive testing for Huntington's disease. N Engl J Med 327:1401, 1992.

Bateman D, et al: A follow-up study of isolated cases of suspected Huntington's disease. Ann Neurol 31:293–298, 1992.

The Huntington's Disease Collaborative Research Group: A novel gene containing a trinucleotide repeat that is expanded and unstable on Huntington's disease chromosomes. Cell 72:971, 1993.

69. What are the neuropathologic findings in HD?

The most important pathologic findings in HD are neuronal loss and gliosis in the cortex and the striatum, particularly the caudate nucleus. Chorea seems to be primarily related to loss of medium spiny striatal neurons projecting to the lateral pallidum. This results in functional hypoactivity of the subthalamic nucleus with consequent hyperactivity of the thalamic tier.

Albin RL, et al: Striatal and nigral neuron subpopulations in rigid Huntington's disease: Implications for the functional anatomy of chorea and rigidity-akinesia. Ann Neurol 27:357, 1990.

70. Is there any protective treatment in HD?

Unfortunately, to date there is no therapeutic intervention capable of halting the relentless progression of HD. In the adult form of HD, death occurs after a mean duration of 15 years, whereas in the juvenile variant the mean survival is 9 years.

The current treatment relies on neuroleptics, which temporarily relieve chorea and psychosis by interfering with dopaminergic transmission. However, these drugs cause several side effects, including tardive dyskinesia. An alternative approach is to use medications that deplete presynaptic dopamine, such as reserpine, which have not been reported to cause tardive dyskinesia. Benzodiazepines and antidepressants are also commonly used for anxiety and depression associated with HD.

Martin JB, Gusella JF: Huntington's disease: Pathogenesis and management. N Engl J Med 315:1267, 1986.

Shoulson I, et al: A controlled trial of baclofen as protective therapy in early Huntington's disease. Ann Neurol 25:252, 1989.

Jankovic J, Orman J: Tetrabenazine therapy of dystonia, chorea, tics and other dyskinesias. Neurology 38:391, 1988.

DRUG-INDUCED MOVEMENT DISORDERS

71. What is an acute dystonic reaction (ADR)?

ADR is an abrupt, drug-induced dystonia, especially of the head and neck. About 2.5% of patients treated with neuroleptics develop ADR within the first 48 hours of the treatment. Cocaine use will increase the likelihood of ADR. Despite being one of the first-described neuroleptic induced-movement disorders, the pathophysiology of ADR remains unknown. Because it follows the use of dopamine-receptor block drugs and it improves with anticholinergics, it is presumed that changes in the striatal dopamine and acetylcholine are important in the genesis of ADR.

72. What is the relationship of metoclopramide to drug-induced movement disorders?

Metoclopramide, a powerful dopamine receptor blocking drug, is commonly prescribed for upper GI problems, such as nausea, vomiting, ulcers, and GI reflux. It is well established that it can cause the same movement disorders as other neuroleptics. There are reports of parkinsonism, ADR, acute akathisia, and tardive dyskinesia related to metoclopramide use. One of these studies showed that there was a mean delay of 6 months between the onset of the movement disorders and the discontinuation of the drug, suggesting that the potential of metoclopramide for causing movement disorders is not fully appreciated by physicians.

Miller LG, Jankovic J: Metoclopramide-induced movement disorders. Arch Intern Med 49:2486, 1989.

73. What is tardive dyskinesia (TD)?

TD is a hyperkinetic movement disorder caused by dopamine receptor-blocking drug. According to the current established diagnostic criteria, it is possible to make the diagnosis of TD when the hyperkinesia develops during treatment with neuroleptics or within 6 months of their discontinuation, and it persists for at least 1 month after stopping all neuroleptic agents. It is estimated that 20% of the patients exposed to neuroleptics develop TD, but the values range from 13% to 49%. Severe TD seems to be more common in young males and elderly females.

Miller LG, Jankovic J: Drug-induced movement disorders: An overview. In Joseph AB, Young RR (eds): Movement Disorders in Neurology and Psychiatry. Cambridge, Blackwell Scientific, 1992, p 5.

74. What is the importance of recognizing stereotypy in an adult patient?

Stereotypy is defined as a seemingly purposeful, coordinated, but involuntary, repetitive, ritualistic gesture, mannerism, posture, or utterance. Examples of stereotypies include repetitive grimacing, lip smacking, tongue protruding, and chewing movements. The tongue may also move laterally in the mouth ("bon-bon sign"). In addition, patients with tardive dyskinesias, the most common form of adult-onset stereotypy, often exhibit head bobbing, body rocking, leg crossing and uncrossing, picking at clothing, shifting weight, and marching in place.

Stereotypy is the most common form of TD, seen in 78% of patients with TD. The second most common form of TD is dystonia, identified in 75% of the patients. The presence of stereotypies in an adult without mental retardation or untreated schizophrenia strongly suggests the diagnosis of TD, especially if associated with other movement disorders commonly present in TD (akathisia, tremor, myoclonus, chorea, and tics).

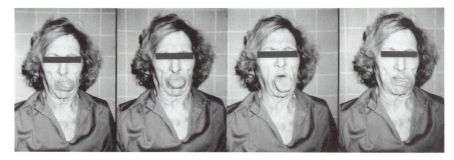

Patient with tardive dyskinesias manifesting stereotypic orolingual movements.

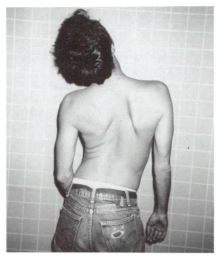

Patient with axial tardive dystonia.

75. What is the pathogenesis of TD?

Because medications that cause TD block the dopamine receptors, dysfunction of striatal dopaminergic systems has been implicated in the pathogenesis of these dyskinesias. However, the mechanism of production of TD is still not understood. Clinical and experimental evidence suggests that TD and levodopa-induced dyskinesias share a common pathogenetic mechanism. These studies suggest that TD ultimately results from disruption of the lateral pallidal-subthalamic GABAergic projection, leading to inhibition of the subthalamic nucleus. Recent evidence supports the notion that dopamine receptor-blocking drugs exert a neurotoxic effect, resulting in neuronal damage. There is, however, no explanation for the diversity of movement disorders in TD. The relatively specific pharmacologic profile of each of these dyskinesias suggests that different mechanisms are involved in their generation.

Crossman AR: A hypothesis on the pathophysiological mechanisms that underlie levodopa or dopamine agonist-induced dyskinesia in Parkinson's disease: Implications for future strategies in treatment. Mov Disord 5:100, 1990.

Miller LG, Jankovic J: Drug-induced movement disorders: An overview. In Joseph AB, Young RR (eds): Movement Disorders in Neurology and Psychiatry. Cambridge, Blackwell Scientific, 1992, p 5.

76. How is TD treated?

The first step in treatment is to stop the offending drug, which will result in spontaneous remission of the TD in approximately 60% of cases. Drugs that deplete dopamine, such as reserpine, are the most effective agents. Tardive dystonia has a less satisfactory response to systemic treatment than other forms of TD. Tardive dystonia may improve with anticholinergic agents, whereas the other types, including stereotypy, may worsen with these medications. In patients with focal forms of dystonia, such as cranial and cervical dystonia, injections of botulinum toxin into the affected musculature is a useful and safe alternative.

Jankovic J, Orman J: Tetrabenazine therapy of dystonia, chorea, tics, and other dyskinesias. Neurology 38:391, 1988.

Jankovic J, Brin MF: Therapeutic uses of botulinum toxin. N Engl J Med 324:1186, 1991.

Khott V, et al: Neuroleptics and classic tardive dyskinesia. In Lang AE, Weiner WJ (eds): Drug-induced Movement Disorders. Mt. Kisco, NY, Futura, 1992, p 121.

Burke RE: Neuroleptic-induced tardive dyskinesia variants. In Lang AE, Weiner WJ (eds): Drug Induced Movement Disorders. Mt. Kisco, NY, Futura, 1992, p 167.

OTHER MOVEMENT DISORDERS

77. How can myoclonus be distinguished from chorea and tics?

Myoclonus is defined as a brief, sudden, shocklike jerk that may be caused by active muscle contractions (positive myoclonus) or lapses of muscle contraction (negative myoclonus). Many of the individual movements of chorea are myoclonic but, unlike the movements in myoclonus, they are continuous, occurring in a constant flow. Tics may resemble myoclonus but they are usually preceded by premonitory feelings, and the patient usually has some degree of control over them.

Patel VM, Jankovic J: Myoclonus. In Appel SH (ed): Current Neurology, Vol. 8. Chicago, Year Book, 1988, p 109.

Deuschl G, et al: Symptomatic and essential rhythmic palatal myoclonus. Brain 113:1645, 1990.

Fahn S, Sjaastad O: Hereditary essential myoclonus in a large Norwegian family. Mov Disord 6:237, 1991.

78. How can myoclonus be classified?

Myoclonus can be classified by etiology, pathophysiology, and distribution.

Classification of Myoclonus*

I. Etiology
  Physiologic Myoclonus
    Anxiety
    Benign infantile myoclonus with feeding
    Exercise
    Hiccup
    Nocturnal myoclonus
  Essential Myoclonus
    Autosomal-dominant
    Sporadic
  Epileptic Myoclonus
    Benign familial myoclonic epilepsy
    Childhood myoclonic epilepsies
      Cryptogenic myoclonus epilepsy
      Infantile spasms
      Juvenile myoclonus epilepsy
      Myoclonic astatic epilepsy
    Fragments of epilepsy
      Epilepsia partialis continua
      Isolated epileptic myoclonic jerks
      Myoclonic absences in petit mal
      Photosensitive myoclonus
    Progressive myoclonus epilepsy
  Symptomatic Myoclonus
    Basal ganglia degenerations
      Cortical basal ganglionic degeneration
      Hallervorden-Spatz disease
      Huntington's disease
      Myoclonic dystonia
      Parkinson's disease
      Progressive supranuclear palsy
    Dementias
      Alzheimer's disease
      Creutzfeldt-Jakob disease
      Gerstmann-Sträussler-Schenker
        disease
    Focal lesions
      Dentato-olivary lesions
      Stroke
      Thalamotomy
      Trauma (central or peripheral
        nervous system)
      Tumor
    Metabolic and toxic encephalopathies
      Biotin deficiency
      Bismuth
      DDT
      Drugs, including levodopa
      Dyalisis syndrome
      Heavy metal poisoning
      Hepatic failure
      Hypoglycemia
      Hyponatremia

I. Etiology (Cont.)
  Symptomatic Myoclonus (Cont.)
    Metabolic and toxic encephalopathies
      (Cont.)
      Infantile myoclonic encephalopathy
      Methyl bromide
      Mitochondrial encephalopathy
      Multiple carboxylase deficiency
      Nonketotic hyperglycemia
    Physical encephalopathies
      Decompression injury
      Electric shock
      Heat stroke
      Post-hypoxia
    Spinocerebellar degeneration
    Storage disease
      Ceroid lipofuscinosis
      Lafora body disease
      Lipidoses
        GM1-gangliosidosis
        GM2-gangliosidosis
        Krabbe's disease
        Tay-Sachs disease
    Viral encephalopathies
      Arbor virus encephalitis
      Encephalitis lethargica
      Herpes simplex encephalitis
      Postinfectious encephalitis
      Subacute sclerosing
        panencephalitis

II. Distribution
  Axial
  Focal
  Generalized
  Multifocal
  Segmental

III. Pathophysiology
  Cortical
    Epilepsia partial continua
    Focal
    Generalized
    Multifocal
  Thalamic
  Brainstem
    Palatal
      Essential
      Symptomatic
    Reticular
    Startle
  Spinal
    Propriospinal
    Segmental
  Peripheral

---

* Adapted from Marsden CD: Myoclonus: Classification and treatment. Syllabus for the Movement of Disorders Course, AAN, 1992, p 93.

79. How is myoclonus treated?

Recognition of the different types of myoclonus has practical implications, because each of the categories has a unique pathophysiologic mechanism and specific treatment. Myoclonus related to metabolic encephalopathies improves with treatment of the metabolic disturbance. Epileptic myoclonus is initially treated with sodium valproate. If toxic reactions occur or the patient is still symptomatic, either clonazepam or primidone can be added. Clonazepam is the first choice in myoclonus arising from the brainstem, but 5-hydroxytryptophan, clomipramine, and fluoxetine are useful alternatives. Spinal and other segmental myoclonus may also respond to clonazepam or to drugs that enhance serotonergic transmission, but injections of botulinum toxin in the affected musculature has been the most useful treatment for this type of myoclonus.

80. What is asterixis?

Asterixis is a form of negative myoclonus mainly associated with metabolic encephalopathies and electrophysiologically characterized by the presence of brief silences of electric muscular activity. Although originally described in patients with hepatic encephalopathy, many other conditions may cause it. In the early stages of the metabolic dysfunction, this movement disorder assumes a rhythmic aspect, resembling tremor. With the progression of the underlying cause, when patients hold their arms outstretched, the wrists display a characteristic flexion (caused by electric silence in the antigravity muscles).

Causes of Asterixis

Hepatic failure	Drugs	Lesions in the CNS
Respiratory failure	Anticonvulsants	Medial frontal cortex
Renal failure	Salicylates	Parietal lobe
Cardiac failure	Levodopa	Internal capsule
Chronic hemodyalisis	Polycythemia	Thalamus
		Rostral midbrain

81. What is the stiff-person syndrome (SPS)?

Patients with this rare disorder have progressive, usually symmetric, rigidity of the axial muscles that may fluctuate in intensity. Motion, tactile stimulation, emotion, and startle are common triggering factors of the spasms. EMG shows continuous normal motor unit potentials in the affected muscles despite the patient's attempts to relax. The diagnosis is supported by relief of the rigidity with general and spinal anesthesia, peripheral nerve blocks, and diazepam, which is still the first-line treatment of SPS.

An insight into the pathophysiology of this condition was provided by the finding that, in a series of 33 patients with SPS, 20 had autoantibodies against glutamic acid decarboxylase (GAD). The hypothesis of an autoimmune etiology of SPS is further supported by the presence of other autoantibodies (to islet cells and gastric parietal cells, for example), coexistent autoimmune diseases such as insulin-dependent diabetes mellitus, vitiligo, thyroid disease, family history of presumed autoimmune conditions, and improvement with plasmapheresis and corticosteroid drugs.

Blum P, Jankovic J: Stiff-person syndrome: An autoimmune disease. Mov Disord 6:12, 1990.

82. What is Wilson's disease?

Wilson's disease is an autosomal recessive disease whose gene is linked to markers located in the q14–21 region on chromosome 13. The prevalence of the disease is estimated to be 1 in 30,000. There is impaired incorporation of copper into ceruloplasmin, as well as impaired biliary excretion of copper, resulting in copper-overloading in the liver, cornea, and brain, particularly in the basal ganglia. Virtually all patients display laboratory and/or clinical evidence of liver insufficiency. The most useful laboratory screening test is plasma ceruloplasmin, usually less than 20 mg/dl (normal: 24–45).

The most common neurologic findings are parkinsonism, bulbar signs such as dysarthria and dysphagia, dystonia, postural tremor, and ataxia. Psychiatric symptoms, such as depression and psychosis, are particularly common among adults.

MRI of the head may display either decreased or increased signal intensity in the striatum on T2-weighted images. MRI of the midbrain may show a specific "face of a giant panda" appearance, which is produced by reversal of the normal hypodensity of the substantia nigra, midbrain tegmentum, and hypointensity in the superior colliculi.

83. What is the treatment for Wilson's disease?

Early diagnosis is essential, because treatment with copper-chelating agents often completely reverses the neurologic and hepatic symptoms. All siblings and cousins should be screened because presymptomatic patients require treatment to prevent the development of symptoms. Penicillamine is the drug of choice for Wilson's disease and the typical dose is 250 mg QID in combination with pyridoxine (25 mg/day). Side effects are initial exacerbation of the symptoms, rash, optic neuritis, thrombocytopenia, leukopenia, and nephrotoxicity. Other options to dcrease copper overload are triethylene tetramine dihydrochloride, zinc sulphate, and tetrathiomolybdate. Symptomatic treatment of neurologic symptoms includes levodopa, anticholinergics, and injections of botulinum toxin. Liver transplant may be necessary in terminal cases of hepatic insufficiency.

Stremmel W, et al: Wilson disease: Clinical presentation, treatment, and survival. Ann Intern Med 115:720, 1991.

Brewer GJ, Yuzbasiyan-Gurkan V: Wilson disease. Medicine 71:139, 1992.

Walshe JM, Yealland M: Wilson's disease: The problem of delayed diagnosis. J Neurol Neurosurg Psychiatry 55:692, 1992.

84. Are there paraneoplastic movement disorders?

Opsoclonus-myoclonus designates a combination of rapid, erratic, involuntary movements of the eyes, with multifocal myoclonus (dancing eyes-dancing feet syndrome). The majority of the cases occur between ages 6 and 18 months. Fifty percent of the cases of opsoclonus-myoclonus are related to an underlying neoplasm, especially neuroblastoma. This syndrome also occurs in adults with brainstem encephalitis, either paraneoplastic or infectious (Whipple's disease). Steroids dramatically improve this form of myoclonus.

Ataxia is another well-established paraneoplastic movement disorder. The mechanism is cerebellar degeneration related to anti-Purkinje cell antibodies. There are also reports of parkinsonism, chorea, dystonia, segmental rigidity, and action and segmental myoclonus occurring as remote effect of neoplasm.

Albin RL, et al: Chorea and dystonia: A remote effect of carcinoma. Mov Disord 2:162, 1988.

Pranzatelli MR: The neurobiology of the opsoclonus-myoclonus syndrome. Clin Neuropharmacol 15:186, 1992.

BIBLIOGRAPHY

1. Jankovic J: The extrapyramidal disorders. In Wyngaarden JB, Smith LH, Bennett JC (eds): Cecil Textbook of Medicine, 19th ed. Philadelphia, W.B. Saunders, 1992, p 2128.
2. Jankovic J, Tolosa E (eds): Parkinson's Disease and Movement Disorders, 2nd ed. Baltimore, Williams & Wilkins, 1993.
3. Johnston MV, MacDonald RL, Young AB (eds): Principles of Drug Therapy in Neurology. Philadelphia, F.A. Davis, 1992.
4. Marsden CD, Fahn S (eds): Movement Disorders 3. London, Butterworths, 1993.

11. AUTONOMIC NERVOUS SYSTEM

Yadollah Harati, M.D., FACP

1. What are the physiologic responses to stimulation of the sympathetic and parasympathetic systems?

Sympathetic Stimulation
Tachycardia
Hypertension
Bronchodilation
Mydriasis
Vasoconstriction
Decreased peristalsis
Piloerection
Sphincter constriction
Ejaculation

Parasympathetic Stimulation
Bradycardia
Hypotension
Bronchoconstriction
Miosis
Vasodilation
Increased peristalsis
Exocrine gland secretion
Bladder contraction
Penile erection

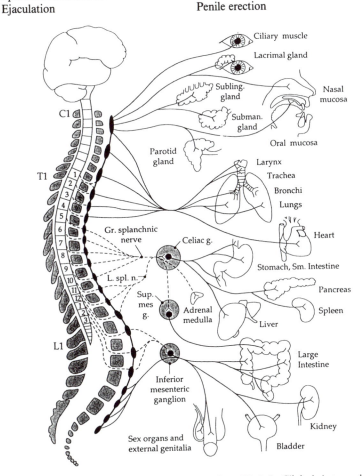

Diagram of the sympathetic nervous system. (From Low PA (ed): Clinical Autonomic Disorders. Boston, Little, Brown and Co., 1992, with permission.)

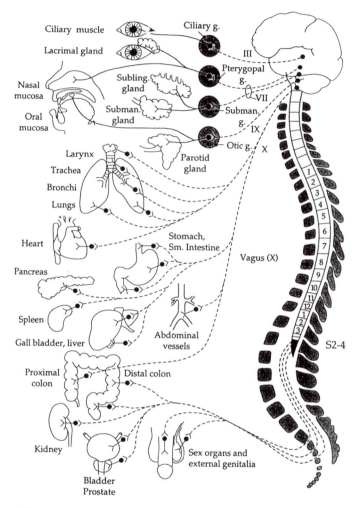

Diagram of the parasympathetic nervous system. (From Low PA (ed): Clinical Autonomic Disorders. Boston, Little, Brown and Co., 1992, with permission.)

2. What features of the history must always be asked in a patient with suspected autonomic dysfunction?

Special attention to symptoms involving the following systems is essential when obtaining a history:

1. **Cardiovascular**—Orthostatic lightheadedness, dizziness, blurred vision, syncope or near-syncope, fatigue, headache and neck ache after prolonged standing, postprandial-postexercise lightheadedness, fainting following alcohol ingestion or insulin injection, palpitations, resting tachycardia, orthostatic cerebral transient ischemic attack symptoms, angina pectoris.

2. **Sudomotor and vasomotor**—Partial or complete loss of sweating, heat intolerance (hot, flush, dizzy, and weak without sweating), excessive sweating (partial or total), facial and upper trunk gustatory sweating (especially when food incites salivation, or with ingestion of cheese), nocturnal sweating, skin cracks on distal extremity, dry and shiny skin, unusually cold or warm feet, and peripheral edema.

3. **Secretomotor**—Dry mouth and eyes.

4. **Genitourinary**—History of urinary tract infections, lengthened interval between micturition, increased volume of first-morning void, need for straining to initiate and maintain voiding, weakness of stream, postvoid dribbling, sensation of incomplete emptying and overflow incontinence, frequency and urgency with or without dysuria (with superimposed infection), impotence (difficulty in initiating and/or maintaining erection), reduced nocturnal tumescence and waking erection, diminished libido, retrograde ejaculation, decreased volume of ejaculation, reduced vaginal lubrication.

5. **Respiratory**—Irregular breathing or apnea during sleep.

6. **Gastrointestinal**—Dysphagia, retrosternal discomfort, heartburn, anorexia, epigastric fullness during or following meals, recurrent episodes of nausea and vomiting (fasting and/ or postprandial) associated with upper abdominal pain, constipation, diarrhea (especially nocturnal), or fecal incontinence (especially at night).

7. **Ocular**—Blurring of vision, photophobia, asymmetric pupils, drooping of eyelids.

3. What physical examination must always be performed in patients with suspected autonomic dysfunction?

Particular attention should be given to acral vasomotor and trophic changes of the skin; pupillary shape, size, and response to light and accommodation; and the heart rate at rest and in response to deep breathing and Valsalva maneuver. Supine blood pressure and heart rate after 5–10 minutes of rest followed by measurement after active standing for 2 minutes should be checked in every patient with suspected dysautonomia. If orthostatic hypotension (systolic and diastolic drop >30 mmHg, or mean arterial BP drop >20 mmHg) is not noted in a patient who nevertheless has symptoms of orthostatic hypotension, the patient should be asked to do 12 squats (orthostatic stress test), after which the standing BP repeated. Another orthostatic stress test is performed by repeating the BP measurement after the patient takes one sublingual nitroglycerin tablet.

4. What are the major anatomic differences between the sympathetic and parasympathetic nervous systems?

Because of the close proximity of sympathetic ganglia to the primary efferent sympathetic neurons (IML, IMM), the sympathetic preganglionic fibers are short: the postganglionic fibers may extend a long way to their target organs. The parasympathetic preganglionic neurons, on the other hand, are relatively long myelinated fibers that synapse with postganglionic neurons in the many small ganglia located near or within the wall of individual innervated organs. The postganglionic parasympathetic fibers are therefore short (1 mm to several cm).

The ratio of preganglionic to postganglionic neurons is usually much smaller in the parasympathetic nervous system, where it is 1:15 to 1:20. The large number of postganglionic neurons in the sympathetic system explains the wide range of sympathetic autonomic effects and the massive sympathetic outflow that occurs during strenuous and stressful situations. Many simultaneous diverse responses may occur as a result of sympathetic activation, including raised arterial blood pressure, increased blood flow to active muscles, increased muscle glycolysis and blood glucose level, enhanced mental activity and muscular strength, increased sphincter contraction and decreased gastrointestinal peristalsis. A disorder that predominately affects the sympathetic nervous system may therefore render the body incapable of dealing appropriately with strenuous physical or emotional stimulation. In contrast, the small proportion between the number of preganglionic and postganglionic neurons in the parasympathetic system promotes a more localized response, and allows for a very specific, controlled function of the parasympathetic system.

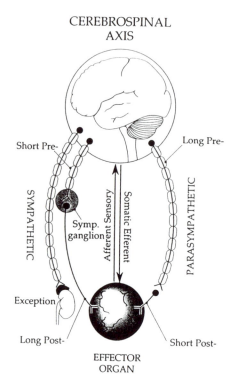

CEREBROSPINAL
AXIS

Schematic diagram comparing the sympathetic and parasympathetic nervous systems. (From Low PA (ed): Clinical Autonomic Disorders. Boston, Little, Brown and Co., 1992, with permission.)

5. What are the receptors in the autonomic nervous system?

The sympathetic effects are determined by two types of adrenergic receptors, alpha and beta, and their subtypes. The parasympathetic effects are mediated by several muscarinic (M_1, M_2, and M_3 and possibly more) and nicotinic receptors.

6. How useful is the measurement of plasma catecholamines in the evaluation of dysautonomia?

Measurement of plasma norepinephrine is a useful, though crude, index of postganglionic sympathetic activity. The origin of plasma norepinephrine is primarily a spillover from postganglionic sympathetic junctional clefts. The measured norepinephrine, however, is a small portion of the released sympathetic nerve terminal norepinephrine that has escaped the enzymatic catabolism or re-uptake and diffuses out of the junctional cleft into the bloodstream. The plasma level is determined by various processes that affect release, re-uptake, or metabolism and removal from the plasma, including emotion, exercise, eating, smoking, caffeine, time of day, blood volume, hypoglycemia, etc. Because norepinephrine is relatively unstable in plasma, care must be taken during sample collection, storage, and processing. The accuracy of plasma norepinephrine levels, therefore, greatly depends on rigorous attention to numerous factors capable of influencing plasma catecholamine levels.

7. What is the normal catecholamine response?

In normal subjects, the plasma level of norepinephrine after 30 minutes in the supine position is 150 to 170 pg/ml and increases 50–100% above supine values after 5 minutes of standing, and remains constant after 10 minutes of standing.

8. How does age affect catecholamine measurements?

Because plasma norepinephrine increases with age, the value must be corrected for age. The mechanism for increase with age is controversial; both reduced clearance and increased release have been suggested. Using microneurographic recordings, there is an increase in muscle sympathetic activity with age, supporting the hypothesis of increased norepinephrine release.

9. Can catecholamine measurements localize the site of autonomic dysfunction?

Patients with a neuropathy causing a primarily postganglionic autonomic abnormality have subnormal plasma norepinephrine in the supine position that fails to increase normally during standing. Because there is considerable overlap between preganglionic and postganglionic abnormalities in individual patients with autonomic dysfunction, however, plasma norepinephrine values alone are usually not sufficiently diagnostic for the site of the lesion.

10. What is the role of the nucleus tractus solitarius (NTS) in the central autonomic network?

This important nucleus, situated at the dorsomedial medulla, receives inputs from neocortical regions, and from nuclei of the forebrain, higher brainstem, and diencephalon. The autonomic afferents, which convey information important to the control of cardiac rhythm and motility, peripheral vascular tone, respiration, and gastrointestinal motility and secretion, all terminate at this nucleus. Axons that originate from the NTS end on the neurons of the reticular formation of the ventrolateral medulla, which in turn project to the intermediolateral (IML) cell column of the lateral horn of the spinal cord. The descending projecting fibers to the IML are diffusely dispersed in the spinal cord. Attempts to identify a group of degenerating fibers in the spinal cord following lesions of the brainstem or hypothalamus have generally been unsuccessful. NTS neurons also send efferent fibers to higher brainstem, hypothalamic and limbic structures, the vagus nerves, and neuronal groups of the spinal cord subserving respiration. In addition to autonomic afferent and efferent fibers, the NTS also receives somatic afferents from the spinal cord (dorsolateral horn) and spinal trigeminal lemniscus. This allows the NTS to serve as an integration station for the autonomic and somatic information, playing a vital role in the maintenance of body homeostasis.

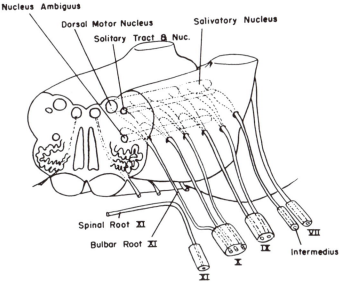

Diagram showing the location of the nucleus tractus solitarius. (From Gilman S (ed): Manter and Gatz's Clinical Neuroanatomy and Physiology, 8th ed. Philadelphia, F.A. Davis, 1991, with permission.)

11. What are the characteristics of the intermediolateral (IML) and intermediomedial (IMM) columns of the spinal cord?

The neurons of the IML and IMM are located in the spinal lateral gray column of the thoracic and upper lumbar regions of the spinal cord. They form the **primary efferent sympathetic neurons** or preganglionic neurons. Their axons, which precede the autonomic ganglia (hence preganglionic fibers), project onto a postganglionic neuron (**secondary efferent sympathetic neurons**) with its cell body in one of the paravertebral sympathetic trunk ganglia or related ganglia. The preganglionic fibers are finely myelinated, contributing to the whitish appearance of the white rami and ventral spinal roots through which they reach the ganglionic neurons. The number of neurons of the human IML and IMM and their axons diminish with age at a rate of 8% per decade. The main neurotransmitter of these neurons is acetylcholine, but they also contain several important neuropeptides.

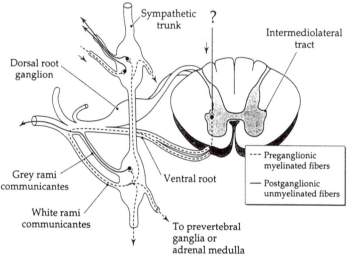

Diagram of the efferent sympathetic connections from the spinal cord, including the intermediolateral columns. (From Low PA (ed): Clinical Autonomic Disorders. Boston, Little, Brown, and Co., 1992, with permission.)

12. What are the most important peripheral neuropathies associated with autonomic dysfunction?

Peripheral Neuropathies Associated with Autonomic Dysfunction

Inherited Peripheral Neuropathies with Dysautonomia
- Hereditary sensory and autonomic neuropathy (HSAN) I, II, III* (Riley-Day syndrome), IV, and V
- Hereditary motor-sensory neuropathies (HMSN) I and II
- Multiple endocrine neoplasia, type 2b (MEN 2b)
- Fabry's disease*
- Amyloidosis* (familial amyloid polyneuropathy types I, II and III)
- Porphyria*

Infectious, Parainfectious, and Immune-mediated Peripheral Neuropathies with Dysautonomia
- Leprosy
- AIDS
- Chagas' disease*
- Systemic lupus erythematosus
- Systemic sclerosis
- Sjogren syndrome
- Rheumatoid arthritis
- Mixed-connective tissue disease
- Guillain-Barré syndrome*
- Chronic inflammatory neuropathy
- Acute pandysautonomia*
- Pure cholinergic dysautonomia*

Table continued on next page

Peripheral Neuropathies Associated with Autonomic Dysfunction (Continued)

Autonomic Neuropathies Associated with Systemic Metabolic Diseases

- Diabetes*
- Chronic renal failure
- Alcoholism
- Non-alcoholic liver disease
- Vitamin B12 deficiency
- Paraneoplastic syndrome
- Primary amyloidosis*

Autonomic Neuropathies Associated with Industrial Agents, Metals, Toxins, and Drugs

- Organic solvents
- Organophosphates
- Vacor
- Heavy metals
- Vincristine*
- Cis-platinum

* Autonomic dysfunction is prominent and clinically important.
From Appel SH (ed): Current Neurology, Vol. 10. Chicago, Year Book, 1990, p 153, with permission.

13. What are the salient manifestations of diabetic autonomic neuropathies?

Manifestations of Diabetic Autonomic Neuropathies

Cardiovascular
  Postural hypotension
  Resting tachycardia
  Painless myocardial infarction
  Sudden death
Gastrointestinal
  Esophageal motor incoordination
  Gastric dysrhythmia, hypomotility
    (gastroparesis diabeticorum)
  Pylorospasm
  Uncoordinated intestinal motility
    ("diabetic diarrhea," spasm)
  Intestinal hypomotility
    (constipation)
  Gallbladder hypocontraction
    (diabetic cholecystopathy)
  Anorectal dysfunction (fecal
    incontinence)
Genitourinary
  Diabetic cystopathy (atonic bladder,
    postmicturition dribbling)
  Male impotence
  Ejaculatory disorders
  Reduced vaginal lubrication,
    dyspareunia

Respiratory
  Impaired breathing control (?)
  Sleep apnea (?)
Thermoregulatory
  Sudomotor (diminished, excessive, or
    gustatory sweating)
  Vasomotor (vasoconstriction, vasodilation,
    neuropathic edema)
Pupillary abnormalities
  Miosis
  Disturbance of dilatation
  "Argyll-Robertson"-like pupils
Neuroendocrine abnormalities
  Reduced pancreatic polypeptide release
  Reduced somatostatin release
  Reduced motilin and gastric inhibitory
    peptide release
  Enhanced gastrin release
  Reduced norepinephrine release (orthostatic,
    exercise, and hypoglycemia induced)
  Reduced parathyroid hormone secretion
    (hypocalcemic induced)
  Elevated atrial natriuretic hormone
  Impaired glucose counterregulation
    (hypoglycemia unawareness)

From Appel SH (ed): Current Neurology, Vol. 10., Chicago, Year Book, 1990, p 153, with permission.

14. How is measurement of catecholamines useful in diabetic autonomic neuropathy?

Measurement of norepinephrine in response to hypoglycemia and exercise has been used in the study of autonomic dysfunction in diabetic neuropathy. Normally, hypoglycemia increases the level of norepinephrine and epinephrine in plasma, but this response is prevented or blunted in diabetics with sympathetic neuropathy and may be responsible for the absence of early symptoms of hypoglycemia (e.g., sweating) in these patients. Plasma norepinephrine during exercise is lower in patients with diabetic autonomic neuropathy than in healthy subjects, or in diabetics without autonomic neuropathy.

15. What is the autonomic dysfunction seen in Guillain-Barré syndrome (GBS)?

About 65% of patients with GBS have some dysautonomia. The incidence is higher when there is more sensory involvement or when axonal damage is extensive. Dysautonomias are important causes of complications, and death due to cardiovascular collapse in the setting of autonomic dysfunction occurs in approximately 3–14% of patients. Afferent baroreflex abnormalities may cause intermittent hypertension associated with orthostatic hypotension. Abrupt fluctuations of blood pressure may precede fatal arrhythmias. Urine and plasma levels of catecholamines and vanillylmandelic acid may be elevated, and fluctuations in blood pressure may correlate with the rise and fall of circulating atrial natriuretic factor in some, but not all, patients.

16. What is the appropriate management for the blood pressure fluctuations seen in GBS?
Blood pressure fluctuations in GBS are best monitored in a medical ICU setting. The ICU staff should be alerted for potential severe and fluctuating episodes of hypotension, hypertension, bradycardia, and tachycardia. Adequate administration of isotonic intravenous fluids should be started, a bladder catheter should be placed, fluid intake and output should be carefully monitored, and blood pressure should be measured frequently. Most importantly, continuous EKG monitoring is mandatory. Additionally, other coexisting causes of cardiovascular instability should be assessed with arterial blood gases, serum electrolyte and glucose measurements, urine osmolality and electrolyte concentration, and evaluation for infection.

Treatment of the autonomic hypotension is aimed at improving venous return to the heart, minimizing vagal reflex slowing of the heart rate, and lessening orthostatic positional changes. Venous return is optimized by the use of isotonic replacement fluids, at times with the aid of Swan-Ganz monitoring of pulmonary capillary wedge pressure, and by mechanical measures to reduce venous distention and edema in the lower extremities (leg warps, elastic stockings, etc.) Vagal stimulation is minimized by reducing positive pressure during artificial ventilation, avoiding sudden postural changes, reducing tracheal stimulation during suctioning, and hyperoxygenating prior to suctioning. If hypotension does not respond to these measures, pressor drugs may be necessary. These must be used with **extreme caution**, as hypersensitivity responses are common. The use of short-acting agents such as dopamine or phenylephrine is recommended. There is often a delay of several minutes in blood pressure response to pressor drugs. For prolonged hypertensive episodes, it is best to use short-acting agents that can be titrated to the blood pressure response. Again, hypersensitivity with resultant hypotension is a potential complication. There may be an exaggerated hypotensive response to even small doses of intravenous drugs (e.g., morphine, furosemide, nitroglycerin, edrophonium chloride, and thiopental).

17. How long do the blood pressure fluctuations persist in GBS?
In most patients, orthostatic hypotension resolves by the time the patient is able to walk. It is important to monitor blood pressure when ambulation or sitting is attempted.

18. What is the appropriate management for the arrhythmias seen in GBS?
Bradycardia of non-sinus origin is probably best treated with a transvenous pacemaker. Sinus tachycardia due to vagal damage occurs in about 50% of patients and usually responds to fluid replacement therapy. Its occurrence in a patient **without infection or circulatory cause** indicates vagal denervation. Absence of beat-to-beat (R-R) variation of heart rate during normal and deep breathing in a patient with early GBS is an important and reliable index of impending cardiovascular dysautonomia due to vagal nerve dysfunction. Acute atrial fibrillation and ventricular tachycardia are best managed by ICU experts, but if beta blockers are used, they must have a rapid onset and offset of action.

19. What is the appropriate management for the other dysautonomias seen in GBS?
Adynamic ileus and atonic bladder may occur. Adynamic ileus requires upper GI tract decompression via a nasogastric tube, and maintenance of NPO status. Urinary retention is treated with an indwelling catheter while the patient is on IV fluids; if present in the rehabilitation phase of GBS, it is treated with sterile intermittent catheterization.

20. What are the clinical features of acute pandysautonomia?
The heterogeneous and usually monophasic and self-limiting syndrome of acute pandysautonomia (acute autonomic neuropathy, acute panautonomic neuropathy) is rare. Pandysautonomia refers to concomitant involvement of both sympathetic and parasympathetic components of the autonomic nervous system, with relative or complete sparing of the somatic nerve fibers. The typical patient has orthostatic hypotension, anhidrosis, cold or heat intolerance, reduced lacrimation and salivation, disturbances of bowel (ileus and abdominal colic, diarrhea, and constipation) and bladder (atony), impotence, and a fixed heart rate. Symptoms evolve over a few days to a few months. Individuals of all ages and of both sexes may be affected, and there is usually no family history. There are usually minimal or no motor, sensory, or coordination abnormalities, but tendon reflexes may be diminished or absent. Occasionally loss of sensation and sensory nerve action potentials, myelopathy, or abnormal electroencephalograms are reported. Cerebrospinal fluid (CSF) protein may be modestly elevated. Recovery is usually prolonged and partial. The syndrome may be indistinguishable from paraneoplastic autonomic neuropathy. No convincingly effective treatment for this condition exists other than supportive therapy for orthostatic hypotension and bowel and bladder symptoms. Because of the possible role of the immune system in the pathogenesis of this syndrome, there may be an indication for corticosteroids, plasma exchange, or high-dose intravenous immunoglobulins in its treatment.

21. What are the pathologic features of acute pandysautonomia?
Sural nerve biopsies demonstrate variable pathologic features, depending on the time during the course of the disease when the specimens were obtained. During the early symptomatic phase of the disease, no abnormalities are found, but reduced numbers of small myelinated and unmyelinated fibers are seen in specimens obtained 6 weeks after the onset of symptoms.

22. What is the cause of acute pandysautonomia?
The pathogenesis of this syndrome is uncertain, although acute and selective immunologic damage to the peripheral autonomic nerves, similar to GBS, has been strongly suggested. Whether this condition is a variant of GBS is controversial. The disease may follow a recognized infection such as rubella, infectious mononucleosis, herpes simplex, or other febrile illnesses. It may also be associated with lung cancer, Hodgkin's disease, or testicular malignancy.

An experimentally induced neuropathy in rabbits sensitized to extracted antigen from human sympathetic nerve and ganglia shows a limited abnormality of vasomotor function occurring 6-8 days after injections. Degeneration of unmyelinated axons in the paravertebral sympathetic chain and serum antibody to the sympathetic antigens are also demonstrated. These findings and the reported association of the syndrome with malignancies and viral infections, its clinical course, and documented recovery are all in keeping with an immunologically mediated process.

Low PA (ed): Clinical Autonomic Disorders. Boston, Little, Brown and Co., 1992, pp 397–401.
Appel SH (ed): Current Neurology, Vol. 10. Chicago, Year Book, 1990, pp 149–150.

23. What are the autonomic abnormalities seen in Sjögren's syndrome?
This autoimmune exocrinopathy, affecting women nine times as frequently as men, is estimated to be second in frequency only to rheumatoid arthritis among collagen vascular diseases. In addition to the clinical presentation, the determination of highly specific autoantibodies Ro and La, directed against small-molecular-weight ribonuclear proteins, aids in the diagnosis of Sjögren's syndrome. All forms of peripheral neuropathy (sensory neuropathy, sensorimotor neuropathy, multiple mononeuropathies, sensory neuronopathy, cranial neuropathy, and entrapment syndromes) may be seen in association with Sjögren's syndrome. Autonomic dysfunction, including Adie's pupil, anhidrosis, orthostatic hypotension, and impaired cardiac parasympathetic function, may be superimposed on a generalized

neuropathy in about 25% of patients. In most patients, sural nerve biopsy shows axonal degeneration, periarteriolar and perivenular inflammatory cell infiltration, and necrotizing vasculitis. Autonomic neuropathy may also be a prominent feature of other autoimmune diseases or mixed connective tissue diseases.

24. Name the four most common paraneoplastic autonomic syndromes.
Lambert-Eaton myasthenic syndrome (LEMS), autonomic neuropathy, intestinal pseudo-obstruction, and subacute sensory neuropathy.

25. What is Lambert-Eaton myasthenic syndrome (LEMS)?
At least half the cases of LEMS occur in patients with a small-cell lung cancer. Antibodies to neuronal voltage-gated calcium channels cross-reacting with antibodies raised against tumor-restricted epitopes are responsible for this syndrome. It is frequently associated with dry mouth (74%), impotence (41%), constipation (18%), blurred vision (8%), and impaired sweating (4%). Some patients may also have orthostatic light-headedness, difficulty with micturition, or tonic pupils. About 57% of patients demonstrate cholinergic and adrenergic supersensitivity of pupils when tested with 2.5% methacholine and 0.5% phenylephrine. Tear production is also reduced. Variations in heart rate and blood pressure may occur with Valsalva maneuver or deep breathing, and sweat tests may also be abnormal.

O'Neil JH, Murray NM, Davis-Newsom J: The Lambert-Eaton myasthenic syndrome: A review of 50 cases. Brain 111:577, 1988.

Clark CV, Davis-Newsom J, Sanderson MD: Ocular autonomic nerve function in Lambert-Eaton myasthenic syndrome. Eye 4:473, 1990.

Khurana RK, Koski, Mayer RF: Autonomic dysfunction in Lambert-Eaton myasthenic syndrome. J Neurol Sci 85:77, 1988.

26. What is the treatment for LEMS?
Treatment of the tumor results in substantial improvement of autonomic dysfunction. In patients who do not have an underlying malignancy, the treatment is directed toward the enhancement of cholinergic function and immunosuppression. Antiacetylcholinesterase agents, guanidine hydrochloride, 4-aminopyridine, and 3-4 diaminopyridine are used to enhance neuromuscular transmission and improve autonomic dysfunction. Of these, 3-4 diaminopyridine is most effective and causes the fewest side effects. It increases the quantal release of acetylcholine by blocking voltage-dependent potassium conductance, prolonging the nerve terminal depolarization, and enhancing voltage-gated calcium influx. Guanidine inhibits the binding and uptake of calcium into mitochondria, thereby increasing the free intracellular calcium level and facilitating acetyl choline release; however, this drug has a number of hematologic (neutropenia, aplastic anemia) and CNS side effects that limit its use. Pyridostigmine and prostigmine provide limited symptomatic relief. Immunosuppression with corticosteroids or plasma exchange may prove beneficial in patients with either the non-neoplastic or neoplastic forms of LEMS. Drugs that adversely affect neuromuscular transmission, particularly those with calcium-channel-blocking properties, should be avoided in patients with this syndrome.

McEvoy KM, Windebank AJ, Daube JR, Low PA: 3, 4-Diaminopyridine in the treatment of Lambert-Eaton myasthenic syndrome. N Engl J Med 321:1567, 1989.

27. What is paraneoplastic autonomic neuropathy?
Some patients with small-cell lung cancer, pancreatic adenocarcinoma, or Hodgkin's disease may develop autonomic symptoms (orthostatic dizziness, impotence, dry mouth, urinary retention, or GI symptoms) that may improve with treatment of the tumor. Patients with autonomic neuropathy may have antineuronal (anti-Hu) autoantibodies. The presentation of autonomic neuropathy may precede or follow the diagnosis of malignancy.

Anderson NE, Rosenblum MK, Graus F, et al: Autoantibodies in paraneoplastic syndromes associated with small-cell lung cancer. Neurology 38:1391, 1988.

28. What is paraneoplastic intestinal pseudo-obstruction?

Pseudo-obstruction of the bowel, with or without other symptoms of autonomic dysfunction, may be seen in association with small-cell lung cancer, pulmonary carcinoid, and undifferentiated epithelioma. These patients may also have gastroparesis and esophageal peristaltic abnormalities. They may subsequently develop other dysautonomic symptoms. The motility disorder may resolve with the treatment of the underlying tumor. The salient GI pathologic features include loss of myenteric plexus neurons, fragmentation and degeneration of axons, and plasma cell and lymphocytic infiltration. Serum IgG antibodies reactive with neurons of the gastric and jejunal myenteric and submucosal plexus have been demonstrated in patients with small-cell lung cancer.

Lennon VA, Sas DF, Busk MF, et al: Enteric neuronal autoantibodies in pseudo-obstruction with small-cell lung carcinoma. Gastroenterology 100:1, 137, 1991.

Sodhi N, Camilleri M, Camoriano JK, et al: Autonomic function and motility in intestinal pseudoobstruction caused by paraneoplastic syndrome. Dig Dis Sci 34:1937, 1989.

29. What is paraneoplastic subacute sensory neuropathy?

Some patients with this syndrome, which usually occurs in association with small-cell lung cancer, may have one or several of the following autonomic dysfunctions: orthostatic hypotension, tonic pupils, hypohidrosis, dry mouth, diminished lacrimation, impotence, urinary retention, and constipation. Serum and CSF of patients with this syndrome frequently contain antineuronal nuclear (anti-HU) antibody, a polyclonal, complement-fixing IgG which also reacts against a 35–40 kda protein of small cell lung cancer cells. The neuronal nuclear antigen has the same molecular weight but lacks the 38 kda band. Treatment of the underlying tumor may result in the partial alleviation of autonomic and somatic symptoms.

Kimmel DW, O'Neil BP, Lennon VA: Subacute sensory neuronopathy associated with small-cell lung carcinoma: Diagnosis aided by autoimmune serology. Mayo Clin Proc 63:29, 1988.

Anderson NE, Rosenblum MK, Graus F, et al: Autoantibodies in paraneoplastic syndromes associated with small-cell lung cancer. Neurology 38:1391, 1988.

Fagius J, Westerberg CE, Olsson Y: Acute pandysautonomia and severe sensory deficit with poor recovery: A clinical neurophysiological and pathological case study. J Neurol Neurosurg Psychiatry 46:725, 1983.

Anderson NE, Rosenblum MK, Graus F, et al: Autoantibodies in paraneoplastic syndromes associated with small-cell lung cancer. Neurology 38:1391, 1988.

30. What is the differential diagnosis of nonpsychogenic causes of male sexual impotence?

1. Penile arterial insufficiency
2. Excessive venous leakage
3. Spinal cord damage
4. Conus medullaris damage
5. Cauda equina damage
6. Sacral plexus damage
7. Peripheral neuropathies
8. Central and peripheral autonomic disorders
9. Drugs
10. Alcohol
11. Hyperprolactinemia
12. Peyronie's disease

31. What are the commonest cardiovascular disturbances associated with CNS disease?

Cardiac arrhythmias, myocardial injury, and changes in blood pressure.

32. What cardiac arrhythmias are associated with CNS disease?

A number of CNS disorders, including subarachnoid hemorrhage, cerebral infarction and hemorrhage, brain tumors, and head injury, may cause a variety of supraventricular and ventricular arrhythmias unrelated to any underlying cardiac disease. These arrhythmias may further compromise the prognosis of the CNS disease: 4–5% of sudden deaths in patients with subarachnoid hemorrhage is attributed to this complication. Arrhythmias occur because of an imbalance between sympathetic and parasympathetic influences on the heart, presumably from an enhanced release of peripheral catecholamines triggered by the central lesion.

Parizel G: On the mechanism of sudden death with subarachnoid hemorrhage. J Neurol 220:71, 1979.

33. What is the nature of the myocardial injury associated with CNS disease?

CNS lesions, particularly intracerebral and subarachnoid hemorrhage, may cause a number of EKG abnormalities suggestive of myocardial ischemia. These changes may closely resemble myocardial infarction and include prolongation of the QT interval, ST segment depression, flattening or inversion of T waves, and the appearance of U waves. With the exception of QT interval prolongation and the U waves, these changes usually revert to normal within 2 weeks after the CNS event. Other less frequently observed EKG changes are increased amplitude of the P wave, development of Q waves, ST segment elevation, and T wave elevation, notching, or peaking. Differentiation between a centrally-induced EKG abnormality and a true myocardial infarction may be difficult, but the patient must be cared for in a monitored setting until a "true" myocardial infarction is excluded. The EKG changes are thought to be due to a neurogenically-mediated excessive release of catecholamines upon cardiac myocytes, resulting in myonecrotic changes. In fact, a higher level of serum catecholamines correlates with a poor outcome in patients with subarachnoid hemorrhage.

Benedict CR, Loach AB: Sympathetic nervous system activity in patients with subarachnoid hemorrhage. Stroke 9:237, 1978.

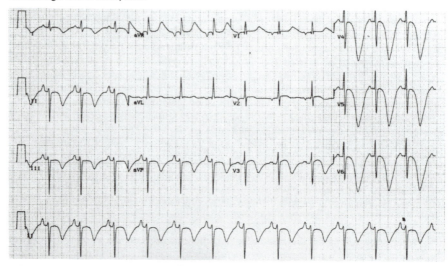

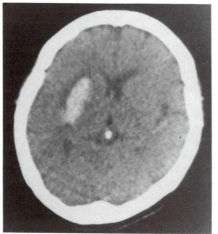

Electrocardiogram of a 41-year-old woman showing typical CNS changes of prolonged QT interval and deep, inverted, peaked T-waves. These EKG changes were secondary to the traumatic basal ganglion hemorrhage shown on her CT scan *(left)*.

34. What is the relationship of changes in blood pressure to CNS disease?

Lesions of the hypothalamus, the medulla oblongata, or tumors of the posterior fossa, may cause arterial hypertension. Ischemic, degenerative, or destructive lesions of the nucleus tractus solitarius in the medulla may result in chronic lability of blood pressure. Cushing's response of hypertension, bradycardia, and apnea, an important sign of increased intracranial pressure and potential herniation, may also develop after ischemic lesions of the dorsal medullary reticular formation along the floor of the fourth ventricle. Hypertension caused by posterior fossa tumors is due to the local distortion of the brainstem. Such an increase in blood pressure may be episodic and indistinguishable from a pheochromocytoma. Patients with normal-pressure hydrocephalus may also have chronic hypertension. Decreased blood pressure is rare with CNS disease, but orthostatic hypotension may accompany brainstem tumors, although the exact mechanism and the specific nuclei involved are not clear.

Low PA (ed): Clinical Autonomic Disorders. Boston, Little, Brown and Co., 1992, p 46.

Reis DJ, Doba N: Hypertension as a localizing sign of mass lesions of brainstem. N Engl J Med 287:1355, 1972.

Micieli G, Martignoni E, Cavallini A, et al: Postprandial and orthostatic hypotension in Parkinson's disease. Neurology 37:686, 1987.

35. What autonomic dysfunctions occur following heart transplantation?

After heart or heart-lung transplantation, which results in afferent and efferent denervation of the transplanted organ, there is a relative resting tachycardia, little or no rise in heart rate after standing, and a delayed increase in heart rate in response to exercise. Also, there are no changes in heart rate with the Valsalva maneuver or carotid sinus massage. In general, the heart rate response in these patients mainly depends on the circulating catecholamines. The cardiovascular abnormalities seen in severe autonomic neuropathies, e.g., diabetes, resemble those seen in a denervated transplanted heart.

36. Which neurologic conditions cause hypothermia?

Based on experimental studies, probably lesions of the anterior hypothalamus cause hyperthermia, of the posterior hypothalamus hypothermia, and of the suprachiasmatic nucleus alterations in the circadian rhythm of temperature. Tumors and degenerative or inflammatory processes involving the hypothalamus may produce hypothermia (core body temperature below 35°C).

Wernicke's encephalopathy, by damaging the posterolateral hypothalamus and the floor of the fourth ventricle, may present with continuous hypothermia. Prompt treatment with thiamine results in normalization of temperature.

Shapiro's syndrome (agenesis of the corpus callosum) may be associated with episodic hypothermia and hyperhidrosis. Lesions of the posterior or anterior hypothalamus, infundibular nuclei, septal region, and cingulate gyrus may be seen on postmortem examination. Anticonvulsants, cyproheptadine, clonidine, or oxybutynin may control the hypothermia and diaphoresis.

Victor M, Adams RD, Collins GN: The Wernicke-Korsakoff Syndrome and Related Neurologic Disorders due to Alcoholism and Malnutrition, 2nd ed. Philadelphia, F.A. Davis, 1989.

LeWitt PA, Newman RP, Greenberg HS, et al: Episodic hyperhidrosis, hypothermia, and agenesis of corpus callosum. Neurology 33:1122, 1983.

LeWitt PA: Hyperhidrosis and hypothermia responsive to oxybutynin. Neurology 38:506, 1988.

37. Which autonomic dysfunctions occur in Parkinson's disease (PD)?

In the classic forms of PD, disturbances in salivation, sweating, and bladder and bowel functions may be seen. Some patients may have orthostatic dizziness, but a significantly lower resting or orthostatic blood pressure is usually not present. The cardiovascular reflexes are generally preserved, although responses may be somewhat reduced. The resting recumbent levels of plasma norepinephrine are slightly lower than in healthy subjects. These subtle autonomic disturbances in PD are thought to be due to a central rather than a peripheral lesion. It is of interest, however, that Lewy bodies may be present in the sympathetic ganglia of patients with PD.

Gross M, Bannister R, Austen-Godwin R: Orthostatic hypotension in Parkinson's disease. Lancet 1:174, 1972.

Bannister R, Mathias CJ (eds): Autonomic Failure, 3rd ed. Oxford, Oxford University Press, 1992, p 543.

Sachs C, Berglund B, Kaijser L: Autonomic cardiovascular responses in parkinsonism: Effect of levodopa with dopa-decarboxylase inhibition. Acta Neurol Scand 71:37, 1985.

Rajput AH, Rozdilsky B: Dysautonomia in parkinsonism: A clinicopathological study. J Neurol Neurosurg Psychiatry 39:1092, 1976.

38. What are the most important genetic causes of autonomic failure?

1. Dopamine/beta-hydroxylase deficiency
2. Familial dysautonomia
3. Fabry's disease
4. Familial amyloidosis
5. Multiple endocrine neoplasia, type 2b
6. Porphyria

39. What is dopamine/beta-hydroxylase (DBH) deficiency?

Congenital deficiency of this enzyme, which converts dopamine into norepinephrine, results in severe orthostatic hypotension due to sympathetic adrenergic failure. Although mild symptoms of orthostatic hypotension, hypothermia, and hypoglycemia may be present from childhood, the prominent clinical picture in adults consists of marked hypotension, bilateral ptosis, decreased sweating, retrograde ejaculation, and hyporeflexia. There is a virtual absence of circulating norepinephrine and epinephrine, while the dopamine level is abnormally elevated.

Bannister R, Mathias CJ (eds): Autonomic Failure, 3rd ed. Oxford, Oxford University Press, 1992, p 721.

40. What is familial dysautonomia (Riley-Day syndrome, hereditary sensory-autonomic neuropathy type II, HSAN-II)?

This syndrome occurs primarily in children of Jewish extraction, being inherited as an autosomal recessive trait and affecting both sexes. Almost all cases occur in Ashkenazic Jews, although a small number of patients have been described in other groups. The frequency of occurrence is 1 in 10,000 live births among the Ashkenazic Jews of the United States. The parents are usually unaffected, but less pronounced autonomic dysfunction has been reported in the parent of a son with familial dysautonomia. The disease affects peripheral autonomic, sensory, and motor neurons, and possibly some populations of CNS neurons.

Clinical manifestations of autonomic dysfunction include diminished lacrimation, hyperhidrosis or erratic sweating, labile blood pressure, postural hypotension, esophageal and GI transit dysfunction (vomiting crises), hypothermia, impaired taste and vestibular reflexes, relative insensitivity to pain and temperature, and transient and emotionally induced skin blotching. The impairment of pain perception may lead to acral mutilation and Charcot joints. Scoliosis may be prominent. Areflexia, corneal insensitivity and abrasions, loss of tongue fungiform papillae, poor motor coordination, and emotional instability also occur. There is absent response to skin scratch and histamine injection. Poor feeding and repeated aspiration-induced pulmonary infections and dehydration are the usual causes of death in infancy and childhood. With early diagnosis and better management of complications, many patients now reach adulthood, and during adolescence most autonomic symptoms (except for postural hypotension) decrease.

41. What are the features of the peripheral neuropathy seen in familial dysautonomia?

Nerve conduction studies show reduced amplitudes of the sensory action potentials, absent H reflexes, and slightly decreased motor nerve conduction velocities. Sural nerve biopsy shows a greatly reduced number of unmyelinated C fibers, consistent with impaired pain and temperature perception, and absent corneal sensation and cutaneous axon reflexes. Morphometric studies have shown reduced neuronal populations in the intermediolateral column of the spinal cord, sympathetic, gasserian, sphenopalatine, and dorsal root ganglia. The ciliary ganglia, on the other hand, show only minor changes, supporting the suggestion that the pupillary hypersensitivity to acetylcholine agonists (e.g., methacholine and pilocarpine) seen in these patients is probably due to local changes in the eye rather than cholinergic denervation.

42. What neurotransmitter changes are seen in familial dysautonomia?

The urinary norepinephrine and epinephrine catabolite, vanillylmandelic acid (VMA), is decreased, while the dopamine product, homovanillic acid (HVA), is normal, resulting in an abnormal HVA/VMA ratio. Absence of dopamine beta-hydroxylase has been shown in 25% of affected children, and decreased levels have been found in their mothers. Consistency of such decreases, however, has been challenged.

43. What is the pathogenesis of familial dysautonomia?

The pathogenesis of familial dysautonomia is thought to be due to an ontogenetic aberration of neural crest cells, resulting in abnormal development and maintenance of certain populations of nerve cells in early life and thereafter. Because nerve growth factor (NGF) plays a critical role in sympathetic autonomic development, both prenatally and postnatally, investigations of familial dysautonomia have centered on whether a defect in NGF exists. Beta-NGF is shown to be reduced in cultured human fibroblasts and serum of patients with familial dysautonomia. This reduction is not due to defective beta-NGF gene structure, but may be due to impaired NGF processing or receptors.

44. What is Fabry's disease?

This X-linked recessive metabolic disorder is due to a deficiency of the lysosomal enzyme alpha-galactosidase, with resulting cell storage of the glycolipid ceramide trihexoside in several organs, including the skin (corpora angiokeratomas), kidneys, cardiovascular and pulmonary systems, blood vessels, and central and peripheral nervous systems. Because the neuropathy is prominent, the disease should be suspected in any boy or young man who presents with episodes of tender feet and painful burning sensations of the lower legs.

There is prominent lipid deposition in the dorsal root and peripheral autonomic ganglia, which are known to have fenestrated blood vessels and a permeable blood-nerve barrier. It appears that much of the stored ceramide trihexoside originates systemically and enters brain and nerve through permeable sites. Storage of lipids within central autonomic nuclei of the brainstem and spinal cord, areas protected by the blood-brain barrier, cannot be readily explained.

The clinical presentation of autonomic dysfunction includes diminished sweating (may be due to lipid accumulation in sweat glands rather than neuropathy), absent skin wrinkling after immersion in warm water, reduced cutaneous flare response, reduced tear and saliva production, disturbed intestinal motility, abnormal cardiovascular responses, and abnormal pupillary response to pilocarpine. Responses to postural change and plasma norepinephrine levels are normal. Peripheral nerve pathology consists of degenerative changes of unmyelinated and small myelinated fibers.

45. What is familial amyloidosis?

Hereditary amyloidosis is a heterogeneous group of familial diseases that have in common the systemic or localized accumulation of polypeptide amyloid fibrils arranged in beta-pleated sheets. Extracellular amyloid deposits result in disruption of normal tissue structure and function. Different subunits of proteins of 10–15 kda form the fibril structure, which has a beta configuration, giving the substance the property of birefringence. The clinical properties of different amyloid protein subunits, as determined by varied amino acid sequences, define the different amyloid diseases. In hereditary amyloidosis, the major component of subunit protein is a prealbumin (transthyretin), a normal constituent of plasma. It is a tetramer composed of four identical subunits, each being a single polypeptide chain of 127 amino acid residues encoded by a single gene on human chromosome 18. It has no structural relationship to albumin, and on electrophoresis migrates faster than albumin—hence, prealbumin. Unlike primary amyloidosis, the amyloid of hereditary amyloidosis is without light chains. Different mutants of the prealbumin protein with single amino acid substitutions are associated with most of the clinical varieties of systemic autosomal dominant amyloidosis. Although some of the mutations correlate with the clinical classification of amyloidosis, clinical pictures may overlap considerably. Future classification of herediatry amyloidosis will take into account the biochemical analysis of the condition.

46. What are the different types of familial amyloid polyneuropathy (FAP)?

FAP has been classified into four types on the basis of clinical manifestations:
1. FAP type I: Onset in lower limbs (Portuguese, Japanese, and Swedish kinships).
2. FAP type II: Onset in upper limbs (Swiss family of Indiana and German family of Maryland).
3. FAP type III: Onset in lower limbs followed by upper limb involvement (mixed family of Iowa).
4. FAP type IV: Cranial nerve involvement with corneal lattice dystrophy (Finnish, Dutch, and French Canadian family).

Of these, only FAP type I manifests with prominent autonomic abnormalities. The substitution of methionine for valine at position 30 in the prealbumin molecule is responsible for the gene mutation in this variety. In addition to a wide range of autonomic symptoms (hypotension, genitourinary, GI, pupillary, and sudomotor), there is involvement of sensory and motor nerves of the lower limbs.

47. What is multiple endocrine neoplasia type 2b (MEN 2b)?

This probably autosomal dominant hereditary syndrome is characterized by multiple mucosal neuromas (conjunctivae, oral cavity, tongue, pharynx, and larynx), medullary thyroid carcinoma, pheochromocytoma, ganglioneuromatosis, bony deformities, marfanoid appearance, muscle underdevelopment, and hypotonia. There are gross and microscopic abnormalities of the peripheral autonomic nervous system, with both sympathetic and parasympathetic systems affected. There are disorganized hypertrophy and proliferation of autonomic nerves and ganglia (ganglioneuromatosis). Neural proliferation of the alimentary tract (Auerbach and Meissner's plexi), upper respiratory tract, bladder, prostate, and skin may also be seen. The clinical autonomic manifestations include impaired lacrimation, orthostatic hypotension, impaired reflex vasodilation of skin, and parasympathetic denervation supersensitivity of pupils, with intact sweating and salivary gland function. Nerve biopsy shows degeneration and regeneration of unmyelinated fibers.

48. What is porphyria?

Acute hepatic porphyrias (acute intermittent porphyria, variegate porphyria, and hereditary coproporphyria) are autosomal dominantly inherited disorders that manifest as acute or subacute, severe, life-threatening neuropathy. The basic genetic defect is a 50% reduction in porphobilinogen deaminase activity (acute intermittent porphyria), protoporphyrinogen-IX oxidase (variegate porphyria), and coproporphyrinogen oxidase (coproporphyria), resulting in abnormalities of heme biosynthesis. In the presence of sufficient endogenous or exogenous stimuli (drugs, hormones, menstruation, starvation, etc.), this partial deficiency may lead to clinical manifestations, including peripheral neuropathy, autonomic dysfunction, skin symptoms, and CNS abnormalities.

Pathologic involvement of the autonomic nervous system (degeneration of the vagus nerve and sympathetic trunk) could explain certain features of acute attacks, including abdominal pain, severe vomiting, constipation, intestinal dilatation and stasis, persistent sinus tachycardia (100–160/minute), labile hypertension, postural hypotension, hyperhidrosis, and sphincteric bladder problems. Persistent tachycardia invariably precedes the development of peripheral neuropathy and respiratory paralysis, and, along with labile hypertension, may be explained by vagus nerve damage. Tachycardia and hypertension may be associated with increased catecholamine release. It has been suggested that autonomic neurons may be more sensitive to the biochemical derangement of porphyria than are somatic neurons. Employment of a battery of baroreflex tests during the acute attack reveals mostly reversible parasympathetic and sympathetic dysfunction. The parasympathetic tests, however, become abnormal earlier and more frequently than the sympathetic tests. The heart rate variation with Valsalva maneuver may be abnormal in asymptomatic subjects with acute intermittent porphyria.

Detailed studies on proximal GI tract motility and circulating gut peptide levels in acute intermittent porphyria suggest the characteristic but rarely reversible disturbances of gut motor activity are due to autonomic and/or enteric nerve damage.

49. What are the major differences between the syndrome of pure autonomic failure (PAF) and multiple-system atrophy (MSA)?

MSA, also called Shy-Drager syndrome, is associated with autonomic dysfunction, particularly orthostatic hypotension, and parkinsonian symptoms of akinesia and rigidity, leading to incapacity in a few years. Clinical features of striatonigral degeneration, olivopontocerebellar atrophy, or pyramidal lesions in various combinations may be present. In PAF, also called idiopathic orthostatic hypotension, there are no other neurologic signs and the natural history is slow progression over 10–15 years.

50. What are the most important factors in the maintenance of normal blood pressure?

Normal blood pressure is a function of:

1. Blood volume
2. Vascular reflexes (e.g., reflex arteriolar-venous constriction, and baroreflex-induced tachycardia and cerebellar reflexes)
3. Hormonal mechanisms (e.g., increased plasma catecholamines, the renin-angiotensin-aldosterone system, arginine-vasopressin, and atrial natriuretic factor activity)

51. What are the baroreceptors? What is their significance?

Baroreceptors are spray-type nerve endings in the walls of blood vessels and the heart that are stimulated by the absolute level of, and changes in, arterial pressure. They are extremely abundant in the wall of bifurcation of the internal carotid arteries (carotid sinus) and in the wall of the aortic arch. The primary site of termination of baroreceptor afferent fibers is the NTS, but the afferent fibers of the carotid sinus, carried by the glossopharyngeal nerve, terminate more caudally near the obex.

The function of the baroreceptors is to maintain systemic blood pressure at a relatively constant level, especially during a change in body position. The system, in general, reduces daily variations in arterial pressure by approximately one-half to one-third of that which would occur if the baroreceptor systems were absent. The relative influence of the carotid sinus and aortic arch baroreceptors on the control of blood pressure is debatable, but data obtained from direct sympathetic nerve recordings in humans indicate that the aortic baroreflex is a more important regulator of efferent sympathetic responses during acute hypotension in healthy subjects than are carotid sinus baroreflexes. Intact baroreceptors are extremely effective in preventing rapid changes in blood pressure from moment to moment or hour to hour, but because of their adaptability to prolonged changes of blood pressure (>2 or 3 days), the system is incapable of long-term regulation of arterial pressure.

Baroreceptors are activated with each arterial pulse wave, and their rate of firing increases with raised arterial pressure and decreases when arterial pressure falls. Stretching of baroreceptors causes them to transmit signals to the NTS, resulting in efferent discharges via sympathetic (decreased signal) and parasympathetic (increased signal) systems to the circulation, to reduce the arterial pressure by vasodilation, venodilation, bradycardia, and decreased cardiac output. In executing such a complex reflex function, several groups of excitatory and inhibitory chemical messengers play major roles. These include amino acids (L-glutamate, gamma-aminobutyric acid [GABA], and glycine), monoamines (norepinephrine, epinephrine, dopamine, serotonin, histamine, and acetylcholine), and neuropeptides. Information obtained largely from experimental animals indicates that inhibition of sympathoexcitatory neurons in the rostral NTS is mediated by GABAergic or noradrenergic mechanisms, whereas L-glutamate is a likely candidate as a primary neurotransmitter for excitatory inputs from these neurons. The monoamines and neuropeptides act mostly as modulators via the descending pathways, setting the level of excitability of sympathetic preganglionic neurons. Interruption of these pathways (e.g., cervical cord transection) results in release of these neurons from suprasegmental control of baroreflexes (autonomic hyperreflexia of chronic tetraplegics).

52. How is baroreceptor function evaluated?

The evaluation of arterial and cardiopulmonary baroreflex function in the clinical setting is indirect and therefore imprecise. Interpretation of overall baroreflex function based on any single test should be cautious unless an abnormality is gross. When different techniques are compared, the correlation is often poor. Apart from disease states, baroreflexes may also be depressed in old age due to both decreased arterial wall distensibility and degenerative changes of the baroreflex arc nerves. During sleep, the baroreflex activity is increased so that arterial blood pressure tends to fall. Five noninvasive tests of baroreflex function have emerged as most popular and fairly reliable. There is now widespread agreement that these tests and other noninvasive cardiovascular reflex tests can provide objective evidence of autonomic involvement:

1. Beat-to-beat heart rate variation
2. Heart rate response to Valsalva's maneuver
3. Heart rate response to standing
4. Blood pressure response to standing
5. Blood pressure response to sustained hand grip

53. What is the difference in orthostatic hypotension caused by autonomic dysfunction and that caused by hypovolemia?

In most autonomic neuropathies associated with orthostatic hypertension, failure of vascular reflexes to increase sympathetic outflow to splanchnic and muscular vasculature results in a drop in both systolic and diastolic pressures. However, there is no increase in plasma norepinephrine (hypoadrenergic response). Conversely, in orthostatic hypotension secondary to hypovolemia, plasma norepinephrine increases excessively in response to standing (hyperadrenergic response).

In orthostatic hypotension secondary to generalized sympathetic failure, a drop in systolic blood pressure is not associated with reflex tachycardia, whereas in orthostatic hypotension secondary to hypovolemia or deconditioning, with intact sympathetic nerves, reflex tachycardia is prominent. A fall in systolic pressure alone is most likely caused by a non-neurologic disturbance (e.g., hypovolemia).

54. What general advice do you extend to a patient with orthostatic hypotension secondary to dysautonomia?

1. Avoid straining, which results in Valsalva maneuvers, by treating and preventing constipation with a high-fiber diet.

2. Avoid severe diurnal variations, particularly morning postural hypotension, by head-up tilt or sleeping in a sitting position at night, sitting for several minutes at the edge of the bed before standing, shaving while sitting, or assuming a squatting position immediately when presyncopal symptoms occur.

3. Avoid exposure to a warm environment to prevent uncompensated vasodilation (travel to warm countries, hot baths, etc.).

4. Avoid postprandial aggravation of orthostatic hypotension by eating smaller and more frequent meals with a reduced carbohydrate content.

5. Avoid a low-sodium diet by increasing the food sodium content to at least 150 mEq.

6. Avoid dehydration by increasing fluid intake to 2.0–2.5 liters per day.

7. Avoid vigorous exercises; moderate isotonic exercises are preferable to isometrics.

8. Avoid prolonged recumbency.

9. Avoid vasodilators such as alcohol.

10. Avoid drugs known to cause vasodilation and/or bradycardia (nitroglycerin or beta blockers).

55. What are the most important non-neurogenic causes of orthostatic hypotension?

1. Volume loss (bleeding, burns, etc.)
2. Dehydration and electrolyte disturbances (vomiting, diarrhea, adrenal insufficiency, diuretic use, etc.)
3. Vasodilation (vasodilator drugs, heat, alcohol, varicose veins, hyperbradykininism, etc.)
4. Cardiac diseases (aortic stenosis, atrial myxoma, pericarditis, and myocarditis)

56. What cardiovascular autonomic changes are seen during rapid eye movement (REM) sleep?

During REM sleep there is decreased sympathetic activity of the splanchnic and renal circulation, but increased activity by skeletal muscles. Whereas the slow phases of sleep are accompanied by hypotension and bradycardia, becoming increasingly more pronounced with the progression of sleep from stage 1 to 4, in REM sleep there are large, transient increases in blood pressure, reversing the hypotension of slow-wave sleep. Direct recording of sympathetic nerve traffic to the skeletal-muscle vascular bed by microneurography shows more than a 50% reduction in sympathetic activity during the slow phases of sleep, but a significant increase to the level of wakefulness during REM. This may suggest that slow-wave sleep provides a protective effect on the cardiovascular and cerebrovascular systems; during REM sleep or immediately afterward, such protective effects may disappear. This could explain why cardiovascular and cerebrovascular events occur more frequently in the early morning hours after awakening.

Somers VK, Dyken ME, Mark AL, Abboud FM: Sympathetic-nerve activity during sleep in normal subjects. N Engl J Med 328:303, 1993.

57. Why does skin turn red (flare) after it is scratched?

The normal skin axon-reflex vasodilation (flare) follows skin stimulation from a simple scratch. The scratch causes activation of unmyelinated sensory nerve terminals (C fibers). The impulse generated by this stimulus travels antidromically, reaches a branch point, then orthodromically arrives at a skin blood vessel, releasing one or more vasodilating peptides or adenosine triphosphate (ATP). The released substance leads to further histamine release, activating other sensory terminals, creating a cascade of spreading flare response. Released histamine also causes itching. Both the flare response and the itching may be reduced by antihistamines. The absence of a flare response provides evidence of dysfunction of unmyelinated sensory fibers in peripheral neuropathies.

58. What is a sudomotor axon reflex?

The sudomotor axon reflex employs the same mechanism as the skin axon-reflex flare, but the neural pathway consists of an axon reflex mediated by the postganglionic sympathetic axon (C fibers) that innervates sweat glands. The axon terminals of these fibers are activated by the local injection of acetylcholine: the generated impulse travels to a branch point where it is deflected, and then travels orthodromically to activate a different sweat gland, releasing acetylcholine, which binds to M3 muscarinic receptors. In other words, in the sudomotor axon reflex, the activation of sweat glands results in the reflex activation of another population of nearby glands, whose sweat output can be quantitatively measured. The quantitative sudomotor axon-reflex test (Q-SART) is, therefore, a sensitive and reproducible test of the integrity of the postganglionic sympathetic sudomotor axon.

59. There is a higher incidence of sudomotor and vasomotor disturbances of the arm with injuries to the lower trunk of the brachial plexus than to the upper trunk. Why?

This is explained by the anatomic fact that there is a higher density of postganglionic sympathetic fibers in the medial cord of the brachial plexus and the median and ulnar nerves.

60. During examination of the external ear canal with an otoscope, the patient developed dry cough and became dizzy. Why?

There is an anatomic explanation. The second branch of the vagus nerve, the auricular nerve, which originates after the vagus nerve has exited from the jugular foramen, is a somatic afferent nerve that provides the sensory fibers for the posterior wall and floor of the external acoustic meatus and the outer surface of the tympanic membrane. Irritation of the external auditory canal and the tympanic membrane by instruments, cerumen, or syringing may therefore cause abnormal vagal reflexes, resulting in coughing, vomiting, slow heart rate, or even cardiac inhibition.

61. What is the syndrome of autonomic dysreflexia observed in tetraplegics?

Traumatic spinal cord lesions result in markedly abnormal cardiovascular, thermoregulatory, bladder, bowel and sexual function. In a recently injured tetraplegic in spinal shock, tactile or painful stimuli originating below the level of the lesion induce no change in blood pressure or heart rate. In the chronic stages of spinal cord injury at a level above T5, however, there is an exaggerated rise in the systolic and diastolic blood pressure, accompanied by bradycardia. The plasma norepinephrine levels are only marginally elevated. The marked hypertension may lead to neurologic complications, including seizures, visual defects, and cerebral hemorrhage. This phenomenon is caused by the increased activity of target organs below the lesion supplied by sympathetic and parasympathetic nerves lacking supraspinal modulation and is called autonomic dysreflexia. Other clinical manifestations of autonomic dysreflexia include headache, chest tightness and dyspnea, pupillary dilation, cold limbs, flushing of face and neck, excessive sweating of the head, penile erection and discharge of seminal fluid, and contraction of bladder and bowel.

Bannister R, Mathias CJ: Autonomic Failure, 3rd ed. Oxford, Oxford University Press, , 1992, pp 850–851.

62. What is the best management of autonomic dysreflexia?

The prolonged episodes of this syndrome may be prevented if the precipitating causes (e.g., painful tactile or visceral urinary and rectal stimuli) are corrected. It is important that the bladder be emptied before performing any procedure on tetraplegics. Blood pressure can often be decreased by elevating the head of the bed. Clonidine, an alpha$_2$ and imidazoline receptor agonist, acting at the level of the medulla, is useful in prophylaxis of autonomic dysreflexia.

63. What are the pathologic causes of hyperhidrosis? How is it treated?

Spinal cord damage or lesions of the peripheral sympathetic nerves may cause localized hyperhidrosis. **Generalized and episodic hyperhidrosis** may occur in patients with infectious diseases (night sweats), malignancies, hypoglycemia, thyrotoxicosis, pheochromocytomas, carcinoid syndrome, acromegaly, or diencephalic epilepsy, and in patients receiving cholinergic agents.

Primary or essential hyperhidrosis usually involves limited areas of the body, particulary the axilla, palms, and plantar regions. Axillary hyperhidrosis predominantly affects younger individuals, and may cause social embarrassment. Essential hyperhidrosis is, however, usually self-limiting by the fourth or fifth decade of life. There is no known cause for essential hyperhidrosis , but in up to half the cases there is a family history of a similar condition. Several studies have demonstrated no abnormalities of the sweat glands themselves, and implicated central and preganglionic sympathetic pathway hyperactivity.

The treatment of essential hyperhidrosis may be difficult and require systemic pharmacotherapy (anticholinergics and diltiazem), topical agents (aluminum chloride), excision of axillary sweat glands, and sympathectomy as the last resort.

64. When your attending physician pimps you on rounds, why do you get sweaty palms but not sweaty armpits?

Anxiety and emotional stress primarily aggravate the hyperhidrosis of the palms and soles, but not of the axilla. This is explained by the fact that the eccrine sweat glands of the palms and soles, as well as those of the forehead, respond to emotional, mental or sensory stimuli, whereas the axillary glands respond primarily to thermal stimuli.

BIBLIOGRAPHY

1. Bannister R, Mathias C: Autonomic Failure, 3rd ed. Oxford, Oxford University Press, 1992.
2. Low PA (ed): Clinical Autonomic Disorders. Boston, Little, Brown, and Co., 1992.

12. DEMYELINATING DISEASE

Loren A. Rolak, M.D.

1. What is myelin?

Myelin is the proteolipid membrane that ensheathes and surrounds nerve axons to improve their ability to conduct electrical action potentials. Oligodendrocytes make myelin and wrap it around axons, leaving gaps called nodes of Ranvier, where membrane ionic channels are heavily concentrated and powerful action potentials can thus be generated.

2. How does demyelination cause symptoms?

When myelin is stripped away from the axon, the underlying membrane does not contain a high enough concentration of sodium, potassium, and other ionic channels to permit a sufficient flow of ions to cause depolarization. The membrane thus becomes inert. The loss of myelin makes it impossible to depolarize the membrane to conduct an action potential, so the nerve is rendered useless.

3. What is multiple sclerosis? What is its incidence?

Multiple sclerosis (MS) is a demyelinating disease, the commonest of all the conditions that destroy myelin in the central nervous system. It affects approximately 250,000 Americans, mostly between the ages of 20 and 40, making it the leading disabling neurologic disease of young people.

4. How does MS cause demyelination?

MS is an inflammatory disease. Lymphocytes, macrophages, and other immunocompetent cells accumulate around venules in the central nervous system and exit into the brain, attacking and destroying the myelin.

5. Are there other demyelinating diseases?

Yes, but they are all very rare. MS is the only common demyelinating disease in adults. Indeed, many clinicians use "demyelinating disease" as a synonym for MS. Other rare conditions include:

    1. **Central pontine myelinolysis,** a syndrome of myelin destruction in the pons, associated with rapid correction of hyponatremia.

    2. **Progressive multifocal leukoencephalopathy,** an opportunistic viral infection of oligodendrocytes, seen most often in patients with AIDS.

    3. **Acute disseminated encephalomyelitis,** a postinfectious, acute, autoimmune demyelination.

    4. **Inborn errors of metabolism,** usually presenting in childhood:

        Metachromatic leukodystrophy, a deficiency of the enzyme aryl sufatase.

        Adrenoleukodystrophy, a defect in metabolism of very long chain fatty acids.

        Krabbe's globoid leukodystrophy, a severe developmental disease of uncertain
           etiology.

6. What is the relationship of optic neuritis to MS?

A patient afflicted with acute inflammatory demyelination of the optic nerve (optic neuritis) has approximately a 30–60% chance of suffering further demyelinating episodes in the CNS—i.e., of developing clinical MS. Many physicians believe that all optic neuritis is MS, and even isolated cases are a forme fruste of the disease. An analogous argument applies to monophasic demyelination of the spinal cord—transverse myelitis.

CLINICAL FEATURES OF MULTIPLE SCLEROSIS

7. What are the commonest symptoms of MS?

Symptoms of Multiple Sclerosis

1. Pyramidal weakness	45%
2. Optic neuritis	40%
3. Sensory loss	35%
4. Brainstem dysfunction	30%
5. Cerebellar ataxia and tremor	25%
6. Sphincter disturbances	20%

8. Are there any symptoms MS does not cause?

Not many. Virtually every neurologic problem has been described in MS, at least as a case report. However, since MS is a disease of myelin (white matter), it only rarely causes neuronal (gray matter) symptoms.

Uncommon Symptoms of Multiple Sclerosis

1. Dementia
2. Aphasia
3. Seizures
4. Pain
5. Extrapyramidal movement disorders

9. What is the clinical course of MS?

Just as the symptoms of MS vary greatly, so does its clinical course. It may present as an indolent, chronic, progressive symptom or as an acute, abrupt deficit. Indeed, different symptoms may present in different fashions in the same patient. Most commonly, MS takes an exacerbating and remitting course, with the sudden onset of neurologic symptoms, usually over a period of several hours to days, lasting for 6–8 weeks, and then gradually resolving completely or nearly back to normal.

10. How often do these "attacks" of MS occur?

These attacks are unpredictable, but average approximately one attack every year and a half. Many exacerbations reproduce previous symptoms.

11. Given the great variability in the signs, symptoms, and clinical course of MS, how can it be accurately diagnosed?

The diagnosis of MS is one of the most difficult in neurology. Nevertheless, careful analysis has shown that certain clinical criteria can accurately diagnose MS.

Schumacher Criteria for Definite Multiple Sclerosis

1. Two separate central nervous system symptoms.
2. Two separate attacks—the onset of symptoms is separated by at least 1 month.
3. Symptoms must involve the white matter.
4. Age 10–50 (although usually age 20–40).
5. Objective deficits are present on the neurologic examination.
6. No other medical problem exists to explain the patient's condition.

The key to the Schumacher criteria for the clinical diagnosis of MS is the first two features—two separate symptoms at two separate times, or lesions disseminated in space and in time.

12. Are laboratory tests useful for diagnosing MS?

Yes—in the proper setting and with proper caution. The principal drawback of the Schumacher criteria is that MS cannot be diagnosed until the second symptom appears. Laboratory tests can facilitate the diagnosis in patients who do not quite meet all of the Schumacher clinical criteria. However, no one test proves the diagnosis, and all laboratory data have sufficient problems with sensitivity and specificity to impair their usefulness in MS.

Poser CM, Paty DW, Scheinberg L, et al: New diagnostic criteria for multiple sclerosis: Guidelines for research protocols. Ann Neurol 13:227–231, 1983.

Paty DW, McFarlin DE, McDonald WI: Magnetic resonance imaging and laboratory aids in the diagnosis of multiple sclerosis. Ann Neurol 29:3–4, 1991.

13. How can the spinal fluid be used to diagnose MS?

Immunoglobulins are increased in the central nervous system in patients with MS, and the CSF often reflects elevations of both total IgG and IgG synthesis rates. Also, when the IgG is examined by electrophoresis, much of it clumps together in specific bands. The finding of several of these bands in the IgG region, called oligoclonal bands, is reasonably sensitive and specific for MS. However, it remains unclear how or why oligoclonal bands are produced in this disease or exactly what they represent.

Muller FA, Hanny PE, Wichman W, et al: Cerebrospinal fluid immunoglobulins and multiple sclerosis. Arch Neurol 46:367–371, 1989.

14. Do other diseases have oligoclonal bands?

Yes, especially inflammatory conditions such as syphilis, meningoencephalitis, and subacute sclerosing panencephalitis (SSPE, a latent measles infection), and autoimmune processes such as Guillain-Barré syndrome.

15. How are evoked potentials used to assist in the diagnosis of MS?

Because evoked potentials measure conduction through the central nervous system, they reveal areas of demyelination by showing slowed conduction through pathways where the myelin has been damaged. MS is the commonest cause of a slowing detected by evoked potentials.

16. What are the evoked potentials usually used to diagnose MS?

1. Visual evoked potentials (VEPs) are performed by flashing a checkered pattern in the patient's eyes while recording the electrical response from the visual cortex in the occipital lobe. Normally, a response appears approximately 100 ms after the stimulus is presented to the eye, and a delay implies demyelination in the visual pathways.

2. Brainstem auditory evoked potentials (BAEPs) are performed by giving an auditory stimulus in the ear, such as a clicking sound while recording from the auditory cortex in the temporal lobe. The sound generates a series of waves as it travels through the brainstem and hemispheres, and a delay in these waves is presumptive evidence of a demyelinating slowing.

3. Somatosensory evoked potentials (SSEPs) are performed by applying an electrical stimulus to the wrist or the ankle while recording from the sensory area of the cortex. Slowing can often be detected in the spinal cord, brainstem, or hemispheres.

17. How valuable are evoked potentials for diagnosing MS?

Studies disagree considerably, but probably about 75% of people with definite MS will have an abnormal VEP, and a similar figure will have abnormal SSEPs. BAEPs are abnormal in about 50%.

Lee, KH, Hashimoto SA, Hodge JP, et al: MRI of the head in the diagnosis of multiple sclerosis: A prospective 2-year follow-up with comparison with clinical evaluation, evoked potentials, oligoclonal banding, and CT. Neurology 41:657–660, 1991.

18. How is magnetic resonance imaging (MRI) used to diagnose MS?

MRI shows abnormalities in approximately 80% of patients with MS. This technique is very sensitive for detecting the inflammatory lesions, or plaques, of MS. Because of this sensitivity and the simplicity and noninvasive nature of the test, MRI has become the most common procedure to confirm the diagnosis of MS.

The drawback to MRI is its lack of specificity. Unfortunately, the scattered subcortical periventricular white-matter abnormalities that characterize MS may occur in a variety of other settings, including some subjects who appear to be normal. For this reason, reliance on the MRI can lead to an overdiagnosis of MS.

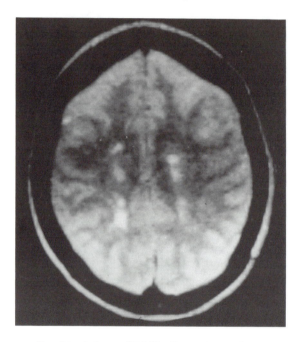

Axial T2-weighted MRI of the brain shows typical confluent, deep white matter signal intensities characteristic of MS.

Kesselring J, Ormerod I, Miller D, et al: Magnetic Resonance Imaging in Multiple Sclerosis. New York, Thieme, 1989

Yetkin FZ, Haughton VM, Papke RA, et al: Multiple sclerosis: Specificity of MR for diagnosis. Radiology 178:447–451, 1991.

19. What is the prognosis of MS?

MS varies greatly, not only in its symptoms and clinical course, but also in its prognosis. Although not a fatal disease, there is a slight statistical shortening of lifespan as a result of secondary complications that can afflict severe sufferers of MS, such as aspiration pneumonia, decubitus ulcers, urinary tract infections, and falls. As a general rule, approximately one-third of patients with MS will do well throughout their life, never accumulating any significant disability. Another one-third will accumulate neurologic deficits sufficient to impair their activities, but not serious enough to prevent them from leading a normal life—holding a job, raising a family, etc. The final third of people with MS become disabled, requiring a walker, a wheelchair, or even total care.

20. What factors allow for a prediction of the course of MS?

The variability of MS makes accurate prediction fallible, but a few factors do portend a good prognosis.

Good Prognostic Factors in Multiple Sclerosis

1. Early age of onset (first symptoms prior to age 40).

2. Sensory symptoms at onset (as opposed to weakness, ataxia, or other motor abnormalities).

3. A pattern of exacerbations and remissions (as opposed to a chronic progressive symptom at onset).

4. Female gender. Women do better than men.

Rolak LA: Multiple sclerosis. In Evans R (ed): Prognosis of Neurological Disorders. New York, Oxford University Press, 1992, pp 295–300.

ETIOLOGY

21. How does the epidemiology of MS provide clues to its cause?

Some unusual features characterize the epidemiology of MS. MS is more common the farther one moves away from the equator. While MS is virtually unheard of in the tropics, its incidence is approximately 15 per 100,000 in Texas and Florida, 80 per 100,000 in Boston, and nearly one per 1,000 in Northern Scotland, Scandinavia, and Iceland.

It most frequently afflicts high socioeconomic classes, such as literate, educated professionals. It is more common in women than men by a ratio of at least 3:2. It primarily strikes people of northern European ancestry, while it is almost unknown in some other racial groups, such as Eskimos and gypsies. This may be related to specific HLA type (i.e., immune functions) in these populations.

The chance of developing MS seems to be set by approximately age 15. A person born in a high-risk area (such as Scandinavia) who leaves for a low-risk area (in the tropics) after age 15 will carry the high risk for developing MS. If he emigrates prior to age 15, he will acquire the low risk of his new home. In short, the risk of MS is determined prior to age 15, even though the disease itself does not appear, on average, until age 30. Unfortunately, none of these tantalizing epidemiologic findings has yet led to a coherent hypothesis for the etiology of MS.

Compston DAS: The dissemination of multiple sclerosis. J Roy Coll Phys 24:207–218, 1990.

22. What is the evidence that MS is an autoimmune disease?

Evidence for an Autoimmune Etiology of Multiple Sclerosis

1. Pathologically, MS is an inflammatory disease involving lymphocytes, phagocytes, and other immune-competent cells.

2. MS is most common in patients with certain HLA types, implying that genes that control the immune system are related to the development of MS.

3. Oligoclonal bands in the spinal fluid imply an abnormality in the immune system.

4. T-cell subsets are abnormal in MS, with most researchers reporting decreased numbers of suppressor T-lymphocytes.

5. There is an animal model of MS, experimental autoimmune encephalomyelitis (EAE), which is an immune-mediated disease. Animals injected with myelin basic protein and immune adjuvants can be induced to mount an immune response against the myelin antigens, which cross-reacts and damages their own myelin.

Hafler D, Weiner HL: MS: A CNS and systemic autoimmune disease. Immunol Today 10:104–107, 1989.

23. What is the evidence that MS is a viral disease?

Evidence for a Viral Causation of Multiple Sclerosis

1. MS is more common in certain parts of the world than others, suggesting an environmental factor. A virus could be this environmental factor.

2. Viral demyelinating diseases are known in animals, some of which serve as a model for MS. Canine distemper virus and Theiler's virus are examples of viral models of MS.

3. Latent viruses and slow viruses are well known in the human central nervous system, fitting the epidemiologic data that suggest latent and relapsing disease as a feature of MS.

4. The immune system in patients with MS reacts abnormally to viral antigens. This is true both of humeral (antibodies) immunity and of cell-mediated immunity.

TREATMENT

24. What treatments are available to alter the course of MS?

No treatment has been proved to cure MS or significantly alter its natural history. Nevertheless, some therapies confer at least short-term benefits and so are useful in the management of the disease.

25. What is the role of steroids in MS?

A number of studies have indicated that steroids are superior to placebo for alleviating attacks of MS. Symptoms resolve more quickly, although it is not clear if treatment of attacks will ultimately prevent disability or mitigate the final outcome of the disease. There remains much controversy about the most appropriate steroid preparation, dosage, route of administration, and duration of treatment.

Beneficial Properties of Steroids in Multiple Sclerosis

1. Immunosuppression
2. Stabilize blood-brain barrier
3. Anti-inflammatory
4. Enhance nerve conduction

26. What is the usual steroid regimen in MS?

The most popular therapy now employs intravenous methylprednisolone (Solu-Medrol) in a dose of 500–1000 mg daily for 3–7 days. This "pulse" of steroids is effective, at least in the short term, for improving MS symptoms.

Milligan NM, Newcombe R, Compston DAS: A double-blind controlled trial of high dose methylprednisolone in patients with multiple sclerosis. J Neurol Neurosurg Psychiatry 50:511–516, 1987.

27. What is the role of immunosuppressants in MS?

Many immune-altering regimens have been used in MS, but prospective, randomized, blinded, controlled, multicentered trials have been few and disappointing. Nevertheless, these agents are still widely employed because of their theoretical benefits for immune-mediated diseases such as MS, and because of the desperate disabilities in the young people afflicted with the disease.

28. What is the role of cyclophosphamide in MS?

Cyclophosphamide (Cytoxan) is the most popular of the powerful immune suppressants used to treat MS. It is generally given in intravenous doses of 500–1000 mg daily, sometimes as single pulses but often in consecutive treatments until immunosuppression is achieved. Complications include alopecia, bone marrow suppression, and hemorrhagic cystitis. Although some trials have reported success in improving or stabilizing the disease, a few carefully controlled trials were unable to confirm any benefit.

Canadian Cooperative Multiple Sclerosis Study Group: The Canadian Cooperative trial of cyclophosphamide and plasma exchange in progressive multiple sclerosis. Lancet 337:441–446, 1991.

29. What is the role of symptomatic treatments for MS?

If MS were cured today, the many sufferers from the disease would still have their neurologic deficits. Management of these deficits is an important part of the treatment of MS. The most disabling symptoms reported by MS patients are fatigue, motor deficits, cerebellar problems, and sphincter disturbance.

Schapiro RT: Symptom Management in Multiple Sclerosis. New York, Demos Publications, 1987.

30. What is the best treatment for fatigue in MS?

Although fatigue seems to be a vague and subjective symptom, it is a very real part of MS. In fact, it is one of the leading reasons for inability to work among MS victims. Amantadine (Symmetrel) has been shown in careful studies to be useful for eliminating fatigue, usually in doses of 100 mg b.i.d. Another helpful drug is pemoline (Cylert), a mild stimulant, which can be given in doses of 18.75 mg b.i.d. or even much higher. Of course, simple common sense measures are also useful, such as resting during the day and reorganizing the home and workplace for better efficiency.

Rolak LA: Fatigue and multiple sclerosis. In Dawson DM, Sabin TD (eds): Chronic Fatigue Syndrome. Boston, Little, Brown, and Co., 1993, pp 153–161.

31. What is the best treatment for motor deficits in MS?

Unfortunately, little can be done to restore muscle strength. However, spasticity often improves with the use of baclofen (Lioresal) in doses of 60 mg or more a day. Dantrolene (Dantrium) and diazepam (Valium) are also useful oral antispasticity agents, although their side effects made them less attractive as first-line drugs. Physical therapy can also minimize spasticity.

Young RR, Delawaide PJ: Spasticity. N Engl J Med 304:28–33, 1981.

32. What is the best treatment for cerebellar tremor and ataxia in MS?

Therapy for cerebellar deficits is frustrating—these are among the hardest symptoms to alleviate. Sometimes simple mechanical measures are helpful, such as attaching weights to the ankles or wrists. Drug treatment usually focuses on agents that increase GABA levels, since this is the primary neurotransmitter of the cerebellum. Benzodiazepines such as clonazepam (Klonopin) may help, in a dose of 0.5 mg b.i.d. or more. Other agents that increase GABA include valproate acid (Depakote) in the usual anticonvulsant dosages, and INH, although this must be used in high doses of 900–1200 mg per day.

Bozek CB, Kastrukoff LF, Wright JM, et al: A controlled trial of isoniazid therapy for action tremor in multiple sclerosis. J Neurol 234:36–39, 1987.

33. What is the best treatment for urologic problems in MS?

Urologic consultation is often useful to manage the neurogenic bladder. The most common problem is a hyperreflexic bladder with a small capacity, early detrusor contraction, urinary frequency, and urgency. It can be managed with medications such as oxybutinin (Ditropan), propantheline (Pro-Banthine), or hyoscyamine (Levsinex). More rarely, there is a flaccid bladder, which may require self-catheterization. When sphincter-detrusor dyssynergia appears, medications to relax the sphincter, such as the alpha-adrenergic blocking agent prazosin (Minipress) may be useful.

BIBLIOGRAPHY

1. Matthews WB: McAlpine's Multiple Sclerosis, 2nd ed. Edinburgh, Churchill Livingstone, 1991.
2. Sibley WA: Therapeutic Claims in Multiple Sclerosis, 3rd ed. New York, Demos Publications, 1993.
3. Rolak LA: Multiple sclerosis. Curr Neurol 9:109–148, 1989.

13. DEMENTIA

Rachelle S. Doody, M.D., Ph.D.

GENERAL CONSIDERATIONS

1. How is dementia defined? How do definitions vary?

Dementia is generally regarded as an acquired loss of cognitive function due to an abnormal brain condition. The National Institute of Health criteria (formerly NINCDS-ADRDA criteria) for the diagnosis of Alzheimer's disease (AD) stress that there must be **progressive** loss of cognitive function, including but not limited to memory loss. The recently proposed State of California criteria for vascular dementia do not require progression of deficits in the definition of dementia. The DSM-III-R general criteria for dementia also include the requirement that there be **functional decline** that interferes with work or usual social activities in addition to cognitive decline.

McKhann G, et al: Clinical diagnosis of Alzheimer's disease: Report of the NINCDS-ADRDA Work Group under the auspices of Department of Health and Human Services Task Force on Alzheimer's Disease. Neurology 34:939–944, 1984.

Spitzer R, Williams J: Diagnostic and Statistical Manual of Mental Disorders, 3rd ed, revised. Washington, DC, American Psychiatric Association, 1987, p 107.

Chui H, et al: Criteria for the diagnosis of ischemic vascular dementia proposed by the State of California Alzheimer's Disease Diagnostic and Treatment Centers. Neurology 42:473–480, 1992.

2. What is pseudodementia?

This term has many meanings and is undergoing reanalysis as a diagnostic entity. It refers to depressed patients who are cognitively impaired and often have motor slowing, but do not have one of the well-defined dementia syndromes. It does not mean that the patient is consciously simulating dementia (malingering) or is cognitively intact but believes himself or herself to be demented (Ganser's syndrome). Some researchers believe that pseudodementia may be a precursor to dementia.

Folstein M, Rabins P: Replacing pseudodementia. Neuropsychiatry Neuropsychol Behav Neurol 4:36–40, 1991.

3. What features are characteristic of pseudodementia associated with depression?

Patients with pseudodementia may or may not have a history of depressive or vegetative symptoms. They do tend to have flat affect, to give up easily when mental status is examined, or to say that they cannot perform a task without even trying it. They often respond surprisingly well when given extra time and encouragement, but they may deny their success. Results are inconsistent on mental examination: for example, they may fail a simple task but perform a similar, more difficult one correctly. Or they may have variable strengths and weaknesses over repeated testing sessions.

4. What is Ganser's syndrome?

It is an involuntary and unconscious simulation of altered mental status (confusion or dementia) in a patient who is not malingering and believes his or her own symptoms.

5. What is delirium?

Delirium is an acute confusional state.

6. What features distinguish delirium from dementia?

Although this distinction cannot always be accomplished with certainty, several features are helpful. Sudden onset suggests delirium, as do findings of altered consciousness, marked problems with attention and concentration out of proportion to other deficits, cognitive fluctuations (e.g., lucid intervals), psychomotor and/or autonomic overactivity, fragmented speech, and marked hallucinations (especially if auditory or tactile). Keep in mind that even chronically demented patients can develop delirium in addition to dementia, which will change the clinical picture.

7. Do all patients with dementia develop psychotic features?
No. Psychosis is a variable finding in all types of dementia and is not even clearly related to the stage or severity of dementia.

8. Which screening instruments are commonly used in diagnosing dementia?
The Folstein Mini-Mental Status Examination (MMSE), Short Blessed, and Mattis Dementia Rating Scale are commonly used clinically and in experimental studies to screen for dementia and to rate severity of dementia.

9. What are the limitations of the MMSE in the assessment of dementia?
Besides the fact that it has both false positives (usually depression) and false negatives (usually early dementia in highly functioning patients), the MMSE also has limitations based on its lack of comprehensiveness. It is particularly insensitive to language dysfunction.

Feher E, et al: Establishing the limits of the mini-mental state. Arch Neurol 49:87–92, 1992.

10. At what point is a patient too demented to require an evaluation?
Patients are never too demented to be evaluated. The need to rule out reversible causes and structural lesions always remains. Neurologic and psychometric examinations can be tailored to the patient's level even in the most profoundly demented patients.

11. What are the most common causes of dementia or conditions resembling dementia?
Alzheimer's disease is the most common form of dementia in adults ($>50\%$ in most series). Depression with pseudodementia is a frequent cause of cognitive loss and must be ruled out in all patients. Other important causes include multi-infarct or vascular dementia, Lewy body dementia, and dementia-like syndromes due to alcohol or the chronic use of certain prescription drugs.

12. What uncommon causes of dementia must be considered in the differential diagnosis of every patient with dementia?

Uncommon Causes of Dementia

1. Toxins (lead, organic mercury)
2. Vitamin deficiencies (B12, B1, and B6, in particular)
3. Endocrine disturbances (hypo- or hyperthyroidism, hyperparathyroidism, Cushing's disease, Addison's disease)
4. Chronic metabolic conditions (hyponatremia, hypercalcemia, chronic hepatic failure, renal failure)
5. Vasculopathies affecting the brain
6. Structural abnormalities (chronic subdural hematomas, normal-pressure hydrocephalus, slow-growing tumors)
7. CNS infections (including AIDS, Creutzfeldt-Jakob, cryptococcal or tuberculous meningitis)

13. Can B12 deficiency cause neurologic symptoms such as dementia in the absence of anemia?
Dementia, paresthesia, sensory loss, ataxia, and psychiatric disorders may all occur without macrocytosis or anemia. They appear to be reversible following repletion of the vitamin.

Lindenbaum J, et al: Neuropsychiatric disorders caused by cobalamin deficiency in the absence of anemia or macrocytosis. N Engl J Med 318:1720–1728, 1988.

14. Which dementia syndromes are associated with alcohol?

The DSM-III-R includes alcohol amnestic syndrome (Korsakoff's syndrome), in which the amnestic disorder predominates, as well as a more generalized dementia associated with alcoholism. Both are associated with some degree of visuospatial impairment, and neither includes aphasia.

ALZHEIMER'S DISEASE

15. How is Alzheimer's disease (AD) diagnosed?

First, the presence of dementia must clearly be established by clinical criteria and confirmed by neuropsychological testing. The clinical manifestations must include impairment of memory and of at least one other area of cognition. There must be no evidence of other systemic or brain disease sufficient to cause the dementia, and the NIH criteria suggest some basic laboratory studies to ensure this (which are not all-inclusive). The diagnosis is both a diagnosis of exclusion and a diagnosis based upon the establishment of certain characteristic features.

McKahn G, et al: Clinical diagnosis of Alzheimer's disease: Report of the NINCDS-ADRDA Work Group under the auspices of Department of Health and Human Services Task Force on Alzheimer's Disease. Neurology 34:939–944, 1984.

16. When should the designations of probable, possible, and definite AD be used?

Probable AD refers to a clinical diagnosis that is made using the NIH criteria. Most patients have this diagnosis.

Possible AD refers to patients with atypical features (progressive isolated memory or language dysfunction, for example) or patients with a concurrent disorder that could cause cognitive impairment, but it is not believed to be the only factor (concomitant cerebrovascular accident, for example).

Definite AD is reserved for those with biopsy- or autopsy-proved AD.

McKahn G, et al: Clinical diagnosis of Alzheimer's disease: Report of the NINCDS-ADRDA Work Group under the auspices of Department of Health and Human Services Task Force on Alzheimer's Disease. Neurology 34:939–944, 1984.

17. How are the alcohol-related dementias differentiated from AD?

There are no absolute features that distinguish these conditions. If the patient has a "systemic disorder" (such as alcoholism) sufficient in the clinician's opinion to cause dementia, the diagnosis should **not** be probable AD. Possible AD may be used if underlying AD is suspected in an actively drinking patient. The patient should stop drinking with the help of appropriate rehabilitative services. If the dementia improves and the improvement continues or persists for a year or more, the diagnosis is not likely to be AD.

18. Which blood tests are typically ordered in a patient with suspected AD to rule out other causes of dementia?

Blood Tests for Dementia

1. Chemistry analysis (including sodium, blood sugar, calcium, liver enzymes, renal function)	9. Serum protein electrophoresis
	10. Serum arterial ammonia
	11. Parathyroid hormone
2. CBC with differential	12. Cortisol levels
3. PT/PTT	13. Rheumatoid factor
4. Thyroid function tests	14. HIV
5. VDRL or equivalent	15. Extractable nuclear antigen panel
6. B12	16. Sed rate
7. Folate	17. Serum (and urine) drug levels
8. ANA	18. Hexosaminidase levels

19. Which ancillary studies (in addition to blood tests) are useful to evaluate patients with suspected AD?

An imaging study (MRI or CT with contrast) and neuropsychological testing to confirm dementia are necessary. EEG, SPECT, or PET studies and lumbar puncture may be useful or even necessary.

20. Under what circumstances is lumbar puncture (LP) necessary in the diagnostic work-up?

When symptoms are of short duration (less than 6 months) or there are atypical features, such as rapid progression or severe confusion, an LP should be performed early. It should also be done if clinical or laboratory features suggest a specific etiology that is an indication for LP, such as CNS meningitis or CNS vasculitis.

21. What are typical symptoms of early AD?

Early symptoms of AD include forgetfulness for recent events or newly acquired information, often causing the patient to repeat himself or herself. Other early features are disorientation, especially to time, and difficulty with complex cognitive functions such as mathematical calculations or organization of activities that require several steps.

22. What are typical symptoms of moderately advanced AD?

Advanced AD includes a history of progression of pervasive memory loss sufficient to impair everyday activities, disorientation to place and/or aspects of person (e.g., age), inability to keep track of time, and problems with personal care (such as forgetting to change clothes). Behavioral changes, such as depression, paranoia, or aggressiveness, are more likely in these stages.

23. Does progression of AD follow a consistent pattern?

Definitely not. There is tremendous variation in salient symptoms and rates of progression.

24. What language disturbances do patients with AD experience?

Early on, most have word-finding difficulties that may cause pauses in spontaneous speech or may be detected by asking the patient to name objects (particularly objects with low frequency in the language). As AD progresses, most develop problems with comprehension with intact repetition (similar to transcortical sensory aphasia); then repetition becomes affected while speech remains fluent (similar to Wernicke's aphasia). Ultimately, some patients develop expressive speech problems in addition to the above symptoms, or they may just stop talking secondary to inanition and apparent lack of anything to say.

25. Does the presence or absence of insight differentiate AD from other dementias?

Lack of insight into one's memory disorder (or anosognosia) occurs in some patients with AD as well as in patients with other dementing disorders. It does not appear to correlate with disease severity and is not useful in differential diagnosis.

Feher E, et al: Mental status assessment of insight and judgment. Clin Geriatr Med 5:477–498, 1989.

26. What motor features may be associated with AD? What is their significance?

Rigidity, bradykinesia, and parkinsonian gait may occur and may be associated with more rapid progression of disease (both cognitive decline and activities of daily living). Tremor is rare, differentiating these patients to some extent from those with Parkinson's disease. Myoclonus may occur, and recent evidence suggests its association with a younger age of onset of AD.

Mayeux R, et al: Heterogeneity in dementia of the Alzheimer's type: Evidence of subgroups. Neurology 35:453–461, 1985.

27. Are there specific clinical subtypes of AD?
This is unclear, but possibilities include early-onset AD, AD with extrapyramidal features, and AD with psychosis. Familial AD is well recognized, occurring in about 10% of cases and characterized by autosomal dominant transmission.

28. What is the genetic defect in familial AD?
In some families with familial AD, there appears to be an abnormality of chromosome 21. In a subset of these families, there may be a defect in the gene that encodes amyloid precursor protein on chromosome 21. In other families, the defect involves chromosome 19 or 14. It is likely that still other genes will be linked to AD in the familial form of the disorder.

29. Is there a genetic component to all cases of AD?
The answer to this question is not clear. Patients with a positive family history for AD in a primary relative appear to be at increased risk, and the risk is higher at younger ages. Yet apparently sporadic cases are common. Genetic factors may account for a predisposition for AD.

30. What other disorders have been associated with AD in epidemiologic surveys?
Patients with Down's syndrome are at high risk for AD. It remains controversial whether or not families of patients with AD have a higher incidence of Down's syndrome. Both Parkinson's disease and a prior history of head trauma have been associated with AD in some large studies but not in others.

31. What are the classic neuropathologic changes in AD?
Senile plaques, neurofibrillary tangles, granulovacuolar degeneration, and amyloid in blood vessels and plaques are classic changes. Plaques and tangles may also be seen in normal brains but are far less numerous.

32. Which neuropathologic changes correlate best with the severity of dementia?
In most studies, senile plaques correlate best with the severity of dementia. More recently, synaptic density has been shown to have an inverse correlation with severity of dementia. Because education seems to increase synaptic density, some have suggested that education may have a protective effect against the manifestation of AD cognitive changes.

Terry R, et al: Physical basis of cognitive alterations in Alzheimer's disease: Synapse loss is the major correlate of cognitive impairment. Ann Neurol 30:572–580, 1991.

33. Which neuropathologic entities overlap with AD?
Besides normal aging, Lewy body dementia, Parkinson's disease, progressive supranuclear palsy, and vascular dementias are sometimes difficult to distinguish from AD, as plaques and tangles can occur with other pathologic changes in these disorders. Clinical correlations are extremely important in such cases.

34. Which neuropathologically distinct entities may be clinically indistinguishable from AD?
Pick's disease, vascular dementias (without plaques and tangles), Lewy body dementia, dementia lacking distinctive histology, and other frontal lobe dementia syndromes may be impossible to separate from AD on clinical grounds alone.

35. What is the clinical picture of "frontal lobe dementia"?
This designation includes a group of entities with variable neuropathologic findings and similar clinical features. Patients have early personality changes, particularly impulsivity and Klüver-Bucy type symptoms or withdrawal/depression. Psychiatric symptoms may precede dementia by several years. Memory and frontal executive tasks (e.g, planning,

set-shifting, set maintenance) are much more impaired than attention, language and visuospatial skills. SPECT studies may show hypofrontality. Neuropathology includes Pick's disease or primary degeneration at multiple brain sites (dementia lacking distinctive histology), usually with gliosis.

36. What is the cholinergic hypothesis?

This hypothesis attempts to explain many of the cognitive deficits seen in AD (particulary the memory disturbance) by a deficiency of cholinergic neurotransmission. Evidence includes the fact that poor memory can be induced in normal people by anticholinergic drugs. There is a loss of cholinergic projection neurons in the nucleus basalis of Meynert and a loss of choline acetyltransferase activity throughout the cortex of patients with AD, which correlate with the severity of memory loss.

37. Besides acetylcholine, which transmitters are affected by AD?

Norepinephrine, somatostatin, dopamine, serotonin, and neuropeptide Y are all decreased. Glutamate dysfunction may also play a role in AD.

Hefti F, Weiner WJ: Nerve growth factor and Alzheimer's disease. Ann Neurol 20:275–281, 1986.

38. What is the role of amyloid in AD?

Clearly there is abnormal accumulation of a breakdown product of the amyloid precursor protein known as beta-amyloid or A4 amyloid. Amyloid appears to be toxic to cells in vitro, and so the abnormal accumulation may actually cause cell loss. No one knows why the A4 amyloid accumulates in the first place, but this may be secondary to abnormal processing within neurons. Substance P may have a protective effect on amyloid toxicity.

Yanker B, Mesulam M-M: β-amyloid and the pathogenesis of Alzheimer's disease. N Engl J Med 325:1849–1857, 1991.

39. What is the role of tau protein in AD?

Tau protein is expressed in association with the cytoskeleton of neuronal cells. In damaged cells (e.g., after heat shock), its expression is increased. Tau appears to be increased in cells destined to develop neurofibrillary tangles. It may be an early marker of cells with abnormal cytoskeletal function and abnormal metabolism.

40. What possible role exists for nerve growth factor (NGF) in AD?

NGF is a trophic hormone that maintains the integrity of cholinergic neurons. A loss of NGF could contribute to the loss of such neurons in AD, and repletion could potentially improve the course or symptoms of the disease by preserving and enhancing the function of remaining cholinergic neurons.

41. What treatments exist for the secondary behavioral effects of AD?

Secondary behavioral effects, such as disturbed sleep, depression, anxiety, psychotic features, agitation and aggressiveness are amenable to treatment. Behavioral modification, such as entraining sleep-wake cycles and increasing daytime activity, should be tried first for sleep disorders, but mild hypnotics such as chloral hydrate may be useful.

Depression, particularly early in the disease, may respond to low doses of antidepressants, but drugs with anticholinergic side effects should be avoided. Drugs that act on the serotonergic system may be better (fluoxetine, trazodone), although controlled studies are lacking for this patient population.

Anxiety and agitation frequently respond to behavioral interventions, such as day center participation, which both engages the patient and reduces caregiver stress. Other respite interventions for caregivers may help to reduce patient stress. If infrequent, anxiety or agitation may be treated with low doses of anxiolytics as needed, such as chloral hydrate or lorazepam (avoid long-acting drugs).

Severe agitation, aggressiveness, and psychotic features that disturb the patient should be treated with neuroleptics, such as haloperidol or thioridazine in the lowest doses possible, as these drugs will further impair cognition (and sometimes motor performance). Psychotic features that do not disturb the patient or disrupt the household need not be treated.

42. What treatments exist for the primary process of AD?

There are currently no licensed treatments specifically for Alzheimer's disease. Experimental studies are under way with cholinesterase inhibitors, antioxidants, vasodilators, drugs that affect lipid metabolism, and growth factors. Many patients can qualify for these studies and should be referred to AD research centers that test medications if they are interested. Available drugs and sites can be identified by calling the National Alzheimer's Disease Association in Chicago, Illinois.

43. What is respite care?

Respite care means any caretaking arrangement for the patient that temporarily relieves the primary caregiver. It can be as informal as a friend or relative coming to the home to care for the patient, part-time in-home aid, or a few days per week at a day center. It could also apply to short-term stays in residential facilities.

44. What responsibilities do physicians and health-care workers have with respect to respite care?

The physician or health-care worker must introduce the concept of respite care and assure every primary caregiver that he or she will need this sooner or later. Many caregivers feel guilty about not being able to care alone for the patient every day and night. They need to know that this condition requires help in caregiving and that this is so for all affected families.

VASCULAR DEMENTIAS

45. What entities constitute the vascular dementias?

Vascular disease likely leads to dementia by several mechanisms:

1. Multiple large infarctions, which usually involve cortical and subcortical tissue, can cause dementia.

2. Multiple smaller infarctions, if they involve critical brain regions, can lead to dementia.

3. It is less clear whether diffuse, chronic vascular processes such as Binswanger's disease, leuko-araiosis, or diffuse changes in white matter due to microinfarcts also cause dementia.

Tatemichi TK: How acute brain failure becomes chronic: A view of the mechanisms of dementia related to stroke. Neurology 40:1652–1659, 1990.

O'Brian MD: Vascular dementia is underdiagnosed. Arch Neurol 45:797–798, 1988.

Brust J: Vascular dementia is overdiagnosed. Arch Neurol 45:799–801, 1988.

46. Can vascular dementia be diagnosed by CT or MRI alone?

No. Patients who have multiple strokes or changes in white matter on scans may be clinically normal. It is not known just how many infarcts or how much change in white matter on a scan translates into dementia for those who do suffer cognitive impairment. Patients with other forms of dementia, such as B12 deficiency, AD, or Parkinson's dementia may have scan changes that are unrelated to the dementing process.

47. Can dementia occur after a single stroke?

Two recent arguments support that it can. One prospective study of patients after acute stroke showed that the risk of dementia after a stroke was 9 to 10 times greater than for matched controls without a stroke.

Tatemichi TK, et al: Dementia after stroke: Baseline frequency, risks, and clinical features in a hospitalized cohort. Neurology 42:1185–1193, 1992.

Chui HC, et al: Criteria for the diagnosis of ischemic vascular dementia proposed by the State of California Alzheimer's Disease Diagnostic and Treatment Centers. Neurology 42:473–480, 1992.

48. What is the Hachinski ischemic score?

Originally the Hachinski score was a 13-item checklist (with each item scored 1 or 2 points if present) to distinguish multi-infarct vascular dementia from AD. The items associated with vascular dementia include:

1. Abrupt onset
2. Stepwise progression
3. Fluctuating course
4. Nocturnal confusion
5. Relative preservation of personality
6. Depression
7. Somatic complaints
8. Emotional incontinence
9. History of hypertension
10. History of strokes
11. Evidence of associated atherosclerosis
12. Focal neurologic symptoms
13. Focal neurologic signs

Scores of 7 or greater are associated with multi-infarct vascular dementia. Shorter versions have also been developed.

49. Can neuropsychological testing differentiate vascular dementia from AD?

Not absolutely. Patchy performances across tests, unilateral motor impairments (e.g., reaction times or finger tapping), and improvements in some but not all areas of cognition over time are typically seen in vascular dementias but not in AD.

50. What basic work-up should be done when vascular dementia is suspected?

The work-up should begin with imaging studies and psychometric testing in addition to the history and physical. In most cases, all of the tests recommended for the diagnosis of AD should be pursued to rule out additional conditions that may cause or contribute to the dementia, including a lipid profile. Some patients, especially those with clear-cut strokes, may benefit from imaging of the carotid arteries, especially when high-grade stenosis or ulcerated plaques are suspected. An echocardiogram is indicated if there is a cardiac history or the patient appears to have had embolic strokes.

51. What ancillary tests might be useful in diagnosing vascular dementia?

The EEG may show multiple slow wave foci, and SPECT or PET scans may show multiple areas of decreased flow or altered metabolism. These tests have not been adequately studied to assess their utility for differentiating the various forms of vascular dementia.

52. Can vascular dementia be diagnosed in patients with aphasia due to a left hemisphere infarct?

Patients should not be tested for dementia in the acute phase of their strokes, whether aphasic or otherwise. Although most tests for cognitive functioning rely heavily on language abilities, tests of nonverbal memory and reasoning can help to support the diagnosis of dementia in an aphasic patient. A history of functional decline not related to language-based tasks is also helpful.

53. What is the treatment of vascular dementia?

As for AD, secondary behavioral effects of dementia are amenable to therapy, and respite care should be introduced early. In addition, it is advisable to control vascular risk factors as much as possible (blood pressure, cholesterol, hypertension). Prophylactic antiplatelet therapy (aspirin or ticlopidine), although not conclusively of proven benefit, may be helpful.

SUBCORTICAL DEMENTIAS

54. What are the characteristics of subcortical dementias?
These dementias lack cortical features, such as aphasia, apraxia, and acalculia. Recall memory is impaired and is worse than recognition memory. Visuospatial skills are often impaired. Frontal executive deficits, bradyphrenia, anomia, personality changes, and psychomotor slowing are prominent. Dysarthria, abnormal posture and coordination, and adventitious movements *may* be present.
Cummings JL: Subcortical Dementia. New York, Oxford Press, 1990.

55. How do the general features of subcortical dementias differ from cortical dementias?
The cortical dementias, such as AD, usually involve language and calculations and may involve apraxia and cortical sensory disturbances (astereognosis, graphesthesia, etc.), whereas subcortical dementias do not. Both recall and recognition memory are usually impaired in cortical dementia, whereas recognition memory is relatively preserved in subcortical dementia. Frontal executive functions are lost in proportion to the overall dementia in cortical processes, but are especially prominently affected in subcortical dementia. Bradykinesia and bradyphrenia, as well as other motor features, are usually absent or late findings in the cortical dementias but occur early in subcortical dementias. Personality changes are variable in both types, but are said to be more prominent early in subcortical dementia.
Cummings JL: Subcortical Dementia. New York, Oxford Press, 1990.

56. In what ways do the specific memory disturbances of subcortical dementias differ from those of cortical dementias?
Problems with short-term spontaneous recall occur in both types, but strategies to enhance encoding and recognition cuing are mainly helpful in the subcortical dementias. Incidental memory (details not related to the task at hand, like what the examiner was wearing) is better in the subcortical dementias. Procedural memory (memory involved in learning tasks) is preserved more in the cortical dementias. Remote memory usually shows a temporal gradient in cortical dementias but not in subcortical dementias.
Cummings JL: Subcortical Dementia. New York, Oxford Press, 1990.

57. Is the distinction between cortical and subcortical dementia a rigid one anatomically? Is it functionally a clear distinction?
No, because so-called subcortical dementias can give rise to, or be associated with, cortical changes and vice versa. Huntington's dementia, like most subcortical dementias, causes disturbances of cortical frontal lobe functioning. Patients with Parkinson's disease may show atrophy of cortical cells. Patients with AD have subcortical changes in deep nuclei, such as the nucleus basalis of Meynert and locus ceruleus.

58. What disorders or clinical syndromes are associated with subcortical dementia?

Common Causes of Subcortical Dementia

1. Parkinson's disease	6. Lewy body disease
2. Huntington's disease	7. Multiple sclerosis
3. Progressive supranuclear palsy	8. Inflammatory conditions involving
4. Spinocerebellar degeneration	the basal ganglia and/or thalamus
5. Idiopathic basal ganglia calcification	9. AIDS

59. What are the clinical features of Parkinson's dementia?

Parkinsonian features sufficient to make a diagnosis of Parkinson's disease usually predate the dementia by at least 1 year. Typically bradyphrenia, dysnomia, and frontal executive dysfunction are present, and depression is common. There may be visuospatial abnormalities, especially upon formal testing.

60. What are the clinical features of Huntington's dementia?

Psychiatric symptoms and/or dementia may occur before or after the features of Huntington's disease (e.g., chorea) are well established. Psychiatric features include personality changes, depression, and psychosis. The memory disorder is typical of the subcortical pattern. Language and speech disorders, including dysarthria, reduced spontaneous speech, impaired syntactic complexity, and impaired comprehension, are common, as are visuospatial abnormalities.

61. What are the clinical features of the dementia associated with progressive supranuclear palsy (PSP)?

PSP is a syndrome characterized by supranuclear gaze palsy, dystonic rigidity of axial musculature, dysarthria, and pseudobulbar palsy. The dementia is not clearly present in all patients and is difficult to characterize because the associated visual scanning disorder interferes with testing. Memory impairments tend to be mild relative to frontal executive functions.

62. What is Lewy body disease?

A spectrum of disorders probably make up Lewy body disease, from Parkinson's disease (with Lewy bodies primarily in the subcortical and brainstem regions) to diffuse Lewy body disease, in which Lewy bodies are present throughout the cortex, subcortex, and brainstem. An intermediate form is Lewy body dementia (senile dementia of the Lewy body type), which is associated with many brainstem and subcortical Lewy bodies, lesser numbers in the hippocampus, and few neocortical Lewy bodies.

63. What are the clinical characteristics of Lewy body dementia?

Patients typically exhibit fluctuating confusion and dementia, often with visual hallucinations and mild extrapyramidal features. The neuropsychological deficits are not well characterized and little is known about the natural history of the disorder.

64. What are the clinical characteristics of diffuse Lewy body disease (DLBD)?

DLBD is not clearly differentiated from Lewy body dementia; it includes dementia, psychiatric features, and extrapyramidal dysfunction. The extrapyramidal symptoms may range from an isolated parkinsonian gait to the full spectrum of abnormalities seen in PSP. One study suggests a characteristic EEG pattern (posterior slowing with a frontally dominant burst pattern), although this has not been confirmed.

Crystal H, et al: Antemortem diagnosis of diffuse Lewy body disease. Neurology 40:1523–1528, 1990.

65. What other disorders are in the differential diagnosis of dementia (not necessarily subcortical) and extrapyramidal features?

Dementias with Extrapyramidal Features

1. Alzheimer's disease	8. Corticobasal ganglionic degeneration
2. Parkinson's disease plus dementia	9. AIDS dementia
3. Creutzfeldt-Jakob disease	10. Hallervorden-Spatz disease
4. Binswanger's disease	11. Neuronal intranuclear inclusion
5. Multi-infarct or vascular dementia	disease
6. Normal pressure hydrocephalus	12. GM1 gangliosidosis type III
7. Dementia lacking distinctive histology	13. Striatonigral degeneration

66. How do patients with corticobasal ganglionic degeneration (CBGD) present?
Patients tend to present either with an alien limb phenomenon with associated motor features (tremor, rigidity, grasp reflex, apraxia, myoclonus) or with an akinetic-rigid syndrome similar to Parkinson's disease. Dementia frequently develops over time and affects cognitive functions pervasively, although the specific deficits have not been well characterized.

Doody RS, Jankovic JJ: The alien hand and related signs. J Neurol Neurosurg Psychiatry 55:806–810, 1992.

BIBLIOGRAPHY

1. Adams RD, Victor M: Principles of Neurology, 4th ed. Hightstown, NJ, McGraw-Hill, 1989.
2. Cummings JL: Subcortical Dementia. New York, Oxford Press, 1990.
3. Rowland LP (ed): Merritt's Textbook of Neurology, 8th ed. Baltimore, Lea & Febiger, 1989.

14. APHASIA AND BEHAVIORAL NEUROLOGY

David B. Rosenfield, M.D.

LANGUAGE DISTURBANCES

1. What is the definition of aphasia?

Aphasia is an acquired disturbance of language. Someone who has been mentally retarded from birth and, in that setting, never developed normal language, is not considered to be aphasic.

2. What is the most common cause of aphasia in adults?

Vascular disease or trauma.

3. What is the difference between language, speech, and phonation?

Language is a set of symbols that are constrained in their interrelationship by perception, production, and central processing rules. Language consists of semantics (meaning of words), phonology (sound of words), and syntax (the rules of the grammer).

Speech is the neuromechanical process of the actual production of the sound, and it depends upon respiratory input, articulatory input, and phonation.

Phonation refers to sounds produced from the larynx.

4. What percentage of individuals are right-handed?

Over 90% of human beings state that they are right-handed. However, if one provides them a list of tasks, ranging from how one strikes a match to what hand is on top of a broom, 60% are strongly right-handed, 35% have a mixed hand preference.

5. What percentage of individuals are left-handed?

Less than 5% of individuals use their left hand for all skilled tasks.

6. What is the effect on aphasia of knowing more than one language?

If one is aphasic in one language, one is aphasic in all others. There might be some differences in the degree of aphasia, depending upon the language: variations have been found in tonal languages such as Thai and Japanese, and in some other languages such as Hebrew. Factors such as the age at which one acquired a language, whether more than one language was simultaneously acquired versus sequentially acquired, skill at both languages, and context of the acquisition when used (such as home or work or school), are all factors that influence the degree of aphasia.

7. What is the rule of Ribot?

Ribot contended that the language that one learns first is the one that is more "automatic" or "over-learned" and, consequently, better preserved if one is rendered aphasic.

8. What is Pitres' law?

Pitres contended that the language most recently learned and used is the one that is best preserved in aphasia. The discrepancy between Ribot's rule and Pitres' law has never been completely resolved.

9. What is the difference between nonfluent aphasia and fluent aphasia?

Aphasics who use short phrases (less than five words) and have a reduced grammatical form are considered to be nonfluent. Those who produce phrases longer than five words and have fairly normal grammatical output are considered to be fluent, although their language may be impaired in other ways. Thus, a nonfluent aphasic may say, "Where is book?" and a fluent aphasic may say, "Where is the paper of the cover?" Most nonfluent aphasics have deficits in articulation as well as in prosody (rhythm of speech). Most fluent aphasics have good articulation and prosody, but this is not always the case.

10. What are the clinical characteristics of nonfluent aphasia?
1. Impaired articulation
2. Impaired melodic production
3. Reduced phrase length (five or less words per phrase)
4. Decreased grammatical complexity

Sometimes patients do not have all of the elements of nonfluency. Thus, some may be nonfluent, partially fluent, or dysarthric.

11. What are the features of Broca's aphasia?

Features of Broca's Aphasia

1. Nonfluency	5. Paraphasic errors (semantic and phonemic)
2. Effortful initiation of speech production	6. Moderately good comprehension but difficulty understanding syntactically complex sentences
3. Poor repetition	
4. Poor ability to name	

Broca's aphasia is usually associated with right hemiparesis, hemisensory loss, buccofacial apraxia, and left limb ideomotor apraxia.

12. Where is the lesion that causes Broca's aphasia?
The lesion that causes Broca's aphasia usually involves the frontal operculum (Brodmann areas 45 and 44) and the deep frontal white matter, sparing the lower motor cortex and the middle paraventricular white matter. Some patients have compromise of the perirolandic cortex, especially in Brodmann's area 4. Still others have compromise in the perirolandic region with extensive subcortical white matter damage. Some contend that damage *only* to Broca's area in the cortex, without compromising surrounding tissue, does not even cause a true aphasia.

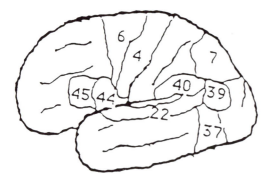

Diagram of the left cerebral cortex, showing the Brodmann's areas important for language function. (From Alexander MP, Benson DF: The aphasias and related disturbances. In Joynt RJ (ed): Clinical Neurology. Philadelphia, J.B. Lippincott, 1992, with permission.)

13. What are paraphasias? Describe the two types.
Paraphasias are substitutions for and within words.
1. A **semantic (verbal) paraphasia** is a substitution of one word for another ("cat" for "dog"). Often, pronouns or prepositions are changed.
2. **Phonemic (literal) paraphasia** is a substitution of one sound for another (e.g., "breen" for "green").

14. What is jargon aphasia?
Jargon aphasia is a fluent, paraphasic output with many phonemic substitutions in a sentence.

15. What are neologisms?
Neologisms are new words ("I am going to the tramechon"). Their use can be considered a type of paraphasia, or word substitution.

16. What is logorrhea?
Logorrhea, or a "press of speech," refers to fluent speech with far too many unnecessary words and frequent neologisms (new words that make no sense). This type of deficit is often seen in Wernicke's aphasia.

17. What are the features of Wernicke's aphasia?

Features of Wernicke's Aphasia

1. Fluent aphasic output	6. Phonemic and semantic paraphasias
2. Normal sentence length	7. Poor auditory and reading
3. Good articulation	comprehension
4. Good (sometimes exaggerated) prosody	8. Impaired repetition
5. Anomia	9. Fluent but empty writing

18. Where is the lesion that causes Wernicke's aphasia?
Classical Wernicke's aphasia usually indicates an extensive lesion of the posterosuperior temporal region, including the superior and middle temporal gyrus, the supramarginal-angular regions, and sometimes part of the laterotemporal-occipital junction. It can also be seen in subcortical lesions that block the inferior afferent signals to the temporal cortex by damaging the temporal isthmus.

19. What are the characteristics of conduction aphasia?

Characteristics of Conduction Aphasia

1. Fluent aphasia	5. Anomic
2. Good comprehension	6. Paraphasic errors
3. Poor repetition	7. Good recitation
4. Paragrammatic	8. Good reading aloud

Most paraphasic distortions are phonemic. Repetition and oral reading frequently exaggerate these errors. Conduction aphasia is usually associated with agraphia and some degree of limited reading comprehension.

20. Where is the lesion that is responsible for conduction aphasia?
The lesion usually involves the left inferior parietal lobule, especially the anterior supramarginal gyrus. Often, the lesion is in the subcortical white matter, deep to the inferior parietal cortex, affecting the arcuate fasciculus or the extreme capsule immediately below the arcuate fasciculus, both of which are connected to the temporal and frontal cortex.

21. What is word deafness?
Pure word deafness is a disturbance in which auditory comprehension is compromised, but there are no other disturbances of hearing. Patients are "deaf" only for words.

22. Describe the three types of pure word deafness.

1. Language is fluent, grammar may be normal or slightly abnormal, and speech is rather empty. Reading comprehension is normal or near normal. Writing is similar to speech. These patients frequently initially present with Wernicke's aphasia.

2. As above, but greater deficits in auditory perception. These patients fail to recognize many sounds (e.g., guitar, piano, bells chimes, buzz saw), and thus have auditory agnosia.

3. Patients have an impairment in sequencing a rapid array of sounds.

All three groups behave as though they they were deaf. All have better comprehension when the rate of speech is slowed, but all still have difficulty. Many have a questioning type of echolalia, repeating what the examiner says, but adding a pitch intonation that implies a question.

23. Where are the lesions for the three types of pure word deafness?

1. In the first group (see above), the lesion involves the left superior temporal gyrus, usually the anterior portion of the classic Wernicke's aphasia lesion. Often there is damage to the left auditory cortex and partial damage to connections with the posterosuperior temporal gyrus, presumably underlying the disordered auditory processing, mild anomia, and paraphasia. It is the sparing of the posterior temporal and parietal regions that accounts for the generally spared reading comprehension. Injuries are unilateral. Prognosis is good.

2. The second type occurs with bilateral superior temporal gyrus damage, at least in part, involving both auditory association cortices. If the lesions are extensive, the patient has cortical deafness. If the lesions are partial, the patient has reduced auditory comprehension.

3. The third type is associated with bilateral lesions, but the left lesion is usually restricted to the auditory cortex and auditory pathways with little, if any, involvement of the posterosuperior temporal gyrus.

24. What are the characteristics of aphemia?

Patients who are aphemic have a slow and halting articulation, altered prosody, and an almost dystonic quality of articulatory movements. Writing is usually normal. Their compromise is fairly modality-limited—the deficit is mainly in speech output, sparing comprehension and writing. When writing is compromised, it resembles speech in that the syntax is normal, although there may be mild anomia. These patients have a right facial paresis and sometimes have mild apraxia.

25. Where is the lesion that causes aphemia?

The location of the classic lesion causing aphemia is not known. When described as cortical dysarthria or cortical dysprosody, involvement has been noted in the white matter, deep to the lower motor cortex. Indeed, some contend that aphemias are a mild form of Broca's aphasia. Aphemia has been described with lesions of the lower motor cortex (cortical dysarthria, cortical dysprosody), subcortical white matter deep to the lower motor cortex (subcortical dysarthria), the middle superior paraventricular white matter, and genu of the internal capsule (capsular dysarthria, dysarthria-clumsy hand syndrome).

26. What are the characteristics of global aphasia?

1. Poor fluency
2. Poor comprehension
3. Poor repetition

The output is often restricted to meaningless speech sounds or stereotypes. Comprehension and repetition are severely compromised.

27. Where are the lesions that cause global aphasia?
These lesions concurrently involve Broca's area and Wernicke's area. They can be cortical-subcortical or purely subcortical.

28. What are the features of transcortical sensory aphasia?

Features of Transcortical Sensory Aphasia

1. Fluent output	5. Echolalia
2. Poor comprehension	6. Impaired auditory and reading comprehension
3. Good repetition	7. Motor and sensory deficits are seldom seen
4. Many phasic disturbances	8. Right visual field deficits are present

29. Where is the lesion that causes transcortical sensory aphasia?
These lesions usually involve the temporal parietal-occipital junction posterior to the superior temporal gyrus and overlapping with the posterior portions of Wernicke's area. Some investigators believe that compromise to Brodmann's area 37, the posteroinferior temporal gyrus, is the critical lesion.

30. What are the features of transcortical motor aphasia?

Features of Transcortical Motor Aphasia

1. Nonfluent	5. Brief utterances
2. Good comprehension	6. Semantic paraphasia
3. Good repetition	7. Echolalia
4. Delayed initiation of output	

These patients usually do not have impaired articulation or dysprosody of the classic nonfluent (e.g., Broca's aphasia); nor do they have the agrammatical speech output.

31. Where is the lesion that is responsible for transcortical motor aphasia?
These lesions have been associated just about anywhere in the left frontal lobe, from the operculum to the supplementary motor area.

32. What are the features of mixed transcortical aphsia?

Features of Mixed Transcortical Aphasia

1. Nonfluency	4. Stock phrases (e.g., "you know,"
2. Poor comprehension	"the thing is") and echolalia
3. Good repetition	are pronounced.

33. Where is the lesion that is responsible for mixed transcortical aphasia?
The lesion responsible for mixed transcortical aphasia overlaps lesions that cause transcortical motor aphasia and trancortical sensory aphasia: the dorsolateral frontal region anterior to the motor cortex, and the temporal-parietal-occipital junction. This syndrome frequently follows anoxia.

34. What are the characteristics of anomic aphasia?

Fluent output	Good repetition
Good comprehension	Word-finding deficits

The term "anomic aphasia" indicates that the word-finding deficit is the only significant impairment in spoken language. Output is fluent and grammar is good, although grammar may be better in some parts of the sentence than in others.

35. Where is the lesion that is responsible for anomic aphasia?
These lesions usually involve the temporal-parietal-occipital junction association cortex, Brodmann's area 37, 39, 40, 19, or 7.

36. What is a useful algorithm for classifying the cortical aphasias?

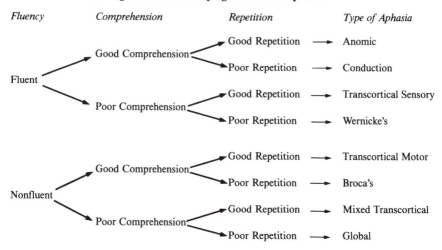

Fluency	Comprehension	Repetition	Type of Aphasia

37. What are the characteristics of subcortical aphasias?
Subcortical aphasias are a set of syndromes that have been recently defined in patients whose lesions are primarily restricted to subcortical regions, such as basal ganglia and the deep white matter pathways. The justification for this nosology is that heretofore neurologists presumed that only cortical lesions were responsible for aphasic syndromes. However, it is a mistake to view aphasia based strictly upon the anatomy, as opposed to the clinical deficit. There are two main types of subcortical aphasia: one due to nonthalamic subcortical lesions and the other due to thalamic lesions.

38. What are the nonthalamic subcortical aphasias?
Nonthalamic subcortical aphasics have mixed fluency, good comprehension, and good repetition. Output is terse and poorly elaborated, but sentence structure is fairly correct. A speech motor deficit (articulation/prosody) usually exists. Comprehension is fairly good for simple tasks but patients have difficulty with more complex syntax. The lesion causing this syndrome involves deep capsular-striatal and mid-paraventricular white matter, with little or no extension into the frontal or temporal white matter. It is unclear whether there needs to be associated damage to the basal ganglia. Most patients also have concurrent damage to the descending dominant hemispheric corticobulbar pathways.

39. What are the thalamic subcortical aphasias?
There are different types of thalamic aphasia. Lesions in the posterior left thalamus produce no definite language impairment. Lesions in the left paramedial thalamic area, including the dorsum medial and centromedian nuclei, as well as the medial intramedullary laminar, produce deficits in attention and memory. When language is compromised, the compromise is limited to anomia; the impairments are probably due to lack of attention. Patients with bilateral paramedian lesions have amnesia and a broader cognitive deficit, mainly due to inattention. These patients can appear grossly normal, but damage to the paramedian mesencephalic area usually produces ocular motor abnormalities (compromise in vertical gaze, partial or complete third nerve damage), intention tremor, or weakness.

Lesions in the anterolateral thalamus cause more specific language compromise. Lesions involving the anterior, ventroanterior, dorsal lateral, ventral lateral, and anterior dorsal medial nuclei or the anterior medial intramedullary region produce an aphasia similar to mixed transcortical or transcortical sensory output. Output is grammatic but terse, with some elements of echolalia. Comprehension is impaired and repetition is fairly good. Severe anomia, agraphia, and impaired reading are usually present, as is right-sided hypokinesia, decreased emotional and facial involvement, and hypophonia. Most patients are apathetic and some are demented.

40. How is aphasia in childhood different from aphasia in adulthood?
Most childhood aphasics are nonfluent. Up until the age of 6 or 7 years, the main fundamentals of phonology, phonemics, lexicon (dictionary of words in our brain), semantics, grammar, syntax, writing, and reading are in the process of being acquired. Brain damage at this time disrupts their acquisition and decreases their capacity. Brain injury during early infancy usually does not cause major compromise in language, although some compromise does occur. Injury after the age of 1 year causes aphasia if the injury is in the dominant hemisphere but not in the nondominant hemisphere. Between the ages of 2 and 9 years, an atypical aphasia profile will occur. Fluent aphasia is rare, even with posterior left hemisphere compromise. After the age of 10, the aphasia profiles are increasingly adult-like.

Recovery is more complete in children than in adults, especially up to the ages of 8–10 years.

41. What is the most common cause of childhood aphasia?
Vascular disease or trauma.

42. What is alexia?
Alexia is the disordered comprehension of written language, i.e., difficulty reading.

43. What is dyslexia?
Alexia is the term commonly used in the United States to describe altered reading comprehension. However, in some countries, the term dyslexia is preferred. In the U.S., however, the term dyslexia generally denotes identified developmental inability to learn to read, either due to inborn deficits or perinatal injury. Alexia refers only to an acquired loss.

44. What are the three different types of alexia?
1. **Posterior alexia**, also known as pure alexia as well as alexia without agraphia, is characterized by inability to read but intact ability to write. These patients cannot read what they have written. Approximately 60% have an associated color anomia. If one spells a word to them, they can usually understand what the word is. They can spell aloud themselves. Usually, a right homonymous visual field deficit is present.

2. **Central alexia** is alexia with agraphia. These patients can neither read nor write. They can comprehend spoken language much better than written language, but cannot recognize words that are spelled aloud. They can neither spell aloud nor produce written language.

3. **Anterior alexia** usually accompanies classic Broca's aphasia. Patients cannot comprehend grammatically significant relational words, such as prepositions or articles. They may comprehend written substantive words. They often fail to read aloud individual letters (literal alexia) but they may read a word that is a homophone for the latter (e.g., "see" for "sea"). Anterior alexia is associated with anterior language compromise, usually Broca's aphasia.

45. Where are the lesions that produce the different types of alexia?
    1. **Posterior alexia.** The lesion usually involves the medial aspect of the dominant occipital lobe as well as to the splenium of the corpus callosum.
    2. **Central alexia.** The lesion involves the dominant angular gyrus.
    3. **Anterior alexia.** The lesion is similar in location to that causing Broca's aphasia.

46. What is agraphia?
Agraphia is compromised production of written language, i.e., difficulty writing.

47. What are the clinical features of Gerstmann's syndrome?
- Acalculia
- Agraphia
- Right/left discrimination
- Finger agnosia

48. Where is the lesion that is responsible for Gerstmann's syndrome?
The dominant angular gyrus.

AGNOSIAS

49. What is agnosia?
Agnosia is the inability to recognize objects despite adequate perception in the modality (e.g., visual, tactile, auditory) in which the object is presented.

50. What are two types of visual agnosia?
    1. **Apperceptive agnosia** is characterized by good acuity, good perception of movement, and good ability to perceive color. Yet the perception of the form is poor and patients complain of poor vision. They are unable to draw objects or copy pictures. They cannot distinguish different shapes. Although they cannot name objects, they can name colors.
    2. **Associative visual agnosia** is not accompanied by complaints of poor vision. Patients can draw, copy, and distinguish shapes. They do not describe the object, circumlocute, gesture, or mimic the use, and can neither recognize nor name the object. Patients with associative visual agnosia cannot recognize objects through vision alone.

51. Pinpoint the location of the lesions responsible for visual agnosia.
Apperceptive visual agnosia usually results from compromise in the calcarine cortex. Patients with associative visual agnosia usually have bilateral, inferior, temporal-occipital lesions that involve the inferior visual association cortex and the white matter pathways into the parahippocampal gyrus. These patients usually have bilateral upper visual field compromise, mild general anomia, severe alexia, and memory impairment.

52. What is prosopagnosia?
Prosopagnosia is the inability to recognize familiar faces. It is frequently associated with achromatopsia or agraphia, and is always associated with unilateral or bilateral visual field deficits.

53. Where is the lesion that is responsible for prosopagnosia?
Prosopagnosia is associated with bilateral occipital-temporal lesions.

54. What is anosognosia?
Anosognosia refers to denial of illness. There are two types. One type is a verbal, explicit denial of illness; the other type is lack of concern regarding the deficit.

55. In which four different behavioral syndromes can anosognosia occur?
Wernicke's aphasia, Anton's syndrome, left hemianopsia, and left hemiplegia. Also, it may occur in patients with Korsakoff's syndrome or with frontal lobe dysfunction.

Behavioral Syndromes Associated with Anosognia

1. Wernicke's aphasia	4. Left hemianopsia
2. Anton's syndrome	5. Left hemiplegia
3. Korsakoff's syndrome	6. Frontal lobe dysfunction

56. What is Anton's syndrome?
It is a syndrome of cortical blindness in which patients deny being blind and confabulate responses when confronted with their errors, making excuses. They may have simple or complex visual hallucinations. The syndrome is usually associated with bilateral cerebral infarcts in the distributions of the posterior cerebral arteries that involve the primary visual areas of the calcarine cortex (Brodmann's area 17) and visual association areas. Parietal and temporal lobes are sometimes injured.

APRAXIAS

57. What is apraxia?
Apraxia is the inability to perform a skilled, learned, purposeful motor act in the absence of a primary disturbance in attention, comprehension, motivation, power, tone, coordination, or sensation that would preclude that act. Individuals must be able to perform the act spontaneously. Thus, an individual might not be able to wave goodbye when so instructed, but can wave goodbye when he spontaneously chooses to do so.

58. What are the three major types of apraxia?
   1. **Motor apraxia** represents a breakdown in the smooth execution of a movement despite preservation of the intended motor pattern. The performance is not affected by the modality of request (e.g., spoken or written). The disturbance is purely one of output.
   2. **Ideomotor apraxia** is the inability to carry out a learned motor pattern to a stimulus that should elicit it (verbal command or gesture for imitation). The errors are usually perseverations or crude undifferentiated movements.
   3. **Ideational apraxia** is due to consternation about how to carry out a movement, but once the patient has been cued, he or she produces the correct response. These patients fail to use everyday objects correctly.

59. Where are the lesions that are responsible for apraxias?
   1. **Motor apraxia** usually results from damage to the motor association cortex, contralateral to the affected limb.
   2. **Ideomotor apraxia** is often associated with large parietal lesions, especially involving the inferior part of the parietal lobe. Large lesions may be deep in the periolandic region, compromising the deep parietal-frontal connections and/or input to the callosal pathways.
   3. **Ideational apraxia** often involves compromise in the dominant parietal lobe, but this has not been well delineated.

60. What is buccofacial apraxia?
Buccofacial apraxia, a type of ideomotor apraxia, usually indicates damage to the frontal operculum in the lower motor cortex, extending deeply into the frontal periventricular white matter. Large striatal capsular periventricular lesions without a cortical lesion can produce buccofacial ideomotor apraxia. Patients with parietal lesions can have transient buccofacial apraxia.

61. What is dressing apraxia?
Dressing apraxia is not a true apraxia. It is an inability to dress that is often associated with left visual field deficits and topographic disorientation. Lesions in the right parietal-occipital-temporal region cause problems with complex perceptual-spatial actions, including dressing. Another problem arising from this region is hemineglect, in which one-half of the body is neither clothed nor groomed. Again, these problems are not true apraxias.

62. What is constructional apraxia?
Constructional apraxia is also a misnomer. Patients have difficulty in copying figures, but this does not imply apraxia. It is also associated with right parietal lobe lesions.

63. What is apraxia of speech?
Apraxia of speech is a controversial term. In its classic concept, it is characterized by articulatory imprecision that worsens with increased phonetic complexity. However, it is not a true apraxia. All of these patients have some deficit in comprehension. The disturbance is thought to represent an interaction of the phonologic errors due to paresis and ataxia of the articulatory system and of phonemic errors due to damage anywhere in the functional system for phonemic production (upper temporal gyrus to the lower motor cortex).

BIBLIOGRAPHY

1. Alexander MP, Benson DF: The aphasias and related disturbances. In Joynt RJ (ed): Clinical Neurology, Vol. 1. Philadelphia, J.B. Lippincott, 1991.
2. Geschwind N: Disconnexion syndromes in animal and man. Brain 88:237, 1965.
3. Mesulam M-M: Principles of Behavioral Neurology. Philadelphia, F.A. Davis, 1985.
4. Rosenfield DB, Barroso AO: Dysarthria, dysfluency, and dysphagia. In Bradley WG, et al (eds): Neurology and Clinical Practice. Boston, Butterworth-Heinemann, 1991.

15. DYSARTHRIA, DYSFLUENCY, AND DYSPHAGIA

David B. Rosenfield, M.D.

DYSARTHRIA

1. Which parts of the brain are involved in speech motor output?

Human speech production involves coordination between respiration, laryngeal activity, and supralaryngeal articulatory movement. The lower motoneurons that control the respiratory movements reside in the anterior portion of the cervical, thoracic, and upper lumbar spinal cord. Motoneurons controlling laryngeal closure reside in the nucleus ambiguus. Neurons directly responsible for the supralaryngeal musculature are the trigeminal motor nucleus, facial nucleus, rostral portion of the nucleus ambiguus, hypoglossal nucleus, and the anterior horn cells at the rostral portion of the cervical spinal cord. These lower motor neurons, and the bilateral inputs from multiple realms (including motor cortex) of both hemispheres to them, constitute the underlying neural input of speech motor production.

2. What is dysphonia?

Dysphonia is an abnormality in phonation (sound output from the larynx).

3. What is the difference between speech compromise and language compromise?

Speech, *a priori*, is motor output. **Speech compromise** is a deficiency in the way speech sounds. It refers to the underlying motor component. **Language compromise** involves errors in syntax, word choice, or how sounds are put together. Talking with food in one's mouth causes speech compromise. An aphasic has acquired language compromise.

4. What is dysarthria?

Dysarthria, although implying a problem of articulation only, is a defect in phonation as well as resonance. Phonation is sound production (from larynx). Resonance is how the sounds are altered in the cavity between the larynx and vocal fold, and the lips/nares (e.g., hyponasal, hypernasal).

5. What are the causes of dysarthria?

Dysarthria can be due to compromise of the brain, brain stem, cerebellum, nerve, neuromuscular junction, or muscle. All diseases that affect these regions, considerable in nature, can cause dysarthria, particularly myopathy, myositis, myasthenia gravis, the neuropathies, motor neuron disease, cerebellar disease, tumors of the brain and brainstem, Parkinson's disease, and various other movement disorders.

6. What determines prognosis in dysarthria when it is caused by damage to the cerebral hemispheres?

Patients with damage in only one hemisphere have a much better prognosis for dysarthria than do patients with damage in both hemispheres.

7. Where can the brain be stimulated during ongoing speech to cause speech arrest?

In right-handed individuals, just about anywhere in the left hemisphere and in the area of the motor strip on the right. Stimulation of the supplementary motor area, bilaterally, induces speech arrest.

8. What happens when Broca's area is electrically stimulated?
If Broca's area is stimulated while someone is talking, the person stops talking. If it is stimulated while a person is not talking, a grunted sound is elicited.

9. What happens when Wernicke's area is electrically stimulated?
If Wernicke's area is electrically stimulated while someone is talking, the person stops talking. If this area is stimulated during silence, a sound may be elicited but not a sentence or word output.

10. What is the Wada test?
The Wada test involves the injection of a short-acting barbiturate into the carotid artery of one hemisphere to render the patient plegic, numb, and blind on the side opposite the injection. If language "resides" on the side being injected, the patient also becomes aphasic. The test is named after Dr. Jun Wada.

11. How does the Wada test relate to handedness?
There is a very good correlation. Over 95% of persons who become aphasic when only one particular hemisphere is injected during the Wada test have handedness pertaining to dominance of that hemisphere.

12. List common brain/brainstem causes of dysarthria.
Structural compromise of the corticobulbar tracts (unilaterally or bilaterally) or cranial nerve nuclei V, VII, X, or XII can cause dysarthria. The common diseases that cause this compromise are stroke, tumor, demyelinating disease, motor neuron disease, and collagen disease.

13. What are the speech signs in Parkinson's disease?
Phonation is weak, pitch varies little, volume is low, and the patient is hoarse. Accelerated rate, repetitive dysfluencies, and imprecise consonants may occur.

14. What are the speech signs in hyperkinetic dysarthria–chorea?
Sudden alterations in pitch and loudness, phonatory arrest, strained harshness, and sudden alterations in precision of vowels and consonants.

15. What are the speech signs in hyperkinetic dysarthria–dystonia?
Slow alterations in pitch and loudness, phonatory arrest, strained harshness, and slow alterations in consonant/vowel precision.

16. What are the speech signs in hyperkinetic dysarthria-palatal-pharyngeal-laryngeal myoclonus?
Rhythmic contractions of intrinsic-extrinsic pharyngeal muscles (1 to 4 per second), rhythmic contractions of palate (1 to 4 per second), and normal or imprecise vowels/consonants.

17. What are the speech signs in hyperkinetic dysarthria–phonatory tremor?
Rhythmic alterations in pitch and loudness, adductor phonatory arrests, and compensatory strain or strangle.

18. What are the speech signs in hyperkinetic dysarthria–Gilles de la Tourette syndrome?
Grunts, barks, squeaks, throat clearing, gurgling, moaning, snorting, sniffing, whistling, clicking, lip smacking, spitting, unintelligible sounds, echolalia, coprolalia, and dysfluencies.

19. What are the speech signs in cerebellar disease?
Phonation may have associated tremor with variations in loudness. Irregular articulatory breakdown, imprecise consonants, and sometimes excessive and equal stress in all syllables of words are present.

20. List the nerve-damage causes of dysarthria.
Collagen disease, viral infection, diabetes, and alcohol.

21. What are the speech signs in motor neuron disease?
Phonation is strained, harsh, wet, and sometimes fluttering during vowel prolongation. Speech is hypernasal. Articulation is slow, consonants are imprecise, phrases are short, and vowels are distorted.

22. What is the effect of a Vth nerve (trigeminal) lesion on speech output?
Phonation and velopharyngeal function are normal, mandibular muscles are weak, and vowels and consonants are imprecise.

23. How does a lesion of the VIIth nerve (facial) affect speech?
Phonation and velopharyngeal function are normal, the orbicularis oris is weak (causing difficulty producing /p/ sounds), vowels are imprecise, and labial consonants are imprecise.

24. How does a Xth nerve (vagus) lesion affect speech?
Phonation is hoarse and breathy, and volume is low. Speech is hypernasal if the lesion is above the pharyngeal branch.

25. What is the effect of a XIIth nerve (hypoglossal) lesion on speech?
Phonation and velopharyngeal function are normal. The tongue is weak, demonstrating atrophy and fasciculation. The patient may have drooling, imprecise vowels, and imprecise lingual consonants.

26. What are the muscles that adduct the vocal folds?
Thyroarytenoid, interarytenoid, lateral cricothyroid, and lateral cricoarytenoid.

27. Which muscles adduct the vocal folds?
Posterior cricoarytenoid.

28. Which nerves innervate which muscles in the larynx?
All of the muscles in the larynx are innervated by branches from the recurrent laryngeal nerve.

29. What are the causes of recurrent laryngeal nerve paralysis?

Causes of Recurrent Laryngeal Nerve Paralysis

1. Inflammation (viral disease, collagen disease, pulmonary tuberculosis, coccidioidomycosis)
2. Polyneuropathy (especially diabetes and alcohol)
3. Trauma (intubation, neck trauma, head trauma, mediastinoscopy, radical neck dissection, carotid endarterectomy, cardiovascular surgery, thyroidectomy, esophageal resection for carcinoma)
4. Neoplasm
5. Syringomyelia
6. Idiopathic

30. List the causes of bilateral abductor vocal cord paralysis in adults.

Causes of Bilateral Abductor Vocal Cord Paralysis

1. Thyroidectomy	6. Demyelinating disease
2. Neck malignancy	7. Central nervous system neoplasm
3. Poliomyelitis	8. Central nervous system infection
4. Brainstem stroke	9. Charcot-Marie-Tooth disease
5. Guillain-Barré syndrome	

Rare causes: foreign bodies near the larynx, bilateral carotid dissection, neck infection, head or neck trauma, substernal thyroid, idiopathic.

31. How does myasthenia affect speech?
Its effects are similar to those of a myopathy, but the speech improves with rest.

32. What is the effect of myopathy/myositis on speech output?
Phonatory output is hoarse, breathy, and diplophonic, and has low volume. The speech is hypernasal and vowels and consonants might be compromised, depending on the muscles involved.

33. Name four muscle disturbances that can cause dysarthria.
Collagen disease, polymyositis, dermatomyositis, hypothyroidism.

34. Define spasmodic dysphonia.
Spasmodic dysphonia is effortful, strained speech that is associated with a sensation of strain and strangle.

35. What is the most common presentation of spasmodic dysphonia?
Strain in the throat, interruption of sound while talking, and difficulty in getting words out, but with no evidence of associated aphasia.

36. What are the neurologic causes of spasmodic dysphonia?
Laryngeal tremor, laryngeal dystonia, and other movement disorders involving the laryngeal neuromotor system. It can also be a symptom of psychiatric disease.

37. What is the prognosis in spasmodic dysphonia?
When there is associated tremor, the prognosis is fairly good with therapy. Many individuals contend that these patients do fairly well with speech therapy; others opt more strongly for various medications, including botulinum toxin injections.

DYSFLUENCY

38. What are the prevalence and characteristics of developmental stuttering?
Developmental stuttering is much more common among males than females (ratio of 4:1). Some argue that everyone stutters, some for just a few minutes or a few hours. The prevalence of stuttering in childhood is 4%, and in adulthood slightly over 1%. Developmental stutterers stutter at the beginning of sentences and phrases, are more fluent when their speech is markedly slowed and drawn out, and do not stutter when they sing. Other fluency-evoking maneuvers include repetitive reading, choral reading, and having loud, broad-band noise to interfere with the hearing of one's own speech. Developmental stutterers are emotionally bothered by their dysfluent output.

39. What are the characteristics of acquired stuttering?

Acquired stutterers have repetitive dysfluencies scattered throughout their sentences, are minimally distraught over their abnormal output, and usually still stutter during fluency-evoking maneuvers (such as singing).

40. Describe the characteristics of cluttering.

The clutterer's speech is characterized by excessive speed, repetitions, interjections, disturbed prosody, and sometimes inconsistent articulatory disturbances. Some contend that these patients have errors in grammar, are hyperactive, and have poor concentration. Although their rate of speech may not always be markedly increased, the listener usually has the sensation that it is. As opposed to developmental stutterers, clutterers frequently are unconcerned about their speech deficit.

41. What are the characteristics of palilalia?

Palilalics compulsively repeat phrases or words with reiteration at increasing speed and with a decrescendo volume.

42. Which diseases are associated with palilalia?

Postencephalitic Parkinson's disease, idiopathic Parkinson's disease, and pseudobulbar palsy.

DYSPHAGIA

43. What is dysphagia?

Dysphagia, or difficulty in swallowing, is a subjective symptom, as opposed to an objective sign, until there is documentation of delay or disruption in the swallowing mechanism. If no objective evidence of dysphagia can be documented, globus hystericus should be considered. Dysphagia may be due to mechanical factors that physically narrow the oropharyngeal lumen and obstruct food passage, or to neuromotor diseases that cause inadequate food bolus propulsion into the stomach.

44. List the three stages of swallowing.

1. Oropreparatory (food passes from mouth into pharynx).
2. Pharyngeal transfer stage (food passes through the pharynx, over the larynx, and into the esophagus).
3. Esophageal stage (food is transported from proximal esophagus, the upper one-third of which contains striated muscle, down to the lower two-thirds, which consists of smooth muscle, across the lower esophageal sphincter, and into the stomach).

45. What is the swallow reflex?

The swallow reflex mediates the first stage of swallowing into the second. It consists of several movements. The soft palate moves upward (velar elevation), closing the passageway between the oral and nasal cavity; the pharyngeal muscles contract (pharyngeal peristalsis), the larynx elevates, and posterior flexion of the epiglottis closes the airway to the trachea. Vocal cord closure occurs, followed by relaxation of the cricopharyngeus muscle, the upper esophageal sphincter.

46. What is the role of the vagus nerve in swallowing?

The vagus nerve supplies motor fibers to the striated muscle of the esophagus. Thus, a serious consequence of damaging the vagus at the origin of the main esophageal branch is dysphagia. A high vagotomy permanently paralyzes the striated muscle at the upper one-third of the esophagus. Peristalsis in the lower two-thirds of the esophagus is an automatic function, mediated by the intrinsic myoenteric plexuses and smooth muscle.

47. Are there different types of dysphagia?

Dysphagia may be due to mechanical problems or neuromotor problems. Each of these realms has an oropharyngeal component and an esophageal component.

48. What are the symptoms of oropharyngeal dysphagia?

The symptoms typically occur immediately upon swallowing and include the sensation of food sticking in the neck, pain while swallowing, nasal regurgitation of food or fluids, and coughing and choking due to aspiration. Discomfort in the mid-neck area may be present.

49. List the causes of oropharyngeal neuromotor dysphagia.

Causes of Oropharyngeal Neuromotor Dysphagia

1. Motor neuron disease	9. Myopathy (including oculopharyngeal
2. Brain tumor	muscular dystrophy, hypothyroidism,
3. Stroke	polymyositis, dermatomyositis)
4. Neuropathy (includes mechanical	10. Parkinson's disease
nerve injury)	11. Cerebral palsy
5. Demyelinating disease	12. Tardive dyskinesia
6. Degenerative disease (especially	13. Cricopharyngeal achalasia
spinocerebellar)	14. Xerostomia (dry mouth)
7. Syringobulbia	15. Sjogren's syndrome
8. Myasthenia gravis	16. Scleroderma

50. What are the causes of oropharyngeal mechanical dysphagia?

Causes of Oropharyngeal Mechanical Dysphagia

1. Oropharyngeal tumor	6. Congenital abnormalities
2. Zenker's diverticulum	7. Tight circumoral tissue due to
3. Cervical osteophytes	scleroderma/burns
4. Dislocation of temporomandibular	8. Neck surgery
joint	9. Retropharyngeal mass
5. Macroglossia	10. Large goiter

51. What are the symptoms of mechanical dysphagia?

Symptoms related to mechanical (oropharyngeal, oroesophageal) dysphagia are usually caused by difficulty in swallowing solid foods, progressing to difficulty in swallowing liquids. When advanced, patients cannot even swallow their own salivary secretions. Symptoms can occur immediately, seconds, or minutes after swallowing, depending on the level and chronicity of the underlying process. More rostral levels of dysfunction cause earlier symptoms.

52. What causes esophageal neuromotor dysphagia?

Causes of Esophageal Neuromotor Dysphagia

1. Scleroderma	6. Postvagotomy dysphagia
2. Achalasia	7. Neuropathy (vagal disease,
3. Diffuse esophageal spasm	especially diabetes)
4. Polymyositis and dermatomyositis	8. Amyloidoses (primary or secondary)
(usually oropharyngeal)	9. Symptomatic esophageal peristalsis
5. Idiopathic autonomic dysfunction	(nutcracker esophagus)

53. List the causes of esophageal mechanical dysphagia.

Causes of Esophageal Mechanical Dysphagia

1. Esophageal carcinoma	8. Postvagotomy hematoma/fibrosis
2. Metastases to esophagus	9. Thoracic aorta aneurysm
3. Benign esophageal tumor	10. Posterior mediastinal mass
4. Inflammation	11. Large hiatal hernia
5. Strictures of the esophagus	12. Dysphagia lusoria (abnormal
6. Pancreatitis with pseudocysts	origin of the right subclavian
7. Pancreatic tumors	artery)

BIBLIOGRAPHY

1. Alexander MP, Benson DF: The aphasia and related disturbances. In Joynt RJ (ed): Clinical Neurology, Vol. 1. Philadelphia, J.B. Lippincott, 1991.
2. Rosenfield DB, Barroso AO: Dysarthria, dysfluency, and dysphagia. In Bradley WG, Daroff RB, Fenichal GM, Marsten CD (eds): Neurology and Clinical Practice. Boston, Butterworth-Heinemann, 1991.

16. VASCULAR DISEASE

John P. Winikates, M.D.

CLINICAL FEATURES

1. What is a stroke?

A stroke is a focal neurologic deficit caused by a disruption of the cerebral circulation. Stroke is a clinical syndrome, like fever or heart failure, with multiple potential causes— chiefly thrombosis, embolism, and hemorrhage. As such, it should be considered a symptom with an underlying etiologic diagnosis, not a diagnosis in itself.

2. How common is stroke?

Stroke is the most common serious neurologic condition in clinical practice. It is the third leading cause of death throughout the industrialized world, after heart disease and cancer. In the United States, about 400,000 strokes occur annually, with about 150,000 deaths. Stroke is also the leading cause of serious neurologic handicap in clinical practice.

3. What is the most common presenting symptom of stroke?

About 70% of strokes present with hemiparesis; another 20% present with aphasia.

4. What are the principal stroke types?

There are four major stroke types: thrombotic, embolic, lacunar, and hemorrhagic.

5. What is the clinical profile of a thrombotic stroke?

The commonly recognized clinical profile of a thrombotic stroke is a gradual, stuttering, or stepwise progression. Thrombotic strokes often occur during sleep, so that the patient awakens with the deficit. This type of stroke is commonly thought to result from in situ thrombosis in an intracranial vessel affected by atherosclerosis. Carotid distribution strokes are generally included in this category, although these strokes (and transient ischemic attacks) are more likely due to artery-to-artery embolism of atherosclerotic material, thrombus, or platelet-fibrin thrombus.

6. What is the clinical profile of an embolic stroke?

The embolic stroke has a sudden onset, often during usual daily activity. The deficit is generally maximal at onset, often with improvement shortly afterward as the embolus breaks up and portions travel farther out into more distal branches of the affected artery. The heart is the generally recognized source of such emboli. Onset may be associated with palpitations, initiation of a cardiac arrhythmia such as atrial fibrillation, or following a Valsalva maneuver, such as during lifting a heavy object or voiding.

7. What is the clinical profile of a lacunar stroke?

There are four classic lacunar stroke syndromes: (1) pure motor hemiparesis, with face, arm, and leg equally affected, (2) pure hemisensory stroke, (3) clumsy hand–dysarthria, in which there is significant disuse of the affected arm out of proportion to the amount of weakness evident, and (4) ataxia with crural paresis. Other lacunar stroke syndromes have been described, but these four are the most widely recognized. Lacunar strokes are associated with hypertension and are thought to result from occlusion of small perforating arterioles as a result of lipohyalinosis of the arterial wall due to hypertension, tortuosity or kinking of the artery, or possibly thrombosis on a substrate of such arterial pathology.

8. What is the clinical profile of a hemorrhagic stroke?

Hemorrhagic strokes are characterized by a deficit that may not be clearly distinguishable as cortical or subcortical, along with a prominent decrease in consciousness early in the course. Fluctuation of mental status is a common feature. Hypertension often occurs, sometimes with bradycardia (the Cushing reflex) or other signs of raised intracranial pressure. Hemorrhagic strokes can result from ruptured cerebral aneurysms with subarachnoid hemorrhage, ruptured arterial venous malformations, or congophilic angiopathy.

9. What percentage of strokes can be attributed to each type?

Types of Strokes

TYPE	% OF ALL STROKES	ONSET	PRECEDING TIAs (%)	ALTERED MENTAL STATUS (%)	MRI OR CT SCAN	OTHER FEATURES
Thrombotic	40	May be gradual	50	5	Ischemic infarction	Carotid bruit stroke during sleep
Embolic	30	Sudden	10	1	Superficial (cortical) infarction	Underlying heart disease, peripheral emboli, or strokes in different vascular territories
Lacunar	20	May be gradual	30	0	Small, deep infarction	Pure motor or pure sensory stroke
Hemorrhagic	10	Sudden	5	25	Hyperdense mass	Nausea and vomiting, decreased mental status

10. What are the main anatomic syndromes in cerebrovascular disease?

The first distinction to make is whether the anterior or posterior circulation is involved. The internal carotid artery supplies the frontal lobes, parietal lobes, most of the temporal lobes, the basal ganglia, and the internal capsule. This is the anterior circulation. The vertebral basilar system supplies the brainstem, thalamus, occipital lobes, and mesial and inferior temporal lobes. This is the posterior circulation.

11. What are the major symptoms of a vascular event affecting the anterior circulation?

Hemiparesis and aphasia are the major symptoms and suggest involvement of the internal carotid artery and its branches. Hemiparesis may be due to either cortical or subcortical ischemia. A pattern of hemiparesis involving the face and arm more than the leg implies cortical localization; when the face, arm, and leg are equally involved, subcortical localization in the internal capsule is more likely.

Other specific signs may also indicate either cortical or subcortical localization. Aphasia, apraxia, and seizures are usually cortical abnormalities. A visual field defect suggests subcortical involvement of the optic radiations. Evaluating the patient for such associated signs may help to clarify clinically (before scanning the patient) whether the lesion will be cortical or subcortical.

12. What are the signs suggesting posterior circulation localization?

Brainstem findings suggest a posterior circulation problem involving the vertebrobasilar system and its branches. These can be summarized as "the four D's with crossed findings." The four D's are diplopia, dysarthria, dysphagia, and dizziness/vertigo. Of these, dizziness is the least specific but the most common. Unless vertigo is combined with other brainstem findings (another of the four D's), it is difficult to attribute it to ischemia. The other main category of posterior circulation symptoms is crossed findings: facial weakness or numbness combined with contralateral extremity weakness or numbness. This pattern stems from involvement of brainstem structures below the crossing of facial fibers but above the decussation of the pyramids or sensory fibers.

13. What are the most important causes of stroke in the anterior circulation?
The most important etiologic possibilities are internal carotid stenosis, cardiac embolism, atherothrombotic disease of the major intracranial branches (especially the middle cerebral artery), and small vessel disease of the penetrating arteries.

14. What are the most important causes of stroke in the posterior circulation?
Posterior circulation symptoms often relate to atherosclerosis of the vertebrobasilar artery or to small vessel disease in the penetrating branches. Cardiac embolism is relatively rare in the posterior circulation because the vertebral arteries are relatively small in diameter and are tortuous, so that an embolus would be unlikely to pass through the vertebral artery and then lodge in the larger basilar artery. The posterior circulation is relatively sensitive to drops in cardiac output, such as from an arrhythmia. Therefore, cardiac evaluation is important in investigating suspected vertebral basilar insufficiency.

15. What is the basic evaluation of a suspected stroke?
The first stage in evaluation is the **history**. The described deficits will suggest the initial localization. The time course of stroke is relatively acute, but some details may be clues to the pathogenesis of the individual event. Onset during sleep or a stuttering progression suggests an atherothrombotic mechanism, whereas sudden onset with maximal deficit at the beginning suggests a cardiac embolism. The **physical examination** includes assessment of the patient's cardiovascular system for the presence of heart murmurs, congestive heart failure, cardiac arrhythmias, carotid bruits, and signs of peripheral vascular disease. The **neurologic exam** focuses on the major deficit and a search for important associated signs that would aid in localization.

16. Which initial laboratory studies should be obtained on patients with a stroke?
Complete blood count (CBC), platelet count, prothrombin time (PT) and partial thromboplastin time (PTT), electrolytes, calcium, glucose, blood urea nitrogen (BUN), creatinine, chest x-ray, and electrocardiogram (EKG) are the most important initial laboratory studies. These provide both general medical assessment and evaluation for some of the complications and underlying risk factors. Subsequent laboratory analysis should include a lipid profile, thyroid profile (thyrotoxicosis may contribute to atrial fibrillation, and hypothyroidism can contribute to hypercholesterolemia), and further assessment of the coagulation system.

Hypercoagulability is suspected initially by a high hematocrit, abnormal PT, prolonged PTT, and elevated fibrinogen. In selected cases, antithrombin III, protein C and protein S may indicate congenital abnormalities in these clotting inhibitors.

If vasculitis is suspected as underlying cause, screening can be accomplished by measurement of erythrocyte sedimentation rate (ESR), rapid plasma reagin (RPR), antinuclear antibody (ANA), rheumatoid factor, serum protein electrophoresis (SPEP), and complement levels C3, C4, and CH50.

17. What initial imaging should be performed in acute stroke?
Noncontrast CT scanning of the brain is the initial imaging study of choice in acute stroke (see figure, top p. 226). Subarachnoid or intracerebral hemorrhage can readily be seen on CT scan, and is not always clear on magnetic resonance imaging (MRI). CT scanning is more readily available than MRI, can be performed more rapidly, and requires less patient

cooperation, and so is preferable in a critically ill, potentially unstable patient. The more sensitive method of MRI can be performed later, if necessary, to assist with uncertain diagnosis and difficult localization (see bottom figure below). MR angiography may be helpful in establishing the mechanism of a particular stroke. New developments in MR scanning, new scan sequences, and new MR angiogram sequences may soon improve the usefulness of MR in the evaluation of acute stroke.

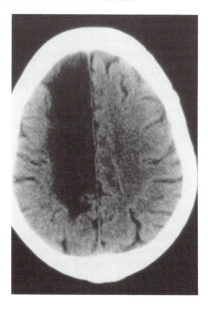

Noncontrast CT scan of the brain showing a well-established ischemic stroke in the territory of the anterior cerebral artery.

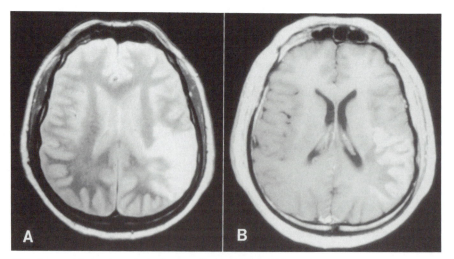

MR of an acute ischemic stroke in the posterior area of the middle cerebral artery territory. The stroke is shown on a proton density technique *(A)* and a gadolinium-enhanced T1 image *(B)*, which demonstrates the gyral enhancement characteristic of many infarcts.

18. What cardiac workup may be useful in stroke?

A cardiac physical exam, EKG, and chest x-ray may be all that is necessary in most cases of stroke. Transthoracic echocardiography (TTE) is frequently performed but is normally negative in the absence of a history, or exam evidence of cardiac disease. Transesophageal echocardiography (TEE) is more sensitive than routine transthoracic echo for the detection of left atrial abnormalities, especially left atrial appendage thrombus.

Although Holter monitoring is frequently performed, it is rarely revealing. It should be ordered only for selected patients in whom cardiac arrhythmia is strongly suspected.

In older patients, myocardial infarction is a common cause of death after a stroke. Cardiac evaluation for coronary artery disease can be performed with a pharmacologic stress thallium cardiac scan, using an agent such as adenosine. Although this may be useful in identifying occult coronary artery disease, its routine use has not yet been established.

19. What other imaging methods may be useful in evaluating stroke?

Carotid Doppler/ultrasound can be useful in screening the extracranial internal carotid arteries for significant stenosis. Its utility depends upon the experience of the laboratory performing the test. Magnetic resonance angiography (MRA) may also be used to evaluate the carotid circulation, the vertebral basilar system, the circle of Willis, and the anterior, middle, and posterior cerebral arteries and their major branches. MRA can provide valuable information on the intracerebral circulation not otherwise available without cerebral angiography. Because of turbulence at a site of stenosis, MRA overestimates the degree of stenosis compared with contrast angiography.

Contrast cerebral angiography provides the most detailed and reliable information on the presence of carotid and intracranial disease. In experienced hands, complications should be less than 1% morbidity and mortality. It is most useful when performed early, because an acute thrombus responsible for a stroke may lyse spontaneously, and the angiogram will be normal days or weeks later (though the lesions of internal carotid stenosis, or vasculitis. would persist).

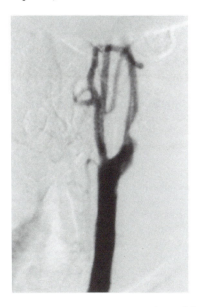

Contrast angiography showing atherosclerotic stenosis of the left internal carotid artery.

20. What is the role of transcranial Doppler imaging in assessment of strokes?
Transcranial Doppler can provide information concerning blood flow in intracranial arteries. Blood flow velocities can be measured in the middle cerebral, anterior cerebral, and basilar arteries by using different ultrasound "windows" in the skull. Decreased flow in the middle cerebral artery may be evidence of stenosis more proximally in the internal carotid; increased flow velocity may be evidence of stenosis or vasospasm in the middle cerebral. The technique can also be used to confirm cross filling of the middle cerebral on one side from the contralateral internal carotid artery via the circle of Willis.

RISK FACTORS

21. What are the major risk factors for stroke?
The most important established risk factor for stroke is age, and second is probably hypertension. Additional well-established risk factors are:

1. Gender (male > female)	7. Carotid bruits
2. Family history	8. Smoking
3. Diabetes mellitus	9. Increased hematocrit
4. Cardiac disease	10. Elevated fibrinogen level
5. Prior stroke	11. Hemoglobinopathy
6. Transient ischemic attacks	12. Drug abuse, such as cocaine

Wolf PA, Kannel WB, Verter J: Current status of risk factors for stroke. Neurol Clin 1:317, 1983.

22. What other risk factors have been described?

1. Hyperlipidemia	6. Peripheral vascular disease	11. Race
2. Diet	7. Hyperuricemia	12. Geographic location
3. Oral contraceptives	8. Infection	13. Season and climate
4. Sedentary life style	9. Homocysteinemia	14. Type A personality
5. Obesity	10. Migraine	15. Alcohol consumption

23. What is the significance of hypertension as a risk factor for stroke?
The risk of stroke relates to the level of systolic hypertension. This applies to both sexes, and at all ages, and to risk for hemorrhagic, atherothrombotic, and lacunar stroke. Interestingly, the risk of stroke at a given level of systolic hypertension is less with advancing age, so it becomes a less powerful, albeit still important (and treatable), risk factor in the elderly. This includes the isolated systolic hypertension of the elderly, once thought to be relatively benign.

24. What forms of cardiac disease have been associated with stroke?
Individuals with heart disease of almost any type have more than twice the risk of stroke compared to those with normal cardiac function. Coronary artery disease is a major association, both as an indicator of the presence of diffuse atherosclerotic vascular disease, and as a potential source of embolli from mural thrombi due to myocardial infarction. Congestive heart failure of any etiology is associated with increased stroke. Hypertensive heart disease, whether detected clinically, by LVH on EKG, or by echocardiogram, is associated with an increased risk of both thromboembolic and hemorrhagic strokes.

Another major cardiac condition is atrial fibrillation, which is strongly associated with embolic stroke. Atrial fibrillation due to rheumatic valvular disease is the strongest association, increasing stroke risk by 17 times. Nonvalvular and lone atrial fibrillation have also been shown to increase stroke risk, especially with advancing age.

Various other cardiac lesions have been associated with stroke, such as mitral valve prolapse. With the increased use of echocardiography, especially TEE, a number of additional lesions have been described. The most clearly associated with stroke risk is left atrial appendage thrombus, poorly seen with transthoracic echo but well seen on transesophageal echo.

Additional lesions associated with stroke, seen primarily with TEE, are patent foramen ovale, atrial septal defect, atrial septal aneurysm, spontaneous atrial contrast, and atherosclerotic and thrombotic lesions of the ascending aorta. The pathophysiologic significance and appropriate therapy of many of these lesions with respect to stroke remain to be clarified.

25. What is the significance of a carotid bruit as a stroke risk?

A carotid bruit does indicate an increased risk of subsequent stroke, although the risk is for stroke in general, and not for stroke specifically in the distribution of the artery with the bruit.

26. Is smoking an established risk factor for stroke?

The Framingham study initially identified smoking as a risk factor for coronary heart disease, but showed only suggestive evidence of its role as a stroke risk factor. The importance of cigarette smoking as a stroke risk remained controversial. Subsequent reports, including meta-analysis of a number of studies, have now shown that cigarette smoking clearly confers an increased risk for stroke, that the degree of risk correlates with the number of cigarettes smoked, and that smoking cessation decreases risk, with risk of stroke reverting to that of nonsmokers by 5 years after smoking cessation. Smoking confers increased risk in all age groups affected by stroke, and to both sexes.

Colditz GA, Bonita R, Stampfer MJ, et al: Cigarette smoking and risk of stroke in middle aged women. N Engl J Med 318:937, 1988.

27. What is the single strongest risk factor for stroke?

Age is the strongest single stroke risk factor. About 30% of strokes occur before the age of 65; 70% occur in those 65 and over. Stroke risk roughly doubles for every decade of age greater than 55 years.

28. What is the role of abnormal lipids in stroke? What is the role of drugs?

Although elevated cholesterol clearly has been related to coronary heart disease, its relation to stroke has been less clear. Elevated cholesterol does appear to be a risk factor for carotid atherosclerosis, especially in males under 55 years. As age advances, the significance of elevated cholesterol diminishes. Low cholesterol may also be a risk factor. Cholesterol below 180, especially below 160, is related to intraparenchymal hemorrhage and possibly also subarachnoid hemorrhage. This was initially shown in Asians, who tend to have low cholesterol levels but a high rate of hemorrhagic stroke. There is no apparent relationship of cholesterol level to lacunar infarction or cerebral embolism.

Drugs of abuse also increase stroke risk. Heroin increases the risk of thrombotic stroke. Cocaine and amphetamines increase the risk of intraparenchymal and subarachnoid hemorrhage.

29. Do oral contraceptives increase stroke risk in women?

The early, high-estrogen oral contraceptives were reported to increase the risk of stroke in young women. Lowering the estrogen content has decreased this problem but not eliminated it altogether. This risk factor is strongest in women over 35 years who are also smokers. The presumed mechanism is an increased coagulation tendency mediated by estrogen stimulation of liver protein production, including clotting factors. An autoimmune mechanism has also been suggested in rare cases.

30. Which clotting system abnormalities are associated with stroke?

Elevated fibrinogen level constitutes a risk factor for thrombotic stroke. Rare abnormalities of the blood clotting system have also been noted, such as antithrombin III deficiency, and deficiencies of protein C and protein S. These are inhibitors and modulators of the activity of the coagulation cascade. They are more commonly associated with venous thrombotic events.

Rebound hypercoagulability following discontinuation of heparin therapy has also been described. This may be the result of heparin-induced thrombocytopenia with rebound thrombocytosis following cessation of therapy, or an effect on antithrombin III, which is consumed by heparin treatment, leading to relative deficiency after discontinuation of therapy.

31. Summarize the most important treatable stroke risk factors.

Clearly the most important treatable risk factor for stroke is hypertension, followed by diabetes, heart disease, and smoking. The presence of prior stroke or TIA has recently become more important as a treatable risk factor. Less powerful treatable risk factors include abnormal serum lipids, alcohol consumption, use of drugs of abuse, use of oral contraceptives, and obesity.

Some treatable stroke risk factors are most important in combination. One of the most important combinations is female sex, age over 35 years, oral contraceptives, and cigarette smoking, with or without migraine. Another important combination is systolic hypertension, diabetes or glucose intolerance, abnormal serum cholesterol, cigarette smoking, and abnormal EKG. In the Framingham study, this combination of risk factors identified a subgroup of patients who had one-third of the observed strokes.

Rokey R, Rolak LA: Epidemiology and risk factors for stroke and myocardial infarction. In Rolak LA, Rokey R: Coronary and Cerebral Vascular Disease. Mt. Kisco, Futura, 1990, pp 83–117.

THERAPY

32. What is the treatment for a completed stroke?

Unfortunately, no therapy has proved beneficial for a stroke, once the ischemia is complete.

33. What are the most comon causes of death in patients admitted to the hospital with a stroke?

The leading causes of mortality in the first month after a stroke are (1) pneumonia, (2) pulmonary embolism, (3) cardiac disease, and (4) the stroke itself. Treatment for a completed stroke is thus largely a matter of treating its medical complications.

34. What is the treatment for a progressing stroke?

A stroke-in-evolution, which is often due to ongoing thrombosis of a vessel, is generally treated with heparin. Although controlled trials have not proved the value of anticoagulation in this setting, some studies have suggested benefits, and this treatment approach is relatively safe.

35. Is heparin beneficial in the treatment of stroke?

Heparin is commonly prescribed in acute ischemic strokes. No controlled study has yet shown conclusive benefit in improving outcome in acute stroke. In current practice, heparin is prescribed for acute cardioembolic stroke to prevent recurrence, and in atherothrombotic stroke-in-evolution to halt progression.

A CT scan is necessary to rule out hemorrhage before intiating therapy. Heparin is begun at 1000 units/hr and titrated to a PTT of 55–65 seconds. Most authorities avoid the use of a bolus to start therapy.

During heparin therapy, the PTT is monitored daily and the platelet count every other day to check for heparin-induced thrombocytopenia. Usually, treatment is for 3–5 days, followed by aspirin, ticlopidine, or warfarin (Coumadin), depending on the clinical situation. The patient should be watched carefully for rebound thrombocytosis and hypercoagulability. Heparin treatment is often delayed for 3–5 days after large, acute cardioembolic strokes, due to the risk of hemorrhagic transformation.

36. What is the role of Coumadin therapy in cerebrovascular disease?

Coumadin should be considered in all patients with cardiogenic emboli. Therapy should be initiated while the patient is acutely heparinized. Coumadin has been shown to be effective in long-term use for the reduction of stroke risk in nonvalvular atrial fibrillation as well as in rheumatic valvular-related atrial fibrillation and intracardiac thrombus. The benefit of Coumadin depends on the risk of stroke versus the risk of a major bleeding event while on Coumadin. The target PT is 18–20 seconds for a higher risk lesion, such as identified left atrial appendage thrombus, and 16–18 seconds for lower risk lesions, such as nonvalvular atrial fibrillation. The bleeding risk is 1–3% per year. The risk of embolic stroke with different cardiac lesions can be stratified as follows:

Risk Stratification for Patients in Atrial Fibrillation

High Risk (≥5% per year)
  Valvular heart disease (e.g., mitral stenosis, prosthetic mechanical valve)
  Recent-onset congestive heart failure (within 3 months)
  Prior thromboembolism
  Thyrotoxicosis
  Systolic hypertension
  Severe left ventricular dysfunction by echocardiogram
  Demonstration of intracardial thrombus

Moderate Risk (3% to 5% per year)
  Age ≥60 years
  Mitral annulus calcification
  Diuretic therapy
  Silent cerebral infarction by CT

Low Risk (<3% per year)
  Lone atrial fibrillation, chronic or paroxysmal, age <60 years

Uncertain Risk
  Diabetes mellitus
  Left atrial enlargement
  Coexistent carotid artery disease
  Recent-onset versus chronic atrial fibrillation
  Reduced cerebral blood flow

From Halperin JL, Hart RG: Atrial fibrillation and stroke: New ideas, persisting dilemmas. Stroke 19:937, 1988, with permission.

37. What is the role of thrombolytic therapy in stroke?

The role of thrombolytic therapy is currently under investigation in clinical trials. Streptokinase, urokinase, and tissue plasminogen activator (tPA), administered both intraarterially and intravenously, have all been under study. Early therapy is necessary to minimize hemorrhages and perhaps also to achieve benefit. The risks, benefits, and optimal modes of delivery and dosage are still under investigation.

38. What is the treatment to prevent a stroke?

The best way to prevent a stroke is to lower the blood pressure. Management of risk factors can reduce the incidence of stroke. Primary prevention of stroke by using antiplatelet agents such as aspirin does not seem to be possible.

39. What is the treatment to prevent a stroke in patients with TIA or prior stroke?

Aspirin may confer some protection for the secondary prevention of stroke in these patients, at least in men. Aspirin, in a dose of one tablet (325 mg) or less daily, has become the established therapy for such patients, but its benefits are probably weak. Statistical meta-analysis suggests it is effective, but some large, careful, controlled trials could not show that aspirin prevented subsequent strokes.

UK-TIA Study Group: United Kingdom transient ischemic attack aspirin trial: Interim results. Br Med J 296:316–320, 1988.

Sze PC, Reitman D, Pincus MM, et al: Anti-platelet agents in the secondary prevention of stroke: Meta-analysis of the randomized controlled trials. Stroke 19:436–442, 1988.

40. Which antiplatelet agents other than aspirin are useful for the prevention of stroke?
Neither sulfinpyrazone (Anturane) nor dipyridamole (Persantine) has any value for the prevention of stroke. Ticlopidine (Ticlid) does reduce the incidence of stroke in patients with prior TIAs.

41. What is the role of ticlopidine in the treatment of cerebrovascular disease?
Ticlopidine, in a dose of 250 mg BID, can reduce the risk of stroke by 20–30%, a performance superior to that of aspirin. However, it is expensive and toxic, with major side effects of neutropenia, rash, diarrhea, and hypercholesterolemia, and for these reasons is generally given only to patients who seem particularly likely to benefit, such as aspirin failures, diabetics, hypertensives, women, and patients with posterior circulation ischemia.

Hass WK, et al: A randomized trial composing ticlopidine hydrochloride with aspirin for the prevention of stroke in high risk patients. N Engl J Med 321:501–507, 1989.

Gent IM, et al: Canadian-American ticlopidine study (CATS) in thromboembolic stroke. Lancet 1:1215–1220, 1988.

42. What is the role of carotid endarterectomy in cerebrovascular disease?
Carotid endarterectomy has been shown to be useful in stroke prevention in three recent trials—the NASCET, ECST, and VA cooperative studies. If TIA or nondisabling stroke is due to an internal carotid artery stenosis of 70% or greater, surgery reduces the risk of subsequent stroke. Lesions less than 30% do not benefit from surgery. Asymptomatic lesion and symptomatic lesion between 30 and 70% are under investigation currently.

Carotid endarterectomy is not effective in the course of an acute stroke. Acute endarterectomy is associated with a high risk of bleeding complications. It is useful only in selected cases of unstable TIAs with risk of major stroke without surgery.

43. Which factors affect the benefit of carotid endarterectomy?
Surgical morbidity/mortality is the key factor determining benefit in carotid surgery. The risk of major stroke was decreased by 81% with endarterectomy if surgical morbidity and mortality is 3%. The benefit of surgery is lost when surgical morbidity and mortality reaches 10%. A knowledge of how the neuroradiologist reads the angiogram and the complication rates with angiography and with surgery are key factors when deciding for or against surgery in an individual case.

44. What other procedures are available for severe cerebrovascular disease?
Angioplasty of distal carotid or middle cerebral artery lesions is currently being performed as an investigational technique for critical symptomatic lesions not amenable to surgical treatment.

SUBARACHNOID HEMORRHAGE

45. What percentage of strokes are due to hemorrhage?
About 15–20% of strokes are due to hemorrhage; roughly half of these are due to subarachnoid hemorrhage (SAH). Subarachnoid hemorrhage is a relatively more common cause of stroke in the young. The actual incidence of subarachnoid hemorrhage increases with age, but becomes a less important cause of stroke overall as atherothrombotic stroke incidence rises.

46. What predisposes to SAH?

SAH is common after trauma. SAH due to ruptured arterial aneurysm is the most serious type, with the greatest morbidity and mortality. SAH may also be a consequence of rupture of an arteriovenous malformation (AVM). Ingestion of cocaine or amphetamines may be associated with SAH. Hypertension and alcohol consumption are also risk factors.

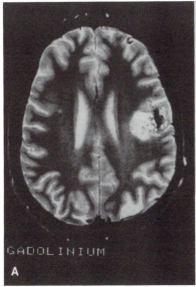

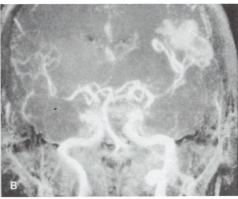

MR appearance of a left fronto-parietal arteriovenous malformation *(A)*. *B* shows the characteristic appearance on an MR angiogram.

47. Where are most intracerebral aneurysms located?

Eighty percent of aneurysms occur in the anterior circulation and 20% in the posterior circulation. The most common locations are (1) the anterior communicating artery (30%); (2) the junction of the posterior communicating artery with the internal carotid artery (25%); and (3) the bifurcation of the internal carotid and middle cerebral artery (20–25%). Aneurysms are multiple in about 25% of patients. About 3% of intracerebral aneurysms are associated with polycystic kidney disease. Fibromuscular dysplasia of the internal carotid artery is accompanied by intracranial aneurysms in about 25% of cases.

48. What is the clinical profile of SAH?

SAH is characterized by sudden severe headache, often described as "the worst headache of my life," with or without focal neurologic deficit, and often with altered mental status. Aneurysmal SAH may evolve over days, beginning with a moderately severe headache caused by an initial bleeding episode, the "sentinel bleed." This may be followed in 3–5 days by clinical deterioration due to rebleeding. SAH may not be suspected from the initial headache, causing delay in diagnosis and treatment.

49. What is the workup of SAH?

The initial test in suspected SAH is a noncontrast CT scan of the brain. This may reveal blood in the cisterns, sylvian fissure, or in the sulci around the convexities. There may also be intraparenchymal blood, suggesting the location of the ruptured aneurysm responsible for the hemorrhage. The aneurysm itself may be visible. The amount of subarachnoid blood visible on CT scanning correlates with the extent of bleeding and with prognosis.

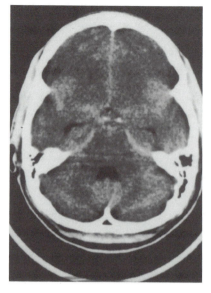

Noncontrast CT scan showing an acute subarachnoid hemorrhage, with blood diffusely filling CSF spaces.

The CT scan may be negative in 10% of SAHs. When SAH is strongly suspected clinically, and the initial CT scan is negative, a lumbar puncture is necessary.

Once SAH is confirmed, neurosurgical consultation should be obtained to plan possible surgical management. Surgical repair of a ruptured aneurysm is considered in patients with a relatively low clinical grade (I or II) within the first 48 hours from onset. Otherwise, surgical care must be delayed due to risk of vasospasm. Cerebral angiography is necesary for identification of the site of bleeding. Angiography should be obtained emergently if early surgical management is a consideration. Angiography may fail to visualize the underlying lesion because of vasospasm, which may prevent visualization of the responsible aneurysm, or because of hemorrhage, which may destroy an AVM or aneurysm responsible for the hemorrhage. Repeat angiography may be necessary if initial angiography fails to identify the bleeding source.

50. What are the treatment options for SAH due to ruptured aneurysm?
Surgical clipping of the aneurysm is the primary definitive treatment. Surgery must be performed within the first 48 hours from onset of symptoms or be postponed 10–14 days due to the risk of vasospasm. Thrombosis of the responsible aneurysm using thrombogenic coils placed via catheter during cerebral angiography may be another option in some cases.

51. What is the basic medical management of SAH?
The general nonsurgical management centers on prevention of rebleeding and prevention of vasospasm. Careful blood pressure control is basic to prevention of rebleeding, and blood pressure should be monitored continuously during the initial phase of treatment.

Nimodipine is administered to prevent vasospasm. The dosage is 60 mg q4h for 3 weeks. If the patient cannot take the medication by mouth, it is administered by nasogastric tube. Nimodipine lowers blood pressure and may cause bradycardia or atrioventricular (AV) block by its effect on the AV node, so the patient's blood pressure and EKG must be monitored during the initiation of therapy.

In the past, the antifibrinolytic agent epsilon-amino-caproic acid (EACA) has been used to promote clot formation within the aneurysm and thereby prevent rebleeding. The dose is 18–36 gm in 500 cc D5W q12h. However, its use may be accompanied by an increased risk of pulmonary embolism and cerebral infarction, and evidence of benefit has been uncertain. The current role of EACA in the treatment of aneurysmal SAH is thus unclear.

52. What is the clinical grading system used to characterize patients with SAH?

Patients with subarachnoid hemorrhage can be graded on a clinical scale of I to V, based primarily on level of consciousness and presence of focal neurologic signs.

Grade I	Awake, with no symptoms, or mild headache and/or nuchal rigidity
Grade II	Awake, with moderate to severe headache, and with nuchal rigidity
Grade III	Drowsy or confused, with or without focal deficits
Grade IV	Stuporous, with moderate to severe hemiparesis, and signs of increased intracranial pressure
Grade V	Comatose with signs of severe increased intracranial pressure

This clinical grading scale has prognostic significance. Grade I or II patients have the best prognosis and should undergo early cerebral angiography and definitive intervention, particularly if evaluation is within the first 48 hours of onset. Grade III patients may undergo angiography early, but then should be managed conservatively until their grade improves and surgical risk decreases. Grade IV and V patients have a poor prognosis and require medical management until their state improves. Angiography may be performed later in such cases if they improve sufficiently to warrant more definitive care.

53. What are the CSF findings expected in SAH?

In fresh subarachnoid hemorrhage, the CSF will be grossly bloody. Initially, the supernatant fluid will be clear. As red cells break down in the CSF, the supernatant fluid becomes xanthochromic due to release of bilirubin. This requires 2 or more hours. One can also look for the "ring sign." [A few drops of bloody CSF are allowed to drop onto the drape used during the procedure. As the fluid spreads on the drape, the outer margin is clear fluid, leaving a ring of bloody fluid behind. This suggests that a traumatic lumbar puncture is likely.]

In acute SAH, the CSF WBC count and protein level correlate with the RBC count: 1 WBC per 700–1,000 RBCs, 1 mg/dl protein per 700 RBCs. As the clinical course progresses, the subarachnoid blood may lead to an inflammatory reaction in the CSF, with an increase in the WBC and a rise in the protein as high as 150–200 mg/dl.

Risk of herniation from lumbar puncture in SAH is low. The opening pressure should be measured, and, if elevated, the minimum amount of fluid to confirm the diagnosis obtained and the needle promptly removed.

54. Which focal neurologic signs commonly accompany SAH? What is their mechanism?

The most common focal neurologic sign in acute SAH is third nerve palsy with ptosis, pupillary dilatation, and impaired extraocular movements. These signs are due to compression of the third nerve by an aneurysm of the posterior communicating artery. Pupillary dilatation suggests external compression of the third nerve because the fibers for pupillary constriction are superficial, whereas those for the extraocular muscles are deeper in the nerve. Development of focal neurologic signs may be a consequence of intraparenchymal bleeding, or ischemia due to vasospasm. Such vasospasm may cause an ischemic stroke.

55. What systemic complications are common in SAH?

Fever may occur in SAH due to infection, especially pneumonia or urinary tract infection. An inflammatory response to the blood in the CSF may also lead to fever, and the clinical picture may mimic acute meningitis. Hyponatremia may occur due to syndrome of inappropriate secretion of antidiuretic hormone. SAH may cause acute EKG changes, especially prolongation of the QT interval, T-wave inversion, and arrhythmia. An EKG should be obtained during the initial evaluation, and the cardiac rhythm monitored continuously in the ICU, with rhythm disturbances treated as necessary. A rare complication of SAH is neurogenic pulmonary edema. Development of congestive heart failure due to underlying heart disease or respiratory failure due to acute respiratory distress syndrome may also occur.

56. What CNS complications occur in SAH?

Rebleeding can cause worsening headache or declining level of consciousness. **Intraparenchymal extension** can cause focal deficits due to the mass effect, including development of cerebral edema and herniation.

Vasospasm occurs with aneurysmal SAH, but not usually from other causes of SAH. It can lead to focal ischemic injury and infarction. Transcranial Doppler (TCD) can be used to monitor the flow velocity of the middle cerebral artery; vasospasm leads to a characteristic increase in the measured flow velocity.

Acute hydrocephalus may develop, usually communicating hydrocephalus due to obstruction of the pacchionian granulations in the venous sinuses by subarachnoid blood. This can be treated temporarily by ventriculostomy or permanently by ventriculoperitoneal shunt, if necessary. Patients in higher clinical grade are more likely to experience further deterioration.

Seizures are another complication of SAH, because blood is an irritant that can induce neuronal firing.

57. What is the prognosis in patients with SAH?

The prognosis of SAH correlates with the clinical grade. Prognosis is best in grade I or II. Five to fifteen percent of patients may rebleed and worsen, but the majority recover well. Deterioration occurs in 25% of patients in grade III, 50% in grade IV, and 80% in grade V.

Grade	Deterioration	Rebleed	Death
I	5%	10–15%	3–5%
II	20%	10–15%	6–10%
III	25%	10–20%	10–15%
IV	50%	20–25%	40–50%
V	80%	25–30%	50–70%

BIBLIOGRAPHY

1. Grotta JC, et al: Prevention of stroke with ticlopidine: Who benefits most? Neurology 42:111–115, 1992.
2. NASCET Collaborators: Beneficial effect of carotid endarterectomy in symptomatic patients with high-grade carotid stenosis. N Engl J Med 325:445–453, 1991.
3. Peterson P, Boysen G, Godtfredsen J, et al: Placebo-controlled, randomized trial of warfarin and aspirin for prevention of thromboembolic complications in chronic atrial fibrillation. The Copenhagen AFASAK Study. Lancet 1:175, 1989.

17. NEURO-ONCOLOGY

Everton A. Edmondson, M.D.

NEUROLOGIC COMPLICATIONS RELATED TO SYSTEMIC CANCER

1. How often are neurologic problems encountered in cancer patients? Name several common and uncommon examples.
Neurologic complications are seen in approximately 30% of cancer patients. The most common problem is metabolic encephalopathy, followed by metastatic disease to the CNS. Unique neurologic complications of cancer include paraneoplastic syndromes, and complications related to cancer therapy (e.g., radiation encephalopathy and radionecrosis, chemotherapy-induced neuropathies, psychosis, cerebellar dysfunction, leukoencepathy). It is not uncommon to find multiple neurologic problems in the same patient. Multifocal structural disease may coexist with metabolic or infectious complications, creating a major diagnostic challenge for the clinician.

Patchell RA, Posner JB: Neurologic complications of systemic cancer. Neurol Clin 3:729–750, 1985.

2. What are the most important paraneoplastic syndromes affecting the nervous system?

1. Lambert-Eaton syndrome
2. Dermatomyositis
3. Carcinomatous neuromyopathy
4. Acute necrotizing myopathy
5. Subacute/chronic sensorimotor polyneuropathy
6. Sensory neuronopathy
7. Autonomic neuronopathy
8. Polyradiculopathy
9. Subacute motor neuronopathy
10. Retinal degeneration
11. Opsoclonus-myoclonus
12. Myelitis
13. Necrotizing myelopathy
14. Limbic encephalitis/encephalomyelitis
15. Cerebellar degeneration

3. How common are paraneoplastic syndromes?
If one excludes coexisting problems such as nutritional deficiencies and complications related to cancer treatment, the incidence of a true remote effect of cancer on the nervous system is less than 1%.

Posner JB: Paraneoplastic syndromes. Neurol Clin 9:919–936, 1991.

4. What are the characteristic features of Lambert-Eaton syndrome?
This is a disorder of the neuromuscular junction characterized by fatigability, limb-girdle weakness (usually more in the legs than arms, but not invariably), marked incremental response to 20–50 Hz of repetitive electrical stimulation, and, in roughly half of cases, dryness of the mouth and impotence due to cholinergic interference. **Ptosis and extraocular dysmotility are not features of this syndrome.**

5. How frequently is dermatomyositis seen as a paraneoplastic problem in adults?
Roughly 10% of cases are associated with underlying malignancy. The most common sources are lung, breast, ovaries, and GI tract. The index of suspicion should be higher in patients over 40 years of age.

6. What is carcinomatous neuromyopathy?
This is not a discrete entity. Commonly weakness and reduced reflexes are accompanied by muscle atrophy, but the problem could be primarily a neuropathy or neuronopathy, or a

combination of myopathy and neuropathy. There is a significant amount of variability with regard to findings on neurodiagnostic studies.

7. Which neoplasms are associated with cerebellar degeneration?

Oat-cell carcinoma and other lung cancers, breast cancer, and ovarian carcinoma are the most common, although other solid tumors can be associated with this entity. Antibodies against Purkinje cells have been demonstrated in this disease. Anti-Yo antibody is the best characterized, and is associated with gynecologic malignancies.

8. What is the anti-Hu antibody associated with?

This antibody is commonly seen in the setting of oat-cell carcinoma with either a sensory neuronopathy or encephalomyelitis.

9. Retinal degeneration is associated with which tumor and antibody?

Retinal degeneration can occur with oat-cell carcinoma. The anti-Ri antibody is associated with this entity.

10. Opsoclonus-myoclonus is associated with which neoplasms?

This syndrome of myoclonic jerks and abnormal eye movements is seen with neuroblastoma in children, but in adults lung cancer is the usual underlying neoplasm.

NEURO-ONCOLOGIC EMERGENCIES

11. What are the clinical features of epidural spinal cord compression? How is it diagnosed and treated?

The most common presentation is acute or subacute back pain, which occurs in over 90% of cases. The pain may even be radicular, such as a shooting dermatomal pain or a bandlike aching in the trunk. A sensory level is a very strong indicator of a myelopathy. Paraparesis and bowel/bladder dysfunction usually indicate a more serious cord compression (with a worse prognosis).

Plain films should be obtained in cancer patients who present with any of the above signs or symptoms. MRI of the spine or myelogram/CT is indicated in any patient whose presenting symptoms include back pain with corresponding x-ray or bone scan lesions or neurologic deficits consistent with radiculopathy or myelopathy. Rodichok et al. found that epidural disease was confirmed in 80% of patients who had back pain and a corresponding lesion on plain films, even if clinically they had no neurologic deficit.

From a prognostic standpoint, patients whose deficits are minimal and who are ambulatory at the time of the diagnosis of epidural cord compression have the best prognosis following institution of treatment. In contrast, only 13% of patients who were paraplegic at the time of diagnosis demonstrated significant neurologic improvement with radiation therapy or surgery. Most studies indicate that surgery is no better than radiotherapy for epidural cord compression; therefore, oncologists regard radiation therapy as the treatment of choice except for two circumstances. Patients with radioresistant tumors or patients who have previously received radiation at the involved site are candidates for surgery.

When the diagnosis of acute epidural cord compression is entertained as a significant possibility, IV dexamethasone 100 mg should be given stat over ½ to 1 hour, and subsequently 4 mg every 6 hours if the diagnosis is confirmed by neuroimaging.

Gilbert RW, et al: Epidural spinal cord compression from metastatic tumors: Diagnosis and treatment. Ann Neurol 3:40–51, 1978.

Rodichok LD, et al: Early detection of spinal epidural metastases: Role of myelography. Ann Neurol 20:696–701, 1986.

12. Excluding spinal cord compression, what other common conditions may present with acute weakness in the cancer patient?

A myriad of conditions may present as acute weakness. The most common are stroke, metabolic insult such as severe hypokalemia, Guillain-Barré syndrome, hemorrhage or necrosis within a CNS mass, or an acutely expanding mass lesion. Also, myasthenia gravis occurs in roughly half of patients who have a thymoma.

13. Which infectious disease can present as Guillain-Barré syndrome in the cancer population?

Cytomegalovirus (CMV) infection is more common in immunocompromised individuals, especially patients on bone marrow transplantation units. CMV can cause acute infectious polyradiculitis.

14. What condition is most commonly perceived as nonemergent? When is it actually a crisis?

Acute cancer pain is unfortunately seldom regarded as an emergency in and of itself. It is not uncommon to witness a tremendous focus on diagnosis but failure to treat the intense pain and suffering with a sense of primary urgency.

15. What situations that are relatively unique to the cancer population can result in acute altered mental status?

Altered mental status may occur as a complication of chemotherapy with agents such as ifosfamide, procarbazine, 5-fluorouracil, methotrexate, Ara-C, and methylmelamine. Leptomeningeal disease may result in chronic, subacute, or abrupt changes in mental status. A common cause of abrupt mental obtundation in a patient with leptomeningeal disease is hydrocephalus. Subclinical seizures or status epilepticus may also occur.

16. Stroke and other cerebrovascular complications are the third most common problem in the CNS in the cancer population. What are the differences between cancer and noncancer populations with regard to stroke presentation? Which complications are relatively unique to the cancer population?

Cancer patients present with many other CNS diseases, such as metastasis, meningitis, and opportunistic infections, which overshadow the cerebrovascular events. **Symptomatic** atherosclerotic and hypertensive cerebrovascular complications are actually less common in the cancer patient than in the general population.

Stroke may occur as a result of **disseminated intravascular coagulation with or without accompanying sepsis. Venous occlusion** may arise from dehydration, direct tumor invasion, or side effects of treatment such as L-asparaginase. **Embolic complications** include non-bacterial thrombotic endocarditis (NBTE), a disorder characterized by sterile platelet-fibrin debris on endocardium and valves. **Septic emboli** are due to pathogens such as fungi, staphylo-cocci, and gram-negative agents, and occur most frequently in patients who have indwelling lines and are neutropenic or in bone marrow recipients. **Tumor emboli** most commonly result from atrial myxoma, but may occur with lung tumors. Serial neuroimaging is often required to confirm that a tumor embolus is present. **Sludging due to leukostasis** may result in altered mental status, seizures, and waxing and waning focal/multifocal signs secondary to leukemic crisis. **Multifocal cerebral hemorrhage** may be seen with acute promyelocytic leukemia. Necrotizing infections such as mucor may cause a stroke by **direct invasion of the artery.**

NEUROLOGIC INFECTIONS IN CANCER PATIENTS

17. What is progressive multifocal leukoencephalopathy (PML)?

PML is a multifocal demyelinating disease caused by JC or SV-40 virus infection. It is a progressive disorder most commonly found in immunocompromised hosts such as cancer patients, AIDS victims, and transplant recipients. Strokelike events are common.

18. What are the three most common neurologic complications related to CMV infection?
CMV can cause Guillain-Barré syndrome, retinitis, and encephalitis.

19. Is cryptococcal meningitis restricted to patients with AIDS or cancer or other immuno-compromised patients?
No. Although it is more common in such patients, it can occur in individuals who are immunocompetent.

20. How common is varicella zoster infection in patients with lymphoma?
The incidence is estimated to be about 15%. Dissemination is relatively common in cancer patients. Rarely, stroke or a necrotizing CNS lesion may result from varicella zoster infection.

Pruitt AA: Central nervous system infections in cancer patients. Neurol Clin 9:867–888, 1991.

COMPLICATIONS OF CANCER THERAPY

21. What are the potential neurologic complications of chemotherapy and biologic response modifiers?

Side Effects of Chemotherapy and Immunotherapy

SIDE EFFECTS	COMMENTS
Drugs Causing Encephalopathy	
Alpha-interferon	
Ara-C	
Cisplatin	Commonly from electrolyte imbalance
5-FU	
Hexamethylmelamine	
Ifosfamide	
Interleukin-2	
L-asparaginase	Can cause hemorrhage or thrombotic insults as well as reversible encephalopathy without parenchymal insult
Methotrexate	
Nitrogen mustard	
Procarbazine	
VP-16 (high dose)	
Drugs Causing Neuropathy	
Adriamycin	Rare
Ara-C	Rare
Cisplatin	Ototoxicity and sensory neuropathy
Procarbazine	
Taxol	
Vincristine	
Drugs Causing Myelopathy	
Ara-C	Administered intrathecally
Methotrexate	Administered intrathecally
Thiotepa	Administered intrathecally
Drugs Causing Cerebellar Dysfunction	
Ara-C	
5-FU	
Ifosfamide	
Procarbazine	

MacDonald DR: Neurologic complications of chemotherapy. Neurol Clin 9:955–967, 1991.
Patchell RA, Posner JB: Neurologic complications of systemic cancer. Neurol Clin 3:729–750, 1985.

22. Name two chemotherapeutic agents that may cause parkinsonism.
The interleukins (alpha-interferon and IL-2) and hexamethylmelamine can cause parkinsonism.

23. Which hormonal drug may cause retinopathy?
Tamoxifen may result in retinopathy after prolonged use.

24. Name three chemotherapeutic agents that can induce TTP.
Seizures and encephalopathy are commonly seen in thrombotic thrombocytopenic purpura (TTP), which is accompanied by renal failure, hemolysis, schistocytes, fever, and thrombocytopenia. Bleomycin, cisplatin, and mitomycin C have been reported to trigger TTP.

25. Name two drugs that enhance leukoencephalopathic changes induced by radiation therapy.
Methotrexate and Ara-C may enhance leukoencephalopathy. Both drugs may induce this problem without prior radiation therapy.

26. What is the peak time course to note radiation myelopathy?
Delayed progressive myelopathy peaks at 9–18 months after radiation therapy, although a transient myelopathy can occur within the first month to the first 2 years. Progressive myelopathy increases in incidence as the radiation dose increases, and is much more common when doses exceed 4400 rads.

27. What are early symptoms of cranial radiation therapy?
Within the first few days of radiation treatment, cerebral edema occurs and may result in headache, lethargy, nausea, vomiting, and exacerbation of preexisting neurologic deficits. Dexamethasone ameliorates these symptoms and should be started prophylactically to minimize early ill effects from radiation.

28. How soon may delayed symptoms of cranial radiation occur?
Delayed signs may appear as soon as 1–4 months after completing radiation therapy and resemble early symptoms—somnolence, worsening of preexisting deficits, headache.

29. When is the peak incidence for focal cerebral radionecrosis?
Radionecrosis peaks at 18 months after radiotherapy but may occur many years later.

30. Name two tumors induced by radiation therapy.
The peripheral nerves and plexus within the radiation port can develop painful nerve sheath tumors years after radiation therapy. Children treated with whole-brain radiation for lymphoblastic leukemia are at risk for developing gliomas if they are long survivors.

PRIMARY BRAIN TUMORS: DIAGNOSIS AND MANAGEMENT

31. Are supratentorial brain tumors more common in adults or children?
Two-thirds of the brain tumors in adults present supratentorially, whereas in children the reverse is true.

32. Metastic disease accounts for what percentage of CNS tumors?
It is estimated that 20–40% of tumors seen in the CNS are metastatic.
   Pathcell RA: Brain metastases. Neurol Clin 9:817–824, 1991.

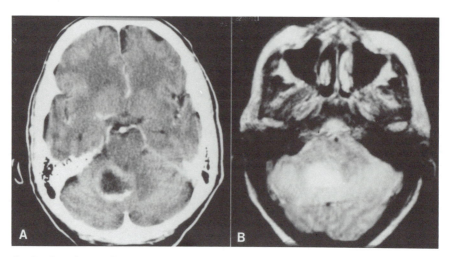

Small-cell carcinoma of the lung metastatic to the cerebellum shown on contrast-enhanced CT scan *(A)* and proton-density MRI *(B)*.

33. What is the most common category of brain tumors?

Gliomas account for 50–60% of primary brain tumors. Low-grade glioma is most common in the first decade and decreases progressively with age. Astrocytoma peaks in incidence in the third decade. Anaplastic astrocytoma has a bimodal peak in the first and third decades. Glioblastoma multiforme (GBM) becomes progressively more frequent with age, representing only 1% of gliomas in the first decade but over 50% after the age of 60.

    Levin VA, Sheline GE, Gutin PH: Neoplasms of the central nervous system. In DeVita VT, Hellman S, Rosenberg SA (eds): Cancer: Principles and Practice of Oncology. Philadelphia, J.B. Lippincott, 1989, pp 1557–1611.

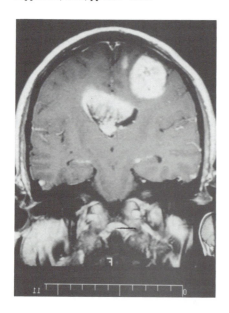

Gadolinium-enhanced T1-weighted MRI of the brain showing a malignant glioblastoma multiforme, with characteristic extension across the corpus callosum.

34. What is the mean survival rate associated with various gliomas?

Mean Survival Rate for Gliomas

TUMOR TYPE	TREATMENT MODALITY	MEAN SURVIVAL
Low-grade glioma*	Gross total resection	5–7 yr
	Biopsy/subtotal surgery	35% at 5 yr
	Subtotal surgery + XRT	46% at 5 yr
Cerebellar microcystic astrocytoma	Surgery	High cure rate
Optic glioma	Surgery	>10 yr
	Surgery + XRT	>10 yr
Anaplastic astrocytoma	Surgery alone	1 yr
	Surgery + XRT	2–3 yr
	Surgery + XRT + chemo	3–5 yr
Glioblastoma	Surgery	4 mo
	Surgery + XRT	9 mo
	Surgery + XRT + chemo	9–10 mo
Oligodendroglioma	Surgery	30% at 5 yr
	Surgery + XRT	85% at 5 yr
		55% at 10 yr
		10 yr
Ependymoma (differentiated) (anaplastic)	Surgery + XRT	2–5 yr[†]

* Location and resectability dictate survival.
[†] Malignant ependymoma with subtotal resection and CSF spread dictates a poor prognosis, whereas gross total resection of a supratentorial ependymoma with negative CSF findings dictates longer survival.

Adapted from Levin VA, Sheline GE, Gutin PH: Neoplasms of the central nervous system. In DeVita VT, Hellman S, Rosenberg SA (eds): Cancer: Principles and Practice of Oncology. Philadelphia, J.B. Lippincott, 1989, pp 1557–1611; and Kornblith PL, Walker MD, Cassady JR: Neurologic Oncology. Philadelphia, J.B. Lippincott, 1987.

35. What are the most common primitive neuroectodermal tumors (PNETs) in children?
Medulloblastoma and ependymoblastoma are two PNETs seen more commonly in children. Others include pineoblastoma, neuroblastoma, medulloepithelioma, and spongioblastoma.

36. What are the prognostic indices that determine poor risk for survival with a diagnosis of medulloblastoma?
Poor prognostic features include (1) subtotal resection, (2) malignant cells in CSF, (3) documented spinal cord metastasis on neuroimaging, and (4) age less than 4 years.

37. What is the 5-year survival rate for good-risk medulloblastoma patients (i.e., negative CSF, greater than 75% resection, over 4 years of age, no metastases)?
Survival is 70% with maximal treatment. The 5-year survival rate for poor-risk patients is only 25%.

38. Which CNS tumors are more likely to metastasize?
PNETs such as medulloblastoma have a high propensity to metastasize within the CSF pathway and may metastasize outside the CNS (e.g., bone marrow invasion).

39. What is the risk of spread into the CSF with astrocytoma, epidermoid tumor, and oligodendroglioma?
There is a 10% incidence of CSF spread with oligodendroglioma, which is significantly more than astrocytoma. Epidermoid tumors are unlikely to seed the CSF.

40. The incidence of meningioma increases with age. True or false.
True. Meningioma is rare in the first two decades and increases progressively thereafter.

41. What are the sites of predilection for meningiomas?
The parasagittal and convexity region has the highest incidence, followed by sphenoid ridge, olfactory groove, suprasellar region, posterior fossa, spine, periorbital, temporal fossa and falx—in that order.

42. What is the treatment of choice for a meningioma?
If the tumor is resectable, surgery is the treatment of choice. Radiation and chemotherapy are of limited value. Unresectable, large meningiomas can be irradiated, and shrinkage may occur, but transformation to a sarcoma or higher malignant grade is a risk. Chemotherapy is limited to the treatment of meningeal sarcoma.

43. The frequency of oligodendroglioma is highest in which decade?
The population between 30 and 39 years of age represents the peak age group affected by oligodendroglioma. The frequency is vanishingly small before age 10 and after the fifth decade.

44. Which tumors have a high incidence of calcification on neuroimaging?
Calcifications are seen in over 50% of oligodendrogliomas, and with high frequency in craniopharyngiomas and meningiomas. Metastatic melanoma and renal cell carcinoma are hemorrhagic tumors that may exhibit exuberant calcific changes on neuroimaging.

45. What population is most at risk for ependymoma?
These tumors are most common in the first decade, and the frequency drops significantly after age 30.

46. Neurofibromatosis is associated with what types of CNS tumors?
Acoustic neuroma and optic glioma.

47. Which tumors occur in the pineal area?
Tumors in the pineal region include astrocytoma, embryonal carcinoma, teratoma, choriocarcinoma, and pineoblastoma.

48. Alpha-fetoprotein and human chorionic gonadotropin (HCG) are markers utilized when tumors are present in what area of the brain?
Tumors in the pineal region may secrete HCG if they are of trophoblastic origin, and alpha-fetoprotein if they are of yolk sac origin.

49. Which tumor is likely to present in the region of the clivus with evidence of bony erosion?
Chordomas occur in the region of the clivus (or the sacrum). Bony erosion results from direct tumor invasion and enzymatic digestion.

50. What is primary CNS lymphoma?
This is a histiocytic lymphoma in the CNS that occurs without evidence of systemic lymphoma. There is much controversy concerning the site of origin of this tumor. More than half of these tumors present in the hemispheres, with a cortical predilection. One-third of these tumors are multicentric. Males are affected more than females. Because of the higher prevalence in AIDS patients, what was once a rare tumor is now increasingly common.

51. Are pituitary tumors more likely to produce hormone when they are intrasellar or extrasellar in extent?
Intrasellar tumors are more likely to be hormone-producing, whereas chromophobe adenoma, the most common pituitary tumor, is large, extends outside the sella frequently, and seldom produces hormone.

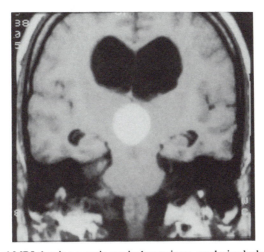

T1-weighted MRI showing a cystic craniopharyngioma, producing hydrocephalus.

52. What are the signs of a large pituitary tumor on plain skull film?
A large sella turcica, with or without erosion and double-density sign, suggests pituitary adenoma.

53. What oral medication is commonly used to treat prolactinoma?
Bromocriptine can be administered to reduce prolactin secretion and is useful in many instances in effecting shrinkage of an intrasellar pituitary prolactinoma.

54. What are the commonest tumors arising from the cerebellopontine angle?
The most common tumors in this area include acoustic neuroma and meningioma; others seen in this region include cholesteatoma and metastatic diseases.

55. What are the commonest tumors of the foramen magnum and skull base?
Meningioma, glomus jugulare, and nasopharyngeal carcinoma.

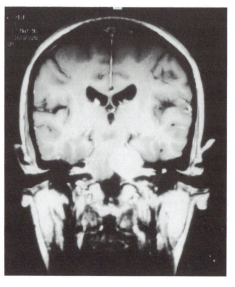

This T1-weighted MRI shows a gadolinium-enhancing tumor of the left glomus jugulare, arising at the skull base and compressing the brainstem.

56. What is von Hippel-Lindau syndrome?
This is an autosomal dominantly inherited condition that includes hemangioblastoma of the cerebellum or retina, and associated systemic disorders—polycystic kidney/hypernephroma, pheochromocytoma, pancreatic cysts, or polycythemia.

57. What is the origin of most extradural spinal tumors?
Metastatic disease is the most common reason for an extradural mass.

58. What types of tumors are found in the intradural, extramedullary region?
Schwannoma and meningioma.

59. Which tumors arise in the intradural intramedullary region?
By far, the most common tumors occurring within the substance of the spinal cord parenchyma are astrocytomas and ependymomas. Ependymomas may also occur in the cauda equina, although the primary site of origin is in the spine.

60. What is the customary total radiation dose administered to the brain for primary tumors?
The usual dose is 5500–6000 rads delivered in fractions over a period of 6 weeks.

61. The nitrosoureas are the most active chemotherapeutic agents for astrocytoma, malignant oligodendroglioma, and glioblastoma multiforme (GBM). How are these agents used?
BCNU is administered intravenously in doses of 225 mg/m^2 as a single dose or 80 mg/m^2 for 3 days. CCNU is delivered orally once every 6 weeks at 110 mg/m^2. These are the most commonly used nitrosoureas in brain tumor therapy. These may be combined with other agents such as procarbazine, vincristine, or hydroxyurea. Bone marrow, hepatic, pulmonary, and renal toxicity may occur as dose-limiting side effects.

62. Are primary brain tumors uniformly fatal?
No. Resectability, location, age of the patient, and tumor histology dictate survival. Aggressive treatment is warranted in patients presenting with primary brain tumors.

Treatment may result, albeit rarely, in a cure for glioblastoma. It is therefore prudent to offer patients the option of all ranges of approaches to management.

63. What percentage of cancer patients die unrelieved of pain?
It is estimated that 25% of cancer patients die without adequate pain relief.
Foley KM: The treatment of pain in patients with cancer. Cancer 36:194–215, 1986.

64. What factors preclude adequate treatment of cancer pain?
Ironically, it is not lack of treatment options or technology that hampers pain treatment, but factors such as opiophobia (fear to use narcotics), inadequate understanding of the origin of the pain (is it nociceptive or neuropathic?), and failure to prioritize pain and suffering as an urgent symptom requiring treatment.

65. What is nociceptive pain?
Nociceptive pain arises from injury or disease in soft-tissue or other somatic structures. Neural structures are not affected.

66. What is neuropathic pain?
Pain emanating from neural injury or dysfunction is neuropathic pain.

67. What is deafferentation pain?
Deafferentation pain is pain resulting from aberrant neural function after the sensory pathway has been interrupted or damaged. Examples include phantom limb pain, post-thoracotomy syndrome, and postherpetic neuralgia.

68. Is nociceptive pain responsive to opiate medication?
Yes. Adequate dose titration should relieve this type of pain.

69. Mild nociceptive pain may be treated adequately with which types of medications?
Nonsteroidal anti-inflammatory drugs (NSAIDs) and acetaminophen can adequately relieve mild nociceptive pain.

70. How is neuropathic pain recognized?
This type of pain usually has bizarre or unfamiliar qualities to the patient, such as intense burning provoked by light innocuous touch (allodynia), electric sensations, or intense numbness associated with deep-seated pain. Repetitive stimulation may greatly enhance the pain (temporal summation), or the pain may extend beyond the confines of injury (spatial summation or extension). Paroxysmal, lancinating pain may occur. Itchy, creepy, crawly, intense tingling, or icy hot sensations may be experienced (dysesthesia).

71. How might neuropathic pain develop in the cancer patient?
The cancer patient may experience neuropathic pain from invasion of neural structures by tumor (brachial and lumbosacral plexus, epidural space), or as a byproduct of treatment such as surgical severance (e.g., thoracotomy, mastectomy, amputation), or as a side effect of chemotherapy such as cisplatin.

72. What types of treatment are available for neuropathic pain?
Neuropathic pain may respond to tricyclic antidepressants such as amitriptyline, protriptyline, and doxepin. Anticonvulsant medications such as phenytoin, carbamazepine, and clonazepam may relieve lancinating paroxysmal pain. Oral anesthetic drugs such as mexiletine may provide relief when tricyclics and anticonvulsants fail. Steroids are sometimes useful as a temporizing measure, and in conditions such as acute causalgia, they may be curative if

begun early in the course. Nerve blocks may be used if there is a focal source amenable to this measure. Chronic epidural infusion may be used in cases of lumbosacral plexopathy, intractable neuropathic limb pain, or post-thoracotomy pain.

73. If you have a patient who is taking morphine 30 mg every 4 hours and you want to change to the equivalent effective dose (equianalgesic dose) of hydromorphone, what would the dose be?
The correct dose is 7.5 mg every 4 hours. Because hydromorphone is available in 4-mg tablets, a dose of 8 mg every 4 hours is appropriate.

Opiate Dose Conversion

DRUG	ROUTE	EQUIANALGESIC DOSE (mg)	CONVERSION FROM IV TO PO	CONVERSION TO MORPHINE
Morphine	IV/IM	10	3	=
	PO	30		=
Levorphanol	IV/IM	2	2	5
	PO	4		7.5
Methadone	IV/IM	10	2	=
	PO	20		1.5
Fentanyl	IV	0.1 (100 μg)	—	100
Hydromorphone	IV/IM	1.5	5	6.7
	PO	7.5		4
Meperidine	IV/IM	75	4	0.13
	PO	300		0.1
Oxycodone	IV/IM	15	2	0.67
	PO	30		=
Codeine	IM	130	1.5	0.8
	PO	200		0.15
Pentazocine	IM	60	2.5	6
	PO	150		
Butorphanol	IM	2	=	0.2
Nalbuphine	IM	10	=	1

IM, intramuscular; IV, intravenously; PO, orally; =, no conversion needed; mg, milligram; μg, microgram.

74. What is the advantage of MS Contin over immediate-release morphine sulfate?
MS Contin (Purdue-Frederick, Norwalk, CT) is a sustained-release preparation available in 15-, 30-, 60-, and 100-mg tablets. Its duration of action is 12 hours. Immediate-release morphine lasts 3–4 hours. Patients experience less nocturnal breakthrough pain and therefore fewer awakenings because of the extended-release effect.

75. Patient-controlled analgesia (PCA) is an effective parenteral method of delivering analgesics. How does PCA work?
Cancer patients who cannot tolerate oral medication because of nausea and vomiting, bowel obstruction, postoperative status, or marked moment-to-moment fluctuation in pain are candidates for PCA. A computerized pump is used that can deliver opiate analgesics in a variety of permutations: continuous-drip rate (basal rate), intermittent boluses (PCA doses) without a basal drip, or PCA doses superimposed on a basal rate. The physician predetermines the limit of PCA doses allowable per hour and the basal rate (continuous-drip dosage). Patient satisfaction with this modality is high because of self-empowerment,

immediate access to medication rather than waiting for medication upon request, and flexible dosing.

Bruera E, Porenneis G, Michand M, et al: Use of subcutaneous route for the administration of narcotics in patients with cancer pain. Cancer 62:407–411, 1988.

Citron ML, Johnston-Early A, Boyer M, et al: Patient-controlled analgesia for severe cancer pain. Arch Intern Med 146:734–736, 1986.

Edmondson E: Advances in pain control for cancer patients. Clin Consult Obstet Gynecol 3:122–128, 1991.

Swanson G, et al: Patient-controlled analgesia for chronic cancer pain in the ambulatory setting: A report of 117 patients. J Clin Oncol 7:1903–1908, 1989.

76. What types of pain syndromes are relatively opiate resistant?
Patients with metastatic bone pain and those with neuropathic pain are more apt to experience suboptimal relief from opiates.

77. What are the existing alternatives for patients with opiate-resistant cancer pain?
Metastatic bone pain may respond to combination therapy consisting of NSAIDs or corticosteroids in conjunction with an opiate drug. Radiation therapy frequently alleviates metastatic bone pain. Patients with neuropathic pain may require tricyclic antidepressants, anticonvulsants, or oral anesthetic agents (e.g., mexiletine). In some instances, chronic epidural infusion of anesthetic and opioids is necessary.

78. Is intravenous administration of opioid medication superior to the oral route?
Generally, oral medication is just as effective as parenteral injections if the dose is adequately titrated. Intravenous medications work faster but their duration of action is shorter. Intravenous dosing has an advantage in the patient with intractable nausea and vomiting, obstruction, or hyperacute pain who requires delicate but aggressive dose adjustments.

METASTATIC DISEASE AFFECTING THE NERVOUS SYSTEM

79. How can the clinician distinguish between radiation-induced plexopathy and cancerous invasion of the plexus?
Radiation-induced plexopathy is far less likely to present with pain, and weakness occurs early in radiation-induced plexopathy. Also, more than half the reported cases of radiation plexopathy have myokymic discharges on EMG, in contrast to none in cancerous cases.

Thomas JE, et al: Differential diagnosis between radiation and tumor plexopathy of the pelvis. Neurology 35:1–7, 1985.

80. Most tumors that result in epidural spinal cord compression do so by direct extension from bone metastasis. How does lymphoma gain access to the epidural space?
In contrast to lung, breast, colon, and other solid tumors, lymphoma may extend via the foramina into the epidural space. Normal plain x-rays of the spine in the face of epidural lymphoma are not uncommon.

81. Solitary metastasis to the brain occurs in what percentage of brain metastases?
Approximately 50% of patients have one metastasis. However, the majority of these have evidence of systemic disease after investigation, which means that the single brain lesion is not the solitary focus of disease.

82. Does gross total resection of a solitary metastasis improve survival?
Surgical resection followed by radiotherapy improves survival in a selected subpopulation. Reasonable candidates are individuals who have no evidence of disease elsewhere, who are

ambulatory, and in whom gross total resection can be achieved without significant risk of inducing major neurologic deficits.

Galicich JH, et al: Surgical treatment of single brain metastasis. J Neurosurg 53:63–67, 1980.

83. Without radiation therapy, what is the usual life expectancy of a patient with brain metastasis?
The mean life expectancy with steroids alone is 1 month. Radiation therapy extends the mean survival time to 4–6 months.

84. Does prostate carcinoma commonly metastasize to the brain parenchyma?
Prostate carcinoma **rarely** metastasizes to the brain.

85. Which solid tumors most commonly metastasize to the brain?
The lung is the most common, followed by breast and colon.

86. What is the clinical presentation of leptomeningeal carcinomatosis?
Leptomeningeal carcinomatosis (also known as carcinomatous or neoplastic meningitis) may present in a myriad of ways. Altered mental status is common, as are seizures, multiple cranial and root signs, and headache. The onset may be fulminant, such as in lymphoblastic leukemia, or subacute, with stuttering multifocal deficits and deterioration of cognitive function, as seen in some patients with breast cancer with this disease. The prognosis is poor, especially in metastasis from solid tumors.

87. Which cancer is the most common cause of leptomeningeal disease in children?
Leukemia.

88. Which solid tumor has the greatest prevalence of leptomeningeal carcinomatosis?
Breast cancer is the most common source in adults, followed by lung cancer, and melanoma.

89. What is the diagnostic yield of CSF examination to establish the diagnosis of lepto-meningeal disease?
The first tap has a 50% yield, but by the third tap the yield goes up to 85%. The CSF may show elevated protein, increased cells, or positive cytology.

90. What ancillary testing can be done to determine the presence of leptomeningeal disease other than CSF examination?
Enhanced computed tomography (CT scan) of the brain or magnetic resonance imaging may reveal leptomeningeal deposits, meningeal enhancement, or hydrocephalus.

91. Name two chemotherapeutic agents used for the treatment of leptomeningeal disease.
Methotrexate and Ara-C are used intrathecally to treat leptomeningeal carcinomatosis.

BIBLIOGRAPHY

1. Kornblith PL, Walker MD, Cassady JR: Neurologic Oncology. Philadelphia, J.B. Lippincott, 1987.
2. Levin VA, Sheline GE, Gutin PH: Neoplasms of the central nervous system. In DeVita VT, Hellman S, Rosenberg SA (eds): Cancer: Principles and Practice of Oncology. Philadelphia, J.B. Lippincott, 1989, pp 1557–1611.
3. Patchell RA (ed): Neurologic Complications of Systemic Cancer. Neurol Clin 9(4):817–1035, 1991.

18. PAIN SYNDROMES

Steven B. Inbody, M.D.

TAXONOMY AND NEUROPHYSIOLOGY OF PAIN

1. What is the difference between pain and nociception?

The subcommittee on taxonomy of the International Association for the Study of Pain defines pain as an unpleasant sensory and emotional experience associated with actual or potential tissue damage. Nociception is a response specific to potential tissue damage and stimulation. Nociception is not, however, pain perception.

Hoffert MJ: The neurophysiology of pain. Neurol Clin 7:183–203, 1989.

2. Is pain a pathologic process?

Most pain is not pathologic. Acute pain experienced in the setting of real or threatened tissue damage is an appropriate and adaptive mechanism for the survival of the organism. It requires the normal functioning of neural pathways specific for pain-related responses to an acute noxious stimulus. In some patients, however, pain becomes a disease process in itself. Such pathologic pain is usually chronic and can be caused by many mechanisms with highly variable characteristics and different pathophysiologic processes.

Wall PD: Mechanisms of acute and chronic pain. In Kruger L, Liebeskind JC (eds): Advances in Pain Research and Therapy, Vol. 6. New York, Raven Press, 1984, pp 95–104.

3. What is the current proposed taxonomy of chronic pain?

Chronic pain can result from many mechanisms, but recent research suggests that three distinct processes predominate in different painful disorders. These three pathophysiologic mechanisms can be termed nociceptive, neuropathic, and psychogenic.

Russell K, Portenoy MD: Mechanisms of clinical pain. Observations and speculations. Neurol Clin 7:205–230, 1989.

4. What is nociceptive pain?

Nociceptive pain is pain related to ongoing stimulation of nociceptive pathways that clinically parallels the degree of activity in these pathways. Nociceptive pain may have a somatic or visceral origin, distinguished by the clinical quality of the pain and the context in which it occurs. Somatic pain is described as aching, throbbing, or stabbing, whereas visceral pain is often described as dull or crampy.

5. What are the mechanisms of acute and chronic nociceptive pain?

Both acute and chronic pain usually result from the activation of a normally functioning nociceptive system. Most acute and chronic nociceptive pain is associated with some degree of local inflammation after a tissue-damaging stimulus causes local vasodilation and exudation of plasma.

6. What are neuropathic pain and its subtypes?

Neuropathic pain is precipitated by neuronal injury, creating clinically distinctive pain characteristics such as dysesthesias or paresthesias, and may be associated with other neurologic deficits or local autonomic dysregulation. This broad area of chronic pain can be further divided into three subtypes: (1) **deafferentation pain**—caused by activity in central neurons; (2) **sympathetically maintained pain**—caused by the efferent function of the sympathetic nervous system; and (3) **peripheral pain**—caused by ongoing activity in a peripheral focus of efferent neuroactivity.

7. What is the mechanism of neuropathic deafferentation pain?

Deafferentation pain may follow any type of injury to the somatosensory nervous system. Well-defined syndromes of deafferentation pain include those precipitated by peripheral nerve lesions, such as phantom limb pain, or central lesions, such as thalamic pain. Common causes of this large group of pain states include trauma, ischemia, surgical incision, or neoplasm. The strongest clinical evidence that the underlying pathogenesis of this syndrome resides within central nervous system (CNS) processing areas is the failure of peripheral therapeutic interventions, such as nerve blocks or cordotomy, to provide significant long-term efficacy. Further evidence for this hypothesis includes the observation that denervation hypersensitivity occurs in neurons in the dorsal horn of the spinal cord, thalamus, and perhaps cortex following deafferent nerve lesions. The observation that receptive fields following nerve injury spread over time is also consistent with this hypothesis. However, the fact that peripheral nerve blocks can temporarily relieve deafferentation pain demonstrates the central mechanisms involved in these conditions are continually influenced by activity from the periphery.

Davar G, Maciewicz RJ: Deafferentation pain syndromes. Neurol Clin 7:289–304, 1989.

8. What is the mechanism of neuropathic sympathetically maintained pain?

Sympathetically maintained pain represents a group of neuropathic disorders that shares several features, including the occurrence of dysesthesia, local autonomic dysregulation (edema, vasomotor disturbances, sweating abnormalities), and local trophic changes. Evidence for a primarily sympathetic efferent mechanism comes from the significant therapeutic response to interruption of sympathetic efferent activity. Historically, this group of disorders has been referred to as causalgia or, more recently, reflex sympathetic dystrophy (RSD).

The pathophysiology of the pain has been ascribed to both central and peripheral processes. Clinical observations suggesting a central abnormality include the development of the syndrome with lesions of the CNS, such as shoulder-hand syndrome following a stroke. Additionally, the failure of deafferenting procedures, such as neurectomy, rhizotomy, or cordotomy, to provide long-term relief of pain to these patients also suggests a central mechanism. Proponents for a peripheral pathologic process, however, cite the possible sensitization of nociceptors by the inciting trauma by postulating formation of posttraumatic connections (ephapses) between efferent sympathetic nerves and nociceptors. The most accepted hypothesis for sympathetically maintained pain postulates a role played by wide dynamic range (WDR) neurons in the dorsal horn of the spinal cord. It is speculated that peripheral injury activates nociceptive fibers, which in turn sensitize these WDR neurons. Activity in non-nociceptive afferents may then stimulate the sensitized WDR neurons, producing patterns similar to those produced by the noxious stimulus. Reflex connections between the WDR neurons and segmental sympathetic pathways are presumed to underlie the autonomic disturbances that accompany the pain.

9. What is the mechanism of neuropathic peripheral pain?

The clinical observation that some patients gain permanent relief following a peripheral nerve injection or resection suggests a peripheral mechanism in maintaining this type of neuropathic pain. Peripheral neuropathic pain may be divided into that caused by normal activation of nociceptive nervi nervorum and that related to the development of neuroma. The stimulation of nociceptive nervi nervorum (the small nerve fibers innervating larger nerves) may account for the pain in compressive neuropathies, such as carpal tunnel syndrome, in which the patient describes aching or stabbing pain (nerve sheath pain). The second category of neuropathic peripheral pain relates to the aberrant sprouting of an injured nerve, also known as a neuroma. Neuroma pain is often associated with a burning discomfort, which has been labeled dysesthetic pain. This peripheral origin of neuropathic pain can be differentiated from both sympathetically maintained pain and deafferentation pain by the observation that the precipitating causes of the latter conditions may be induced by lesions of either the peripheral or CNS. Support for a peripheral mechanism in neuroma pain comes from the observation that ectopic discharges are produced by neuromas, and that injecting these neuromas eradicates these discharges and simultaneously relieves the patient's neuropathic pain. The presence of Tinel's sign following peripheral nerve injury demonstrates the mechanical sensitivity of regenerating axons.

10. What is psychogenic pain?
Patients with psychogenic pain can be divided into those without evidence of an associated organic process, and those with a pathologic process, both of whose complaints of pain are judged clinically to be in excess of the organic lesion. Profound behavioral and psychosocial disturbances usually accompany these pains. Although psychological factors are commonly seen in patients with nociceptive or neuropathic pain, the predominating pathophysiology for the pain is the organic lesion. Although there is an association between depression and chronic pain, unifying mechanisms relating the neurochemical hypothesis for depression and that which underlies the development of pain remain speculative.

11. What is the difference between hyperalgesia and allodynia?
Hyperalgesia (hyperpathia) is defined as a lower pain threshold or an exaggerated pain response to a noxious stimulus. Although related, allodynia refers to pain following a non-noxious stimulus. These two related phenomena may simply represent a continuum characterized by enhanced pain response to a stimulus.

12. What is meant by the terms paresthesia, dysesthesia, and hyperesthesia?
Paresthesia is described by the patient as a pins-and-needles-like sensation, whereas dysesthesia is described as a burning sensation. Either may or may not also be associated with loss of primary sensory functions. Hyperesthesia reflects an abnormal increase in sensitivity to stimuli.

13. What is referred pain?
Pain experienced in a region remote from the site of the initiating organic lesion is defined as referred pain. Nociceptive injuries associated with referred pain include visceral pain, which is typically ill-defined, poorly localized, and experienced deeply within the body; and somatic pain, which is better localized, experienced in superficial structures, and described as aching or throbbing. Referred pain commonly develops in neuropathic disorders, either in a clearly defined pattern of pain such as a radiculopathy, or outside of a recognizable dermatome, as in RSD.

MYOFASCIAL PAIN SYNDROME AND FIBROMYALGIA

14. What is the myofascial pain syndrome (MPS)?
MPS is a frequently encountered soft tissue disorder that is one of the least understood causes of chronic pain and disability. Much of the confusion regarding MPS stems from the lack of obvious organic findings in patients with this disorder. The clinical characteristics include pain in a zone of reference, trigger points in muscles, and symptoms that long outlast the initiating events. In its most recognized form (cervical whiplash injury), symptoms develop after rapid hyperextension of the neck. Patients in this condition report painful regions and tight bands of muscle that refer pain to distant areas when palpated. Generally no neurologic deficits are associated with MPS. Other synonyms for MPS include muscular rheumatism, myalgia, myogelosis, interstitial myofibrositis, fibromyositis, and myofascitis.

Friction JR: Myofascial pain syndrome. Neurol Clin 7:413–428, 1989.

15. What is the role of trigger points in myofascial pain syndrome?

The presence or absence of trigger points determines whether a clinical presentation qualifies as MPS. Muscle trigger points are the central elements of MPS and are characterized by tight bands within the muscle that manifest a local twitch reponse on direct palpitation. Trigger points are generally classified as either active or latent. Active trigger points cause ongoing pain and restricted motion of the muscle in which they occur. Latent trigger points are quiescent and result primarily in muscle tightness, shortening, and dysfunction, without the presence of persistent pain. Trigger points have specific patterns of pain radiation during palpation, depending on the location of the trigger point. These pain reference zones may mimic more traditionally recognized dermatomal or myotomal referred pain patterns. Active trigger points can "metastasize" with the activation of satellite or secondary trigger points, resulting in the gradual transformation from an initial regional myofascial presentation to a subsequent global fibromyalgic picture.

16. What is the proposed pathophysiology of MPS?

Pathophysiologic explanations for the development of trigger points in MPS remain hypothetical. Presumably an initiating event such as direct trauma or cumulative noxious input results in disruption of the sarcoplasmic reticulum, stimulating a local contractile cycle mediated by calcium and adenosine triphosphate (ATP). The cycle may exceed local circulatory aerobic support and lead to relative ischemia with increased production of anaerobic byproducts and interstitial serotonin, histamine, kinins, and prostaglandins. Noxious stimulation of free nerve endings ensues, resulting in a centrally mediated referred pain syndrome via the dorsal horn cells. Perpetuating factors then prohibit closing of the sensory neuronal circuit. The prolonged contraction of specific muscle filaments in the absence of neuromuscular junction stimulation further consumes ATP and calcium substrates and increases local anaerobic byproducts. Muscle filaments initially contracted at the onset of trauma are unable to lengthen to original dimensions once ATP is depleted in this environment of relative ischemia. Ultimate dissolution of the muscle filaments into granular ground substrate results in localized fibrosis.

17. What are common perpetuating factors in MPS?

Perpetuating factors include many structural, metabolic, nutritional, psychological and infectious conditions that facilitate either reinjury of the affected muscle group or propagation of the neuromuscular feedback loop theorized to result in chronic trigger-point activity. Mechanical stressors include structural asymmetry such as leg length discrepancy, scoliosis, or poor posture. Neurologic disorders associated with MPS include radiculopathy, entrapment neuropathies, peripheral neuropathy, plexopathy, and multiple sclerosis. Rheumatologic disorders, including osteoarthritis, rheumatoid arthritis, and systemic lupus erythematosus, have been associated with MPS. Secondary psychosocial factors, including secondary gain issues, psychosomatic or somatoform disorders, and adjustment disorders with depression or anxiety, also commonly perpetuate MPS.

18. Which common neurologic pain syndromes share similarities with MPS?

1. Mixed tension-vascular headaches have been associated with trigger points in the sternocleidomastoid, suboccipital, temporalis, posterior cervical, and scalene muscles.

2. Thoracic outlet syndrome (TOS) has also been associated with trigger points in the scalene and pectoralis minor muscles, producing classic TOS symptoms, which may explain failures in TOS surgery.

3. Similarly, the controversies surrounding the diagnosis of temporomandibular joint (TMJ) dysfunction may be explained by recent work suggesting that TMJ conditions often

are primarily myofascial in origin, with particular trigger-point involvement of the temporalis, masseter, and pterygoid muscles.

4. Trigger points have also been identified within the piriformis muscle, resulting in pseudosciatica with entrapment of the sciatic nerve by the involved piriformis muscle.

19. What is fibromyalgia?

Fibromyalgia represents a pathologic process affecting primarily soft tissues. The American College of Rheumatology in 1990 set criteria for the classification of fibromyalgia that includes at least 3 months of widespread pain and the presence of at least 11 of 18 specific tender points on palpation. The distinction between active trigger points in MPS and less specific tender points in fibromyalgia is an important one. Tender points in the fibromyalgia syndrome may be associated with tough banding or nodularity within the muscle but will not manifest a local twitch response or characteristic pain reference zone on palpation.

20. How do MPS and fibromyalgia compare?

The distinction between MPS and fibromyalgia is important with respect to diagnostic criteria and to treatment approach and prognosis.

Myofascial Pain vs. Fibromyalgia

	MYOFASCIAL PAIN	FIBROMYALGIA
Sex	Male and female	Predominantly female
Age	All	Age 40–60 years primarily
Pain	Focal	Diffuse
Mediation	Endorphin	Substance P
Duration	Acute or chronic	Chronic
Twitch response	Present	Absent
Pain areas	Distinct reference zones	Nonradiating
Etiology	Generally mechanical	Internal, environmental
Prognosis	Good with elimination of perpetuating factors	Guarded

From Goldman LB, Rosenberg NL: Myofascial pain syndrome in fibromyalgia. Semin Neurol 2:274–280, 1991, with permission.

21. What treatments are now recommended for MPS?

First, trigger points must be identified that stimulate a portion of the patient's pain complaints, and then all pertinent underlying or perpetuating conditions must be addressed. The clinician may then proceed with specific myofascial interventions. Techniques include loosening of the trigger points by spray-and-stretch counterstimulation, myofascial massage, and trigger-point injections. Completion of trigger-point therapy should be followed by a stretching and restrengthening program in order to restore optimal function to the injured muscle and minimize the risk of reinjury.

22. What treatments are now recommended for fibromyalgia?

Numerous treatments may be used for fibromyalgia, including physical therapy, acupuncture, and transcutaneous nerve stimulation. Behavioral therapies include biofeedback and psychotherapy. Medications such as tricyclic antidepressants and nonsteroidal anti-inflammatory agents have been the most extensively studied, with the tricyclic medications appearing to be most effective. Although all of these therapies may produce some initial improvement, long-term benefit in the majority of patients has been disappointing.

SYMPATHETICALLY MAINTAINED PAIN

23. What is reflex sympathetic dystrophy (RSD)?

RSD is a condition of sympathetic hyperactivity causing burning pain, hyperesthesia, swelling, hyperhidrosis, and eventual trophic changes in the skin and bones of the affected extremity. Precipitating causes are numerous including injury to nerve or bone. The diagnosis is primarily clinical; however, sympathetic blockade can help confirm the diagnosis.

Schwartzmann RJ, McLellan TL: Reflex sympathetic dystrophy: A review. Arch Neurol 44:555–561, 1987.

24. What are the clinical features and course in RSD?

RSD is characterized by burning pain, hyperesthesia, vasomotor changes, and dystrophic changes that usually begin gradually days or weeks after the injury but may manifest within a few hours. The patient suffers greatly and protects the affected area. This disorder progresses in stages that have variable lengths, lasting anywhere from weeks to years.

25. What are the clinical stages of RSD?

• **Stage I** (acute) is associated with pain that is disproportionate to the initial injury. The quality of pain is often burning or aching and is increased by dependency of the affected part, physical contact, or emotional upset. Edema, temperature inequality, or increased hair and nail growth may occur in the affected part.

• **Stage II** (dystrophic) is characterized by edematous tissue becoming indurated and the skin cool or hyperhidrotic with libido reticularis or cyanosis present. Hair loss may occur, with nails becoming cracked or brittle. The pain is constant and is increased by any stimulus to the affected part. Roentgenograms may reveal diffuse osteoporosis.

• **Stage III** (atrophic) is typified by paroxysmal spread of pain and irreversible tissue damage. The skin appears thin and shiny and the fascia becomes thickened, with flexion or Dupuytren's contractures. Roentgenograms show marked bony demineralization and ankylosis.

More commonly, RSD fails to progress through classic stages and rather takes on a partial form in which severe pain is associated with a minimal degree of sympathetic hyperactivity, such as a slight or intermittent swelling and mottling in association with the characteristic burning pain. Decreased skin temperature may also occur early. When RSD is precipitated by a peripheral nerve injury, the symptoms quickly spread outside the distribution of the damaged nerve. RSD typically starts distally and spreads proximally, with some cases spreading into additional extremities without a new injury.

26. What are the clinical variants of RSD?

Several similar clinical syndromes have been given different designations because of a predominant clinical feature or precipitating insult. All of these conditions have in common sympathetic hyperactivity with associated persistent pain and response to sympathetic denervation. Today the term RSD is commonly used to encompass all of these variants. Important conditions in this group include:

1. **Causalgia**, which is RSD occurring after a peripheral nerve injury.

2. **Sudeck's atrophy of bone**, which is RSD occurring after soft tissue trauma, with bony atrophy as a predominant finding.

3. **Shoulder-hand syndrome**, which is RSD associated with a frozen shoulder, occurring after myocardial infarction, cerebrovascular accident, or cervical radiculopathy.

27. What precipitating etiologies are associated with RSD?

The frequency of RSD after peripheral nerve injury ranges from 1–15%. The occurrence of RSD after myocardial infarction has dropped to less than 1%. The frequency of RSD after fractures, sprains, and trivial soft tissue injuries has not been ascertained, but these injuries are probably the most common precipitating causes. Central causes of RSD include cerebral infarction, severe head injury, brain tumor, and cervical cord injury. Other associated causes include immobilization, such as prolonged bed rest or casting of injured limbs. The disorder appears to be idiopathic in 30–50% of cases.

28. What is the relationship between emotional disturbance and RSD?
Patients with RSD seem emotionally unstable, anxious, and socially withdrawn. The combination of the emotional impact of the illness and the disparity between the degree of pain and the physical examination lead many physicians to think that the pain is psychogenic. Patients report that anxiety may exacerbate the pain. In patients observed before and after relief of RSD, the emotional disturbance resolves with successful treatment of the condition. No significant differences have been found in the personality traits of patients with RSD compared with patients with nerve injuries without RSD.

29. What diagnostic tests are available for RSD?
The diagnosis of RSD is primarily clinical. Although roentgenographic studies were the first to confirm this disorder, demonstrating patchy demineralization, these changes often do not occur until later stages of the disease. Scintigraphy with agents containing technetium 99 demonstrate increased periarticular uptake in the involved extremity, but this finding also appears only late in the disease. The best diagnostic approach to confirm the presence of RSD in the upper extremities is the use of differential neural blockade, often combined with placebo injections in the ipsilateral stellate ganglion. To ascertain successful sympathetic blockade, temperature monitoring and observation for the presence of a Horner's syndrome are mandatory. Lumbar sympathetic blockade is used to evaluate lower-extremity RSD. Some clinicians, however, favor epidural spinal blocks, titrating anesthetic agents in increasing increments to allow differentiation between primarily sympathetically maintained pain, which would be abolished at low concentrations, and primarily peripheral nerve pain, which would require higher concentrations of anesthesia.

   Roberts WJ: A hypothesis on the physiological basis for causalgia and related pains. Pain 24:297–311, 1986.

30. What is the role of sympathetic blockade in the treatment of RSD?
Paravertebral sympathetic ganglion blockade is now the most widely recommended treatment for RSD. Serial sympathetic ganglion blocks lead to definite if transient improvement in most patients.

31. When is sympathetic ganglionectomy indicated in the treatment of RSD?
Paravertebral sympathetic ganglionectomy is recommended for patients in whom only transient relief occurs with ganglion blocks. Several major series have examined the results of paravertebral sympathectomy, with 58–100% of patients reporting complete relief of symptoms. Patients whose pain is not relieved by ganglionectomy usually have incomplete sympathetic denervation or severe longstanding disease.

32. What other treatments are currently recommended for RSD?
All effective therapies block the effects of sympathetic hyperactivity. The most important factors in the effective treatment of RSD are early recognition and treatment of the disease. Physical therapy alone has been shown to be effective in the treatment of RSD, with exercises directed toward improving the mobility of the affected extremity. Because of significant pain, however, patients are usually unable to participate in meaningful physical therapy. Studies of treatment with corticosteroids have shown variable benefit, and these agents are reserved for patients who refuse or cannot tolerate treatments that directly block

sympathetic activity. Phenoxybenzamine, a sympathetic blocker, provides modest benefit, although most patients have recurrent pain after completing a tapering schedule. Orthostatic hypotension limits the use of this medication in many patients. Bier block, a technique used for regional anesthesia, is helpful in a subpopulation of patients whose symptoms have been present for 9 months or less.

NEUROPATHIC PAIN IN PERIPHERAL AND CENTRAL NERVOUS SYSTEM DISEASE

33. What are the clinical symptoms of painful polyneuropathy?

Despite the variability in the underlying pathophysiology of painful polyneuropathy, the spectrum of pain complaints is markedly uniform, at least among disorders characterized by a generalized axonopathy. Patients usually report a constellation of symptoms that include paresthesias and dysesthesias of the feet, distal legs, and sometimes the hands that are often associated with paroxysmal lancinating pains (spontaneous or provoked), deep aching in the feet and legs, and muscle cramping. Some patients have severe allodynia or hyperpathia, which markedly impairs the ability to walk. They may also report the perception of gross swelling or squeezing of the feet, as if the shoes were too tight, paradoxical cold despite skin that may be red and warm, and a sense of walking on sandpaper or ground glass. Patients with significant dysesthesias typically manifest preserved reflexes, distal pain and temperature sensory loss, relative sparing of proprioception and vibratory sensibility, and an associated autonomic neuropathy. This supports probable small-fiber involvement, as larger-fiber neuropathies such as painless sensory neuropathies tend to have areflexia with distal loss of proprioception and vibratory sense. Virtually all chronically painful neuropathies are distal axonopathies.

Asbury AK, Fields HL: Pain due to peripheral nerve damage: An hypothesis. Neurology 34:1587–1590, 1984.

34. What are the clinical features of postherpetic neuralgia (PHN)?

PHN is a common cause of severe neuropathic pain, especially in the elderly. It is often intractable to conventional pain-relieving approaches and is rarely totally relieved. Herpes zoster is caused by reactivation of the varicella zoster virus, usually contracted in childhood. The virus presumably lies dormant in the trigeminal, geniculate, and dorsal root ganglia until decreased immune surveillance (such as accompanies advancing age or immunocompromised states) causes the virus to re-erupt in the sensory ganglia. The incidence of PHN following herpes zoster has been variously estimated at 9–15%, with 35–55% of patients still having pain 3 months later, and 30% having severe pain persisting for 1 year. The pain has been described both as steady or paroxysmal, with dysesthesia, hyperesthesia, and allodynia reported.

Ragozzino MW, Melton LJ, Kirland LT, et al: Population-based study of herpes zoster and its sequelae. Medicine 21:310–316, 1982.

35. What are the dermatomal frequencies in PHN?

Thoracic dermatomes	55%
Trigeminal distribution	20%
Cervical dermatomes	10%
Lumbar dermatomes	10%
Sacral dermatomes	5%

36. What is phantom limb pain?

Phantom limb pain is a neuropathic deafferent pain syndrome seen after limb amputation. It is often delayed in onset and described as a sharp, shooting, or burning sensation. It develops after limb amputation in up to 80% of patients and may also complicate other traumatic nerve and nerve root lesions, such as nerve root avulsion or traction injuries of the brachial and lumbosacral plexus. Phantom pain may be triggered by touching cutaneous regions that are outside the deafferented zone, or by visceral activities such as urinating or defecating. Phantom pain can also be aggravated by pain or discomfort in the stump of an amputee.

37. What is trigeminal neuralgia?

Trigeminal neuralgia is characterized by recurring paroxysms of sharp, stabbing, burning, or electric-shock-like pain in the distribution of one or more branches of the trigeminal nerve. Attacks only last a few seconds to minutes, with patients pain-free between attacks. It is most common in elderly patients and is due to paroxysmal firing of the trigeminal nerve, in some cases triggered by compression of the nerve from adjacent blood vessels.

   Keller JT, Van Loresen H: Pathophysiology of the pain of trigeminal neuralgia and atypical facial pain: A neuroanatomical prospective. Clin Neurosurg 32:275, 1985.

38. What are the recommended treatments for trigeminal neuralgia?

Medical treatment should be the primary approach, with surgical intervention reserved for patients refractory or intolerant to currently available medications. Almost all patients with typical trigeminal neuralgia respond to carbamazepine, at least initially. Only 25% of patients obtain sustained relief with the use of phenytoin, so its main use is as an adjuvant to carbamazepine. Baclofen, like carbamazepine and phenytoin, facilitates segmental inhibition and depresses excitatory transmission in the spinal trigeminal nucleus. Many investigators feel the treatment of trigeminal neuralgia should start with baclofen because it is so safe, even though it may not be as effective as carbamazepine.

   Patients who become refractory to medications require neurosurgical intervention. Microvascular decompression and radiofrequency rhizotomy are currently the procedures of choice. Microvascular decompression has the advantage of attacking the presumed cause of trigeminal neuralgia, while preserving the trigeminal nerve and producing longer lasting relief in most patients. Radiofrequency rhizotomy avoids the risk of craniotomy but lacks the long-term relief of pain accomplished with microvascular decompression. Recurrent symptoms after surgical intervention should be re-challenged with another trial of medical therapy.

   Jannetta PJ: Observations on the etiology of trigeminal neuralgia, hemifacial spasm, acoustic nerve dysfunction and glossopharyngeal neuralgia. Neurochirurgia 20:145, 1977.

39. What are the clinical features of glossopharyngeal neuralgia?

Patients describe severe paroxysmal jabs of pain in the neck or temporal area, radiating to the ear and mastoid. The pain may cause hypotension and syncopal episodes. Glossopharyngeal neuralgia has been reported in patients with leptomeningeal metastasis or the jugular foramen syndrome, and as a presenting symptom of head and neck malignancy. Carbamazepine or phenytoin provide the best relief.

40. What are the most common causes of atypical facial pain?

   1. **Odontalgia** is characterized by a dull aching, throbbing, or burning pain that is more or less continuous and is triggered by mechanical stimulation of one of the teeth. It is relieved by sympathetic blockade.

   2. **PHN** affecting the first distribution of the trigeminal nerve is preceded by a vesicular eruption. The pain is usually described as a chronic burning feeling. Many patients may experience electric-shock-like paroxysms on touching the eyebrow region on the affected side.

   3. **Temporal arteritis** causes chronic aching over the affected artery, often with marked tenderness on palpation of this artery.

4. **Cluster headaches** cause a burning, boring, piercing, or tearing hemicranial pain lasting minutes to hours, often triggered by the ingestion of alcohol.

5. **TMJ dysfunction** causes aching pain that is triggered and exacerbated by jaw movement and may last for days, weeks, or months.

6. **Myofascial pain** similarly presents as an aching pain lasting from days to months and is elicited by palpation of trigger points in the affected muscle.

7. **Atypical facial neuralgia** causes chronic aching pain involving the whole side of the face or even the head outside the distribution of the trigeminal nerve. This condition is much more common in women than men and is often associated with significant depression.

41. What is the central dysesthesia syndrome associated with spinal cord injury?
Spinal cord injury, whether due to trauma, demyelinating disease, necrotizing myelitis, syringomyelia, spinal cord ischemia, arteriovenous malformation, or spinal cord tumor, often interrupts the central connections of nociceptive neurons in the spinal cord. Despite differences in the site of injury in the central dysesthesia syndrome, phantom body sensations are often perceived below the level of injury, with intermittent lancinating pain occurring on a background of continuous burning pain. Patients frequently have regions of hyperalgesia and allodynia in the deafferented zones. Electrophysiologic studies demonstrate changes in spinothalamic tract conduction with relative sparing of dorsal column conduction.

42. Which brainstem structures can produce a deafferent pain syndrome?
Thrombosis of the posterior inferior cerebellar or vertebral artery (Wallenberg syndrome) often causes damage to the ipsilateral medulla, including the nucleus caudalis and the adjacent spinothalamic tract. Pain may be perceived in the ipsilateral face and may persist despite an improvement in neurologic deficits. There may be an associated loss of pain sensation, usually in the first and second trigeminal dermatomes, and in the contralateral limbs and trunk. Allodynia and hyperaglesia are frequently present in the regions of sensory deficit. The pain in this condition is usually poorly localized and described as a burning or shooting sensation that may not begin until weeks or months after the thrombotic event.

In contrast to patients with vascular injuries, patients who have demyelination of brainstem nociceptive structures often experience sharp, jabbing facial pain that is recognized clinically as trigeminal neuralgia. This pain is believed to result from interruption of the descending fibers of the trigeminal nerve within the brainstem. In addition to lancinating pain, such patients frequently describe constant burning pain in the affected trigeminal dermatomes.

43. What are the clinical features of the thalamic syndrome of Dejerine and Roussy?
Dejerine and Roussy described a painful condition as a result of vascular injury to the ventral posterolateral (VPL) and ventral posteromedial (VPM) nuclei of the thalamus. This condition is characterized by persistent spontaneous burning and occasional sharp pain in the involved extremities, as well as an altered response to cutaneous and deep painful stimuli. Vascular lesions reported to produce this thalamic pain syndrome include ischemic stroke and hypertensive vascular hemorrhage. Thalamic tumors, arteriovenous malformations, and surgical lesions of the VPM may also cause typical thalamic pain.

PRINCIPLES OF PAIN MANAGEMENT

44. What is the mechanism of action of tricyclic antidepressants for chronic pain?
Tricyclic antidepressants have been used for many years in the treatment of persistent pain. Their benefit does not come simply from treatment of depression caused by the pain. The tricyclics prevent the reuptake of serotonin (amitriptyline, imipramine) or noradrenaline (desipramine), and their effect is probably through increasing the effectiveness of descending

adrenergic and serotonergic modulation of spinal segmentation nociception. An additional effect, when given in combination with morphine, is the increase in the plasma concentration of free morphine by competition for protein binding. Sedation and cholinergic side effects may reduce the acceptability of treatment, however.

McQuay HJ: Pharmacologic treatment of neurologic and neuropathic pain. Cancer Surv 7:141–159, 1988.

45. What is the role of anticonvulsant therapy in neuropathic pain?

Anticonvulsant medication is currently recommended as a second-line therapy when treatment with tricyclic antidepressants fail. Their mechanism of action appears to include suppression of excessive discharges from pathologically altered neurons and prevention of normal neurons from becoming involved in the process. Recent anticonvulsant trials in neuropathic pain suggest that carbamazepine appears effective in some patients with brief shooting pain and in patients with steady burning or muscular pain. Results of controlled trials with phenytoin are mixed, with several studies failing to demonstrate any analgesic effect. Two other anticonvulsant drugs, clonazepam and valproic acid, may also minimize lancinating neuropathic pains.

46. What other pharmacologic agents are useful as adjuvant therapy in chronic pain syndromes?

1. Baclofen's proved efficacy in trigeminal neuralgia suggests that it may be effective in the treatment of other lancinating neuropathic pains.

2. Clonidine relieves neuropathic pain in a subpopulation of patients with painful diabetic neuropathy. The hypothesized mechanism of action of this alpha$_2$-adrenergic agonist may involve direct inhibition of spinothalamic neurons or generalized inhibition of CNS sympathetic efferent activity.

3. Use of neuroleptics as independent analgesics has limited efficacy in neuropathic pain states. Although the combined use of an antidepressant and a neuroleptic in painful neuropathy can be beneficial, the minimal supporting data and the potential toxicity of these drugs relegate their use as analgesics to patients with pain that has been refractory to other classes of drugs.

47. What is the mechanism of action of local anesthetics in neuropathic pain?

A number of local anesthetics depress evoked discharges of spinal cord neurons activated by C fibers and might plausibly relieve burning pain by both this central mechanism and by an effect on injured peripheral nerve. An orally available analogue of lidocaine, mexiletine, is efficacious for the pain associated with diabetic neuropathy. Similar to the findings in controlled trials of intravenous lidocaine infusion in this condition, studies show that mexiletine appears capable of ameliorating the continuous dysesthesias that usually characterize the pain associated with peripheral neuropathy.

48. What is the role of opiate analgesics in chronic pain syndromes?

The persistent administration of opioid drugs to patients with chronic nonmalignant pain is controversial. Clinical experience suggests that some patients with painful polyneuropathy or other neuropathic pain syndromes can obtain partial and sustained analgesia without the development of either significant opioid toxicity or aberrant behaviors indicative of psychological dependence/addiction. A trial of regular doses of an opioid under close monitoring may be considered in patients for whom other treatments provide little relief.

49. What is the role of nonsteroidal anti-inflammatory drugs (NSAIDs)?

NSAIDs inhibit prostaglandin production, which normally mediates the inflammation that occurs after tissue damage. Although the role of NSAIDs is well accepted in acute inflammatory states, their use in the treatment of neuropathic or deafferent pain is more speculative. The parenteral form of ketoglutarate may provide significant relief, but this agent has not been tested in chronic deafferent pain conditions.

50. What is the mechanism of action of Capsaicin?
Capsaicin ointment selectively stimulates and then blocks unmyelinated sensory afferents from skin and mucous membranes. Many of the C fibers contain substance P, which is an excitatory neurotransmitter necessary for pain. It is thought that Capsaicin may relieve pain by initially releasing and then depleting substance P. Relief of neuropathic pain associated with postherpetic neuralgia has been shown anecdotally. Burning after application of Capsaicin ointment is the limiting side effect.

51. What are the most important behavioral and cognitive therapies for chronic pain?
If the patient is amenable, referral to a professional to learn relaxation, imagery, hypnosis, or meditation can be a primary or adjuvant treatment for chronic pain. These techniques require practice, and the patient should be committed to work daily on the cognitive techniques for at least one month. Although specific data about the efficacy of these therapies are mixed, in the course of using these methods, a patient's perspective on his or her situation may change and suffering lessen.

52. Which neurostimulatory approaches are currently used for chronic pain?
Neurostimulatory approaches range from noninvasive counterirritation techniques, such as systematic rubbing of the painful part, to transcutaneous electrical nerve stimulation (TENS) and acupuncture. A number of invasive measures such as dorsal column stimulation and deep brain stimulation have been used in patients for whom drug therapy was relatively contraindicated or failed to provide adequate relief. These invasive nerve stimulatory techniques should be considered only in patients with refractory disabling dysesthesias and who have undergone extensive evaluation and treatment by practitioners experienced in chronic pain management.

53. What is the role of implantable drug pumps for the treatment of chronic pain?
A number of technologic advances have made possible the delivery of morphine to selected regions of the CNS. Support for this modality of therapy followed the identification of opiate receptors not only in brain regions but also in the spinal cord, where significant concentrations have been detected in substantia gelatinosa, which receives C fiber input from the dorsal roots. Application of locally administered morphine in this area can significantly reduce discharges form spinal nociceptive neurons. Clinically, local intrathecally applied morphine has been shown to raise the threshold of pain dramatically in the region of application only. The use of epidural administration of morphine has become more commonplace in anesthesia for control of postoperative pain. The most important observation has been that effective relief of pain can occur with regional morphine without central effects such as lethargy, confusion, and respiratory depression.

Choosing patients for implantation of drug pumps requires firm guidelines. The first indication is for patients who fail to control pain with supratherapeutic oral medication. A second indication is for patients who cannot tolerate narcotics because of mental confusion, lethargy, or nausea. The third indication is for patients who have good relief of pain from a single dose of intrathecally administered morphine or from chronically infused morphine by an external pump through an epidural catheter. Chronic infusion of intrathecal spinal morphine does not change the neurologic examination and tolerance has not been a major problem. It therefore appears that implantable morphine pumps may have a specific role in the management of pain when oral medications have failed.

Pawl RP: Surgery for pain. Semin Neurol 9:257–268, 1989.

54. What is the role of neural ablative procedures for chronic pain?
Cordotomy, or technically and more accurately spinal tractotomy, is an ablative procedure aimed at anesthetizing some significant portion of the body rendered painful from disease. Although popular a decade ago, its use has declined steadily. The procedure is performed stereotactically, using a radiofrequency current delivered through a needle or electrode, and resulting in coagulation of neural fibers. This procedure is most easily performed at the C1–2 interspace, where the fibers from ventrolateral spinothalamic tract begin crossing from the anterior cord to the posterior lower brainstem. The presence of intermingled motor fibers at this level has led to unacceptable side effects, such as paresis or urinary incontinence.

Peripheral neuronectomy and rhizotomy are quite limited in scope, producing pain relief by anesthesia of the affected body part, and are no longer used regularly.

Stereotactic ablative and stimulating procedures that target thalamic nuclei or frontal projections of the thalamus remain under study. Deep-brain stereotactic surgery has been advocated to treat patients with the chronic pain that accompanies cerebral damage. With the advent of magnetic resonance imaging, however, it has become apparent that cerebral injury outside the thalamus and even outside the nociceptive pain pathway may be associated with chronic pain.

BIBLIOGRAPHY

1. Horenstein S (ed): Low Back Syndromes. Semin Neurol. New York, Thieme Medical Publishers, 1986.
2. Fields H: Pain. New York, McGraw-Hill, 1987.
3. Portenoy RK (ed): Pain mechanisms and syndromes. Neurol Clin 7(2): 1989.

19. HEADACHES

Howard Derman, M.D.

GENERAL PRINCIPLES

1. What is the incidence of headaches of all types?
A recent study examined a population of 2000 adults, and 45% reported that they had at some time experienced a severe or disabling headache.

2. Are headaches more common in males or females?
Typically, 70% of migraines occur in females and 30% in males. Cluster headaches occur almost entirely in men; 90% of cluster headache patients are male. Muscle contraction headaches have a slightly increased incidence in female patients, but these headaches are seen almost equally in both genders.

3. Does the location of head pain help differentiate headache types?
Typically, migraine occurs on half the face, involving the frontal area, usually in and about the eye and cheek. Cluster headaches are more periorbital in location and patients may report a boring, excruciating pain above and behind the eye. Muscle contraction head pain is classically described as band-like, in the temporal region, occasionally extending back to the occipital region and forward to the forehead.

4. Which cranial structures are sensitive to pain?
Certain pain-sensitive cranial structures are capable of producing headaches. The brain itself is insensitive to pain.

Pain-sensitive Cranial Structures

1. The scalp
2. Scalp blood supply and their appendages
3. Head and neck muscles
4. Great venous sinuses
5. Arteries of the meninges
6. Larger cerebral arteries
7. Pain-sensitive fibers of the fifth, ninth, and tenth cranial nerves
8. Parts of the dura mater at the base of the brain

5. Is there a place for narcotic analgesics in treatment of headaches?
The use of narcotic analgesics for treatment of headaches should be strongly discouraged. For the most part, narcotic analgesics should not be used. A talk with the patient about the issue of narcotic analgesia prior to starting therapy is often helpful.

6. When is a headache a sign of a serious neurologic problem?
Some indications that a headache could be due to a serious underlying illness include:
1. Sudden onset of a severe headache
2. Headache accompanied by impaired mental status, fever, seizures, or focal neurologic signs
3. New headaches beginning after age 50

7. What are some of the more common serious diseases that may present as a headache?

Some Common Serious Diseases That May Present as a Headache

1. Primary brain tumor	7. Meningitis
2. Metastatic brain tumor	8. Temporal arteritis
3. Abscess	9. Hypertension
4. Subdural hematoma	10. Hydrocephalus
5. Intracerebral hemorrhage	11. Glaucoma
6. Subarachnoid hemorrhage	

MIGRAINE HEADACHES

8. What is the age of onset for migraine headaches?
Migraines typically may begin in teenage years and can begin as late as age 40.

9. What is the frequency of attack in migraine headaches?
Migraines usually occur 2–4 times per month. Some migraineurs have headaches more sporadically, 3–4 times per year. In some women there may be a strong association with menstruation.

10. What are the common symptoms of migraine?
   1. Unilateral headache (60% of the time). The pain may begin as a dull ache but then becomes throbbing and possibly incapacitating.
   2. Visual or sensory loss
   3. Anorexia, nausea, vomiting
   4. Photophobia and phonophobia
   5. Mood changes

11. What are the 5 phases of a complete migraine attack?
   1. **Prodrome.** The prodrome occurs hours to days before the headache and consists of changes in mood, behavior, appetite, and cognition.
   2. **Aura.** The aura occurs within an hour of the headache and is most commonly visual or sensory.
   3. **Headache.** The headache itself is commonly unilateral and may be pulsatile.
   4. **Headache termination**
   5. **Post-drome.** Following termination of the headache, the complete migraine attack is ended with the post-drome or hangover phase.

12. How often are migraines accompanied by an aura?
Approximately 35% of migraines are accompanied by an aura. This type of headache is known as a **classic migraine.** Migraine without an aura is known as **common migraine.**

13. What are the common auras of migraine?
Visual auras are the most common and include photopsias, flashing lights, scintillating scotomata, and fortification spectra. Sensory auras are the next most common, especially numbness or paresthesias in a limb. Motor weakness and aphasia are less common.

14. What are the characteristics of migraine with aura?
The patient must have 2 attacks fulfilling a minimum of 3 of the following 4 characteristics:
   1. One or more fully reversible aura symptoms indicating focal cerebral, cortical, or brainstem dysfunction.

2. At least 1 aura symptom developing gradually over 4 minutes, or 2 or more symptoms occurring in succession.

3. No aura symptom lasting more than 60 minutes.

4. The migraine headache must follow the aura within 60 minutes or less.

15. What are the characteristics of migraine without aura?

The patient must have at least 5 attacks that fulfill the following criteria:

1. The duration of the headache must be 4–72 hours.

2. During the headache, the patient must suffer at least 1 of the following: nausea and vomiting or photophobia and phonophobia.

3. The headache must have at least 2 of the following characteristics: unilateral location, pulsating quality, moderate to severe pain that inhibits or prohibits daily activities, and aggravation by routine physical activity.

16. What is the vascular theory of migraine?

The vascular theory of migraine, as elaborated by Wolff, states that the migraine aura is due to cerebral vasoconstriction and that the headache itself is caused by vasodilatation. Recent cerebral blood flow studies cast some doubt on this vascular theory. There is a decrease in cerebral blood flow during migraine with aura, but there is no change in cerebral blood flow during migraine without aura. The role of vascular changes in the pathogenesis of migraine thus remains controversial.

Oleson J, Larsen B, Lawitzea M: Focal hyperemia followed by spreading oligemia and impaired actuation of rCBF in classic migraine. Ann Neurol 9:344–352, 1980.

17. Does serotonin play a role in migraine?

Serotonin is widely distributed throughout the body, with 90% concentrated in the GI tract and the remainder in the brain and platelets. During a migraine attack, the blood level of serotonin may decrease, while urinary concentrations may increase. This shift in serotonin levels may trigger changes in blood vessels and blood flow, and also alter pain perception in the brain. Serotonin may thus play a role (as yet incompletely understood) in the cause of migraine. Certain medications such as amitriptyline, nortriptyline, and sumatriptan, which have an effect on serotonin metabolism, are useful in treatment of migraine headache.

18. Can certain foods bring on migraine?

Certain foods can precipitate a migraine, as some patients will note during history taking. Foods commonly identified as exacerbating migraine include:

- Foods rich in tyramine (cheese, red wine)
- Foods containing monosodium glutamate (Chinese and Mexican food)
- Foods containing nitrates (cold cuts—bologna, salami, smoked meats)
- Pickled, fermented, marinated foods (pasta salads)
- Alcoholic beverages (especially red wine)
- Caffeinated beverages (soft drinks, tea, and coffee)

19. What are the most useful drugs for acute, abortive therapy of migraines?

The most useful abortive migraine treatments are ergotamines, Midrin, or sumatriptan.

20. Is ergotamine helpful therapy for migraines?

Ergotamine derivatives can be useful in patients who have migraine with a clear-cut prodrome. Ergotamine is available in oral, sublingual, suppository, injectable, and inhalation forms. Because of the extreme nausea and vomiting seen with migraines, the suppository and sublingual preparations are the most useful and tolerable. When using sublingual or suppository form, the usual dosage is 2 mg. The patient may take 3 doses per headache, separated by ½ hour, up to 9 doses per week.

21. What is Midrin? Is it useful in headaches?

Midrin is a combination medication that consists of dichloralphenazone (a muscle relaxant), isometheptene (a vasospasm agent), and acetaminophen. It can be used either as a prophylactic medication, in a dose of 1 pill 2–3 times per day, or as abortive therapy in a dose of 2 pills with the onset of the headache and then 1 pill every hour after that, up to 5 pills total.

22. What is sumatriptan?

Sumatriptan (Imitrex) represents a new class of medications—the 5-hydroxytryptamine (5HT) receptor agonist. Early reports show that 6 mg given subcutaneously completely abolishes headache in 71% of migraineurs. Only minor side effects were reported. The drug is currently being tested in an oral preparation. Sumatriptan can be used as abortive therapy in migraine and represents a major new frontier in migraine treatment.

   Cady RK, Wendt JK, et al: Treatment of acute migraine with subcutaneous sumatriptan. JAMA 265:2831–2835, 1991.

23. Which group or groups of drugs represent first-line therapy for migraine prophylaxis?

Tricyclic antidepressants, beta blockers, and calcium channel blockers are the drugs of choice for migraine prophylaxis.

24. What are the indications for prophylactic treatment of migraine?

When headaches occur at a frequency of two or more per month or, more importantly, when the headaches affect the patient's day-to-day life (causing absence from work or school), then prophylactic therapy is indicated.

25. Which tricyclics are the most helpful prophylactic agents?

Tricyclic antidepressants work through an analgesic action independent of their antidepressant effect. Among the many tricyclic antidepressants, amitriptyline (Elavil) is used most often in migraine therapy. Other drugs that have been successful include doxepin (Sinequan), nortriptyline (Pamelor), and imipramine (Tofranil).

26. When prescribing a tricyclic antidepressant for migraine, what dosage should be considered?

In the case of amitriptyline, it is best to start at a dose of 25 mg taken at bedtime because patients often become lethargic with initial dosing. The level can be built to a maximum dose of 200 mg by raising the dose slowly (25 mg per week over 3–4 weeks). However, doses greater than 100 mg are often associated with significant side effects.

27. What are the major side effects of the tricyclic antidepressants?

Dry mouth, constipation, and urinary hesitancy. Patients may also become quite sedated. Finally, weight gain is often an intolerable side effect.

28. Are beta blockers still useful as prophylaxis for migraine?

Beta blockers, especially propranolol, have been used effectively for migraine prophylaxis for many years. Propranolol is safe and has fewer side effects than many drugs, such as methysergide. The usual dose is 80 mg LA (long-acting), increased to 160 mg LA, as indicated. Monitoring of pulse is important and drug dose may be increased to 160 mg if the pulse stays greater than 60.

29. Are beta blockers well tolerated in migraineurs?

For the most part, beta blockers are well tolerated, but several issues need to be discussed with patients before starting the beta blocker. (1) Bronchospasm is a concern in patients with asthma. (2) When starting a beta blocker, find out if the patient participates in an exercise program. The number of patients treated for migraine who are also enrolled in aerobic exercise classes is surprising. Patients often become irate when they see members of their exercise class achieving heart rates of 160 while they are on a drug that keeps their heart rate at 60. (3) Patients often feel miserable exercising while taking a beta blocker.

30. Are calcium channel blockers effective in migraine?
Calcium channel blockers are now considered first-line therapy in migraine. To date, diltiazem, nifedipine, verapamil, and nimodipine are the calcium channel blockers that are currently available, with verapamil being the most useful in migraine.

31. How is verapamil prescribed in migraine?
Verapamil is usually started at a dose of 180 mg at night, increased as necessary to 240 mg at night over a 4-week period. The drug has been very well tolerated and has efficacy in over 70% of migraineurs.

32. Is nimodipine helpful in migraine prophylaxis?
Nimodipine is particularly effective in spasm of cerebral blood vessels and is indicated in the treatment of stroke and subarachnoid hemorrhage. The drug is not being used regularly for migraine headache prophylaxis.

33. How should you decide amongst a beta blocker, a tricyclic antidepressant, or a calcium channel blocker in migraine prophylaxis?
It is essential to consider patients' work habits and other factors in their lives, such as exercise programs, etc., when deciding treatment. Anecdotal reports seem to favor beta blockers for patients who have significant visual problems (flashing lights, zigzag lines, fortification spectra) with their headaches. In patients who are markedly anxious, depressed, or have a sleep problem, a tricyclic antidepressant may be more appropriate.

34. Is sodium valproate successful in migraine prophylaxis?
Studies indicate that sodium valproate (Depakote) may be helpful in migraine prophylaxis. A recent study showed that average doses of 1250 mg, starting at 250 mg twice daily, may be helpful in migraine prophylaxis.

Sorenson KU: Valproate: A new drug in migraine prophylaxis. Acta Neurol Scand 78:346–348, 1988.

35. Is methysergide maleate a drug to consider for migraine?
Methysergide maleate (Sansert) is a selective vasoconstrictor that has been available for many years to treat migraine. It is very effective but is no longer considered a primary or secondary therapy in migraine because of serious side effects attending prolonged use. The most serious side effect is retroperitoneal fibrosis.

36. When using methysergide, what precautions should be taken?
Methysergide can still be used, despite major complications, if 3 months of drug therapy are followed by 1 month of drug holiday, repeated 3 times a year. However, because many other treatment options exist, methysergide should be used only when all other medications have failed.

37. How does pregnancy affect treatment of headache?
When pregnant patients must use some medication for their headaches, then and only then is the use of narcotics justified. Codeine is probably the safest medication to use judiciously for headaches during pregnancy. If this does not work, then either acetaminophen (Tylenol) or aspirin may be helpful, and then finally, a tricyclic antidepressant or cyproheptadine (Periactin) may be used.

38. Are any drugs clearly contraindicated in pregnant patients?
Ergotamine derivatives and any drug with a vasospastic component are contraindicated. Beta blockers are relatively safe but are used only if acetaminophen or codeine fails. Usually, after a heart-to-heart talk with pregnant patients, most are willing to proceed during their entire pregnancy without medication if they are convinced that drugs may in some way harm the fetus.

CLUSTER HEADACHES

39. What is the age of onset for cluster headaches?
Cluster headaches typically start at age 25, and may occur as late as age 45.

40. What symptoms are associated with cluster headaches?
The headache strikes abruptly, without any aura, around and behind one eye. The pain is extremely severe and lasts 20–60 minutes. Patients report nasal stuffiness, rhinorrhea, and redness of the eye ipsilateral to the head pain. There may also be partial Horner's syndrome with ptosis and miosis on the side of the head pain.

41. Why are cluster headaches called cluster headaches?
The headaches all occur during a short time span; this cluster then recurs periodically. A typical cluster of headaches may last 4–8 weeks, with 1–2 headaches per day during the cluster. Patients may go 6 months to 1 year before another cluster occurs.

42. What is the differential diagnosis of cluster headaches?
Trigeminal neuralgia, cyclical migraine, sinus infection, and Raeder's paratrigeminal neuralgia.

43. What is the management for the acute attack of cluster headaches?

Oxygen inhalation	Dihydroergotamine (DHE)
Locally applied anesthetic agents	injections
Ergotamine	Sumatriptan

44. How is oxygen used in cluster headaches?
The average dose of oxygen used is 8 L/min for 10 minutes, which will relieve pain in approximately 80% of patients. Some patients have a rebound headache once the oxygen is stopped, and oxygen therapy must be instituted very early in the head pain.

45. Are steroids helpful in cluster headache?
Steroids can be quite useful and are used in two ways. For the acute attack, a tapering dose of 60 mg, 40 mg, and 20 mg of prednisone over 3 days may be helpful. If the patient is in the midst of a cycle, then a tapering course starting at 60 mg, decreasing to 0 mg over a 3-week period, is recommended.

46. Is lithium useful in cluster headache?
Lithium carbonate may be useful in the prophylactic treatment of cluster headaches. Patients usually benefit from a dose of 600–900 mg per day, maintaining a therapeutic level of 0.4–0.8 mEq/L.

47. What is the treatment for rhinorrhea and lacrimation associated with clusters?
Cyproheptadine (Periactin), a drug that works as an antihistamine and also has an effect on serotonin, can be useful. The dose is usually 2 mg by mouth 3 times a day. Side effects include sedation as well as appetite enhancement, and these issues must be discussed with the patient before starting medication.

TENSION HEADACHES

48. What is a tension headache?
A tension headache is dull, persistent pain that occurs in the temporal region in a band-like distribution and may radiate forward to the frontal region or posteriorly to the occipital region. It is also referred to as a muscle contraction headache.

49. What symptoms are associated with muscle contraction headaches?
Neck stiffness, shoulder tightness, and aching.

50. What causes tension headaches?
The cause of tension headaches is open to debate. It has not been possible to relate them very well to any particular psychological profile. They may arise from tight, tense muscles, but not all studies verify this association. Some authorities suggest they are variants of migraine headaches.

51. Are there different types of tension headaches?
Yes—episodic and chronic.

52. What are the characteristics of an episodic tension-type headache?
The patient must have at least 10 previous headache episodes fulfilling the following diagnostic criteria:
1. The headache must last from 30 minutes to 7 days.
2. A minimum of 2 of the following pain characteristics: pressing or tightening pain, mild to moderate intensity, bilateral location, no aggravation upon physical activity.

53. What are the characteristics of a chronic tension-type headache?
1. Average headache frequency of 15 days per month for 6 months, or 180 days per year
2. Frequently associated with analgesic overuse
3. May have migrainous features superimposed intermittently

54. What is the treatment for tension headache?
The treatment of muscle contraction headache is different from that of migraine. Treatment includes drugs that are primarily analgesics, such as nonsteroidal anti-inflammatory drugs, as well as drugs that help with muscle spasm.

55. Are benzodiazepines useful for the treatment of headaches?
Any drug that helps to relax posterior strap muscles as well as cervical neck muscles will help with muscle contraction headaches. Benzodiazepines such as diazepam (Valium), chlorazepam (Librium), and chlordiazepate (Tranxene) often help with this spasm. Equally effective are drugs such as Soma Compound, Parafon Forte, and Skelaxin, which also help with intense muscle spasm.

SPINAL TAP HEADACHES

56. Are headaches frequent after lumbar puncture?
Approximately 20–25% of patients have a headache after lumbar puncture. Headaches occur whether or not there is a traumatic tap and regardless of the amount of spinal fluid removed.

57. Do patients with postspinal headache have other complaints?
Patients are often severely disabled by nausea and vomiting along with the headaches. Characteristically, the headache is much worse when the patient is upright and improves dramatically when the patient lies flat in bed.

58. What is the treatment for postspinal tap headache?
The first step is to reassure the patient that the headache will eventually go away. The patient must remain flat in bed as much as possible. Simple analgesics are recommended. Finally, if the headache becomes disabling, blood patch therapy with a second spinal tap may be indicated.

POSTCOITAL HEADACHES

59. What is postcoital cephalgia?
Postcoital cephalgia refers to headaches that occur before and after orgasm. They occur with equal frequency in men and women. The pain is usually sudden in onset, pulsatile, fairly intense, and involves the entire head.

60. Are headaches that occur with intercourse a sign of subarachnoid hemorrhage?
Less than 2% of the patients who present with subarachnoid hemorrhage secondary to aneurysm leakage have this leakage occur with intercourse. More often than not, headaches that occur with intercourse are either migraine or muscle contraction in origin.

61. What is the treatment for postcoital cephalgia?
There are two drugs of choice. If one believes the headaches are muscle contraction in origin, then a nonsteroidal anti-inflammatory drug is indicated. If the headaches are thought to be migraine, then a beta blocker is most useful.

HEADACHES FROM BRAIN TUMORS OR MASS LESIONS

62. Are headaches associated with a brain tumor different from other types of headaches?
The headaches associated with a brain tumor may present in much the same fashion as headaches associated with either muscle contraction or migraine headaches. The headaches may be more frequent—daily versus episodically for migraine.

63. What special features in the history and physical should be considered when concerned about a possible brain tumor?
Patients who have headaches associated with brain tumor often awake early in the morning with their headaches. Neurologic examination may reveal focal abnormalities, as well as papilledema on funduscopic examination.

PSEUDOTUMOR CEREBRI

64. What is pseudotumor cerebri?
Pseudotumor cerebri, also known as benign intracranial hypertension, is increased intracranial pressure without evidence of malignancy on neurologic testing. It is manifested primarily by headaches and visual obscuration.

65. Is there a specific type of person in whom to suspect pseudotumor?
Pseudotumor is generally seen in female patients who are quite obese and often have menstrual irregularities.

66. How can one make the diagnosis of pseudotumor cerebri?
The patient is generally obese and female. A neurologic exam is normal. An MRI or CT scan often shows slit-like ventricles with no other abnormality. The pressure is elevated on spinal fluid examination.

67. Name some etiologic factors associated with benign intracranial hypertension.

1. Mastoiditis and lateral sinus thrombosis
2. Head trauma
3. Oral progestational drugs
4. Marantic sinus thrombosis
5. Cryofibrinogenemia
6. Addison's disease
7. Hypoparathyroidism
8. Tetracycline therapy
9. Hypervitaminosis A

68. What are the visual complaints of patients with benign intracranial hypertension?

Visual acuity is usually normal, but patients may report transient obscurations of vision. Their visual fields may show enlargement of the blind spot, and examination may show optic disc edema.

69. Are there any medicines that are useful in benign intracranial hypertension?

Usually, treatment includes the use of acetazolamide at 250 mg 1 or 2 times a day, or prednisone at 20 to 40 mg per day. Patients may need to be on treatment for up to 6 months at a time.

70. Aside from medication, are there any other treatments for benign intracranial hypertension?

Patients are generally treated with repeat spinal taps to maintain pressures in the normal range.

TEMPORAL ARTERITIS

71. What is temporal arteritis?

Temporal arteritis is a granulomatis arteritis affecting large and medium-sized arteries of the upper part of the body, especially the temporal vessels. Histologic studies reveal interval thickening and lymphocytic infiltration of the media and adventitia.

72. What is the clinical setting of temporal arteritis?

Patients generally present after age 60. The headaches are abrupt in onset, and patients also complain of pain and stiffness in the neck, shoulders and back, and sometimes in the pelvic girdle.

73. What is the headache associated with temporal arteritis?

Severe pain may be experienced in one temple, but sometimes occurs in the occipital area, face, jaw, or side of the neck, and may be associated with exquisite hypesthesia throughout the scalp. The pain may have a throbbing character.

74. Are there any serious complications of temporal arteritis?

The most severe complication is impairment of vision, which may result in unilateral loss of vision and may not be reversible.

75. How does one make a diagnosis of temporal arteritis?

In addition to clinical findings, ancillary data include an elevated sedimentation rate and positive temporal artery biopsy.

76. If temporal arteritis is suspected or diagnosed, is there any treatment?

Treatment involves immediate use of large doses (i.e., 40–60 mg) of prednisone daily for the first week, with gradual reduction over the next 4–6 weeks to a maintenance dose of 5–10 mg a day. Sedimentation rates can be followed, and when the sedimentation rate is normal for 4 months, further tapering of medication is justified.

BIBLIOGRAPHY

1. Dalessio DJ: Wolff's Headache and Other Head Pain, 5th ed. Oxford, Oxford University Press, 1986.
2. Diamond S, Dalessio DJ: Migraine headaches. In Diamond S, Dalessio DJ (eds): The Practicing Physician's Approach to Headaches, 4th ed. Baltimore, Williams & Wilkins, 1986, pp 49–65.

20. SEIZURES AND EPILEPSY

Paul Rutecki, M.D.

1. What is a seizure?
Many behaviors are referred to as seizures but the definition of a seizure should be restricted. Seizures are produced by the abnormal synchronization of cortical neurons that results in a change in perception or behavior. Between 7 and 10% of the population will have a seizure at some point in their lives.

2. What is epilepsy?
Epilepsy is the condition of recurrent seizures caused by an inherent brain abnormality. The underlying abnormality may result from a number of etiologies, including hereditary factors, developmental disorders, perinatal injury, infection, trauma, infarction, or neoplasm. Between 0.5 and 1% of the population has epilepsy.

3. How are seizures classified?
Seizures are classified according to their clinical and electroencephalographic (EEG) characteristics. The most recent classification of seizures is summarized below:

Classification of Epileptic Seizures

I. Partial seizures
    A. Simple partial seizures (consciousness not impaired)
    B. Complex partial seizures (consciousness impaired)
        1. Impairment of consciousness at onset
        2. Simple partial seizure onset followed by impaired consciousness
    C. Partial seizures evolving to generalized tonic-clonic convulsions (GTC)
        1. Simple partial evolving to GTC
        2. Complex partial evolving to GTC

II. Generalized seizures
    A. Absence seizures   C. Clonic seizures
        1. Typical   D. Tonic seizures
        2. Atypical, complex   E. Tonic-clonic seizures
    B. Myoclonic seizures   F. Atonic seizures (astatic)

Commission on the Classification and Terminology of the International League Against Epilepsy: Proposal for revised clinical and electroencephalographic classification of epileptic seizures. Epilepsia 22:489–501, 1981.

4. What is the difference between partial and generalized seizures?
Partial seizures start focally and have clinical and electroencephalographic changes that indicate onset from one brain region and in some cases one cerebral hemisphere. Impaired consciousness is the inability to respond normally to the environment because of altered awareness. Generalized seizures begin in both hemispheres at the same time. The clinician should try to classify all of the patient's seizure types because appropriate treatment depends on correct seizure classification.

5. What causes primary generalized seizures? At what age do they usually start?
Primary generalized seizures, i.e., seizures that cannot be localized to one cerebral hemisphere at onset, usually have a genetic predisposition. The seizures usually begin before the age of 20. These seizures are not associated with well-defined auras (an aura is the first subjective symptom of the seizure).

6. What does the EEG show in primary generalized seizures?

The interictal EEG signature of generalized seizures is the frontocentral dominant spike and wave discharge or polyspike and wave pattern. There may be shifting asymmetry of voltage, but there is not a consistent lateralizing feature.

7. What are the features of the different types of primary generalized seizures?

The shortest generalized seizures consist of a single myoclonic jerk during which consciousness is not lost. Associated with the jerk is a generalized spike or polyspike and wave discharge in the EEG. **Absence seizures** consist of 3-Hz spike and wave discharges in the EEG associated with a brief (usually less than 30 seconds) episode of unresponsiveness that may be accompanied by eyelid fluttering, decreased tone, increased tone, automatisms, autonomic components, or a combination of the above. **Atypical or complex absence seizures** are longer in duration and are associated with more automatisms and motor signs. The EEG shows a 1.5–2.5-Hz spike and wave discharge during the seizure. **Tonic seizures** are associated with generalized 10-Hz or faster activity. **Generalized tonic-clonic seizures** begin with an initial tonic component that is followed by a clonic component. At the end of the seizure the person is unresponsive and gradually regains consciousness. The EEG initially shows generalized 10-Hz activity during the tonic phase followed by slow waves or sharp and slow waves during the clonic phase **Atonic seizures** are associated with low-voltage fast activity, attenuation, or polyspike and wave discharges.

8. What are the characteristics of simple partial seizures?

The manifestations of partial seizures depend on the area of the brain involved. The more restricted the brain region involved, the more limited the symptoms and the less likely that consciousness will be impaired. Often simple partial seizures are referred to as auras, which may consist of an abnormal sensation (smells, flashing lights, somatosensory symptoms, etc.) or experimental phenomena (déjà vu, well-formed hallucinations). If the seizure is restricted to a small area of motor cortex, there is associated focal clonic activity. As the seizure activity spreads, the person may develop impaired consciousness and a complex partial seizure.

9. What are the characteristics of complex partial seizures?

Complex partial seizures are characterized by abnormal responsiveness to the environment, automatisms, autonomic features (pupillary dilatation, salivation), and amnesia for the seizure. Either simple partial or complex partial seizures may progress to a generalized tonic-clonic seizure.

10. How can complex partial seizures and absence seizures be differentiated clinically?

Three main features may help to differentiate complex partial from absence seizures. (1) Complex partial seizures, unlike absence seizures, may be preceded by a well-defined aura. (2) On average, complex partial seizures last 90 seconds, whereas absence seizures usually last only 10–15 seconds. (3) Following complex partial seizures, the patient is usually confused or has some postictal cognitive problem. Absence seizures are not associated with a postictal state and patients return to their baseline cognitive state at the end of the seizure. Automatisms are common with both absence and complex partial seizures.

Penry JK, Porter RJ, Dreifuss FE: Simultaneous recording of absence seizures with video tape and electroencephalography. Brain 98:427–440, 1985.

11. What are epileptic syndromes? How are they classified?

An epileptic syndrome is a composite of signs and symptoms associated with certain pathologies or etiologies (symptomatic) or lack of identifiable pathology or etiology (idiopathic). Many of the idiopathic syndromes are inherited. Syndromic classification of patients is useful because some of the syndromes have well-defined prognoses.

Classification of Epileptic Syndromes

I. Localization-related epilepsies and syndromes
   A. Idiopathic with age-related onset
      1. Benign childhood epilepsy with centrotemporal spike
      2. Childhood epilepsy with occipital paroxysms
   B. Symptomatic: Related to area of onset and clinical and EEG features (this encompasses most partial seizures)

II. Generalized epilepsies and syndromes
   A. Idiopathic, with age-related onset, listed in order of age.
      1. Benign neonatal familial convulsions
      2. Benign neonatal convulsions
      3. Benign myoclonic epilepsy in infancy
      4. Childhood absence epilepsy (pyknoepilepsy)
      5. Juvenile absence epilepsy
      6. Juvenile myoclonic epilepsy (impulsive petit mal)
      7. Epilepsy with grand mal seizures (GTCS) on awakening
   B. Idiopathic and/or symptomatic, in order of age
      1. West syndrome (infantile spasms)
      2. Lennox-Gastaut syndrome
      3. Epilepsy with myoclonic-astatic seizures
      4. Epilepsy with myoclonic absences
   C. Symptomatic-epileptic seizures as the presenting or dominant feature, i.e., malformations or degenerative diseases, with or without a metabolic etiology, that present with seizures as part of the clinical picture

III. Epilepsies and syndromes undetermined as to whether they are focal or generalized
   A. Both generalized and focal seizures
      1. Neonatal seizures
      2. Severe myoclonic epilepsy in infancy
      3. Epilepsy with continuous-spike waves during slow-wave sleep
      4. Acquired epileptic aphasia (Landau-Kleffner syndrome)
   B. Without unequivocal generalized of focal features—GTCS in which a focal or generalized onset cannot be determined by clinical or EEG features

IV. Special syndromes
   A. Situation-related seizures
      1. Febrile convulsions
      2. Seizures related to other identifiable situations such as stress, hormonal changes, drugs, alcohol, or sleep deprivation
   B. Isolated, apparently unprovoked epileptic events
   C. Epilepsies with specific modes of seizure precipitation, e.g., reading epilepsy
   D. Chronic progressive epilepsia partialis continua of childhood

Commission on the Classification and Terminology of the International League Against Epilepsy: Proposal for the classification of epilepsies and epileptic syndromes. Epilepsia 26:268–278, 1985.

12. What are the pathologic features of brains from people with epilepsy?

The answer depends on the etiology of the seizures. Obviously, patients who have seizures from cerebral infarctions, brain tumors, or congenital malformations will show these pathologic abnormalities. Hamartomas and heterotopias have also been associated with focal (partial) seizures. Patients with temporal lobe seizures of uncertain etiology or following prolonged febrile seizures most commonly have Ammon's horn sclerosis or hippocampal sclerosis. Patients with primary generalized epilepsy, particularly those with generalized tonic-clonic seizures, and patients with partial seizures have been noted to have subpial gliosis and areas of microdysgenesis. These areas of microdysgenesis consist of abnormal cortical architecture or small areas of ectopic gray matter.

Margerison JH, Corsellis JAN: Epilepsy and the temporal lobes. Brain 89:499–530, 1966.

13. What systemic physiologic changes occur during a seizure?

The systemic and CNS physiologic changes depend on the type of seizure. For both absence and complex partial seizures, the patient may have a variety of autonomic alterations, including changes in pulse rate, sweating, salivation, pupillary dilatation, and incontinence. The most dramatic systemic changes occur during generalized tonic-clonic seizures or prolonged tonic, myoclonic, or clonic seizures. Generalized tonic-clonic seizures are associated with an increase in blood pressure and pulse rate, increased autonomic nervous system activation, a metabolic acidosis, a drop in PO_2 and an increase in PCO_2 during the apneic tonic phase, and, rarely, hyperkalemia or rhabdomyolysis. Following an isolated generalized tonic-clonic seizure, these abnormalities usually return to baseline within an hour. With prolonged generalized tonic-clonic seizures, these systemic problems intensify and can have serious consequences.

14. Describe CNS physiologic changes that occur during a seizure.

During a seizure, blood flow and glucose utilization in the brain are increased. Accompanying the neuronal activity may be changes in lactate and pH, alterations in the concentration of neurotransmitters, an increase in extracellular potassium, and a decrease in extracellular calcium. Generalized tonic-clonic seizures and most complex partial seizures activate the hypothalamus and increase serum prolactin, a finding that may help to differentiate epileptic from nonepileptic seizures.

15. What are the identifiable causes of seizures as a function of age?

Common Causes of Seizures by Age

NEONATE TO 3 YRS.	3 TO 20 YRS.	20 TO 60 YRS.	OVER 60 YRS.
Prenatal injury	Genetic	Brain tumors	Vascular disease
Perinatal injury	predisposition	Trauma	Brain tumors, especially
Metabolic defects	Infections	Vascular disease	metastatic tumors
Congenital	Trauma	Infections	Trauma
malformations	Congenital		Systemic metabolic
CNS infections	malformations		derangements
Postnatal trauma	Metabolic defects		Infections

16. What are the metabolic causes of seizures?

Common Metabolic Causes of Seizures

1. Hypocalcemia	6. Anoxia
2. Hyponatremia	7. Nonketotic hyperglycemic states
3. Hypoglycemia	8. Inherited metabolic diseases
4. Liver failure	a. Aminoacidurias
5. Renal failure	b. Urea cycle disorders

17. What drugs are common causes of seizures?

Seizures may be caused by many drugs, both prescribed and illicitly taken medications. Cocaine and amphetamines are the two drugs of abuse most commonly associated with seizures. Some drugs at toxic levels will produce seizures. These include penicillin, lidocaine, aminophylline, and isoniazid. Other drugs, such as phenothiazines and tricyclic antidepressants, appear to lower seizure threshold and, in susceptible individuals, may produce seizures. Whenever a patient presents initially with a seizure, toxicology studies are indicated. The other setting associated with seizures is withdrawal from drugs, particularly alcohol, barbiturates, or benzodiazepines.

18. What are the characteristics of alcohol withdrawal seizures?
Chronic alcohol abuse may be associated with seizures during abstinence. Most seizures occur between 7 and 48 hours after the last drink. The seizures are usually generalized tonic-clonic, although multiple seizures or even status epilepticus may occur. A subset of patients with alcohol withdrawal seizures have epilepsy and require maintenance anticonvulsants. These patients usually have posttraumatic epilepsy. In patients with only alcohol withdrawal seizures, benzodiazepines appear to be the most efficacious therapy, whereas phenytoin does not appear to help.

Porter RJ, Mattson RH, Cramer JA, Diamond I (eds): Alcohol and Seizures: Basic Mechanisms and Clinical Concepts. Philadelphia, F.A. Davis, 1990.

19. What inherited diseases are associated with seizures?
Numerous genetic diseases, including many degenerative neurologic diseases, are associated with seizures. At least 25 autosomal dominant diseases are associated with seizures, including tuberous sclerosis and neurofibromatosis. Approximately 100 autosomal recessive diseases are associated with seizures, many of which have an inborn error of metabolism; for instance, the aminoacidurias and the lipid storage diseases. Finally, some 20 X-linked diseases are associated with seizures, including adrenoleukodystrophy and Pelizaeus-Merzbacher disease.

20. What are the four most common inherited epileptic syndromes?
(1) Febrile convulsions, (2) benign childhood epilepsy with central temporal spikes, (3) childhood absence epilepsy, and (4) juvenile myoclonic epilepsy. The first three syndromes usually are associated with seizures that remit spontaneously. Juvenile myoclonic epilepsy usually responds to treatment with valproate.

21. What are benign febrile convulsions?
Benign febrile convulsions are an inherited predisposition to developing a tonic-clonic seizure with a high fever. The description is limited to convulsions associated with high fever in persons under the age of 5 (usually between 6 and 36 months of age), with no etiology for the seizure other than the fever. Benign febrile seizures are common, occurring in 3–5% of children under the age of 5. Most individuals will have only one or two seizures.

22. What is the consequence of having a febrile seizure?
It is important to differentiate benign febrile convulsions from epilepsy. In general, if there are no other reasons to suspect recurrent seizures, the child is not treated. A single isolated febrile seizure that is short in duration probably does not greatly influence the later development of epilepsy.

Risk Factors for Epilepsy

1. Underlying neurologic or developmental abnormality
2. Family history of nonfebrile seizures
3. Prolonged febrile convulsions
4. Multiple febrile convulsions
5. Atypical or focal features (complex febrile seizures)

Annegers JF, Hauser WA, Shirts SB, Kurland LT: Factors prognostic of unprovoked seizures after febrile convulsions. N Engl J Med 316:493–498, 1987.

Nelson KB, Ellenberg JH: Predictors of epilepsy in children who have experienced febrile seizures. N Engl J Med 295:1029–1033, 1976.

23. Which factors predict the development of epilepsy following head trauma?

Open head trauma produced by bullets or shrapnel is associated with a 50% or greater chance of developing epilepsy. Closed head trauma, such as would occur following automobile accidents or blunt injuries, carries a much lower risk (5% or less). Factors that predispose to the development of epilepsy following head trauma include a seizure within 2 weeks of the injury, a depressed skull fracture, or the presence of a cerebral contusion or subarachnoid blood.

Jennet WB: Epilepsy After Non-Missile Head Injuries. Chicago, Year Book Medical Publishers, 1975.

24. What is the differential diagnosis of progressive myoclonic epilepsy?

The five main causes of progressive myoclonic epilepsy may be differentiated based on their clinical, pathologic, or laboratory features:

1. **Unverricht-Lundborg disease** is a clinical diagnosis. Affected patients begin having myoclonic seizures between the ages of 8 and 13 years. Dementia is not a prominent feature.

2. **Lafora body disease** presents in persons 11–18 years of age. Dementia is a prominent feature. The disease is named for Lafora bodies—eosinophilic inclusions present in skin, liver, or brain biopsies.

3. **Neuronal ceroid lipofuscinosis** may present at any age, is associated with dementia, and has visual loss with characteristic funduscopic findings. It also is associated with inclusion bodies seen on electron microscopy of nerve.

4. **Sialidosis** is associated with dysmorphic features and funduscopic findings (cherry-red spot), and is associated with α-N-acetylneuraminidase deficiency.

5. **Mitochondrial encephalomyopathy with ragged red fibers** (MERRF) on muscle biopsy is often associated with short stature, hearing loss, optic atrophy, neuropathy, and myopathy. Some patients have maternally inherited mitochondrial genome abnormalities.

Berkovic SF, Andermann F, Carpenter S, Wolfe LS: Progressive myoclonic epilepsies: Specific causes and diagnosis. N Engl J Med 315:296–305, 1986.

25. What percentage of persons with epilepsy will have an abnormal EEG during the interictal period?

The answer depends on the type of epilepsy. One study found that only 35–40% of patients with the clinical diagnosis of epilepsy had interictal epileptiform activity on a single EEG. Most of these patients had partial seizures with or without secondary generalization. Multiple EEGs could enhance the yield of positive EEGs to 60%. Untreated patients with absence seizures usually have an abnormal routine EEG. The diagnostic yield of EEG may also be increased by prolonged monitoring, including sleep. An important point is that epilepsy is a clinical diagnosis and cannot be ruled out by normal EEG.

Salinsky M, Kanter R, Dasheiff RM: Effectiveness of multiple EEGs in supporting the diagnosis of epilepsy: An operational curve. Epilepsia 28:331–334, 1987.

26. What is the intracellular correlate of the interictal EEG spike?

In animal models of epilepsy, coincident with an interictal EEG spike, many neurons depolarize and generate a burst of action potentials that are followed by an afterhyper-polarization. The depolarization is known as the paroxysmal depolarizing shift (PDS) and is composed of a large, synchronously occurring compound excitatory postsynaptic potential. This depolarization also activates a number of voltage-dependent ionic currents, including calcium currents, sodium currents, and calcium-activated potassium current, that contribute to the PDS and afterhyperpolarization.

27. Which patients with seizures should have CT or MRI scans?

Patients with partial seizures or focal features on EEG should have CT or MRI scans to look for a brain lesion associated with their seizures. CT scans should be performed with intravenous contrast medium, particularly in adults, because structural lesions are often the cause of the seizures. Patients with clear-cut primary generalized epilepsy based on EEG and clinical features usually do not require CT or MRI scanning.

28. What is the value of PET scanning in patients with epilepsy?

Positron emission tomography (PET) scans have helped us to understand some of the metabolic changes that occur during seizures. PET scans demonstrate hypermetabolism or increased glucose uptake during the seizure. Most patients, however, are studied during the interictal period. In this setting, patients with epilepsy that have focal onset may show an area of hypometabolism in the region of seizure onset and a decrease in glucose uptake. PET scanning has been useful in helping to localize seizure onset in patients with intractable complex partial seizures that are being evaluated for surgical therapy.

29. When should antiepileptic treatment be initiated?

People should be treated with antiepileptic medication when the clinician thinks that the person will probably have another seizure without treatment. The seizure type may help with this decision. For example, absence seizures are rarely isolated and so require therapy, whereas febrile seizures are often isolated and therapy is usually not indicated. Between 20 and 70% of people with an isolated unprovoked generalized tonic-clonic seizure will never have another seizure. Ideally, it would be best not to treat these patients. Seizure recurrence is more likely if the patient has focal neurologic deficits, mental retardation, an EEG that demonstrates epileptiform abnormalities, or a structural brain lesion. In these patients it is reasonable to begin antiepileptic therapy. In patients with well-defined provocative etiology, it is best to treat the underlying process rather than the seizures themselves, particularly in clear-cut cases of alcohol withdrawal seizures and drug-induced seizures.

    Hauser WA, Anderson VA, Loewenson RB, et al: Seizure recurrence after a first unprovoked seizure. N Engl J Med 307:522–528, 1982.

30. When should antiepileptic treatment be stopped? What are the risk factors for recurrence of seizures?

Treatment should be stopped when it is the physician's opinion that the patient probably will not have seizures off medications. Certain seizure types and benign epileptic syndromes will remit. Patients with absence seizures will usually "outgrow" their seizures and therapy will no longer be needed. Benign childhood epilepsy with centrotemporal spikes also remit. Recent studies suggested that approximately one-third of adult patients and one-fourth of children who were seizure free for 2 years will relapse following termination of antiepileptic medication.

Risk factors for recurrence include:

1. Prolonged duration before seizures were controlled
2. High frequency of seizures before control
3. Neurologic abnormalities
4. Mental retardation
5. Complex partial seizures
6. Consistently abnormal EEGs

    Shinnar S, Vining PG, Mellits ED, et al: Discontinuing antiepileptic medication in children with epilepsy after two years without seizures: A prospective study. N Engl J Med 313:976–980, 1985.
    Callaghan N, Garrett A, Goggin T: Withdrawal of anticonvulsant drugs in patients free of seizures for two years: A prospective study. N Engl J Med 318:942–946, 1988.

31. Which antiepileptic medications are most appropriate for different seizure types?

The choice of medication is dictated by the types of seizures the patient has. If possible, monotherapy should be used.

First- and Second-Line Drugs for Specific Seizure Types

	PARTIAL SEIZURES	GENERALIZED SEIZURES			
		Tonic-clonic	Absence	Myclonic	Atonic/Tonic
First-line drugs	Carbamazepine Phenytoin	Carbamazepine Phenytoin Valproate	Ethosuximide Valproate	Valproate Ethosuximide	Valproate Ethosuximide
Second-line drugs	Phenobarbital Primidone Valproate	Phenobarbital Primidone	Clonazepam	Clonazepam	Clonazepam

The selections in this table are based on side effects as well as effectiveness. Phenobarbital and primidone are as efficacious as phenytoin and carbamazepine but are more likely to produce side effects. Tonic and atonic seizures are often resistant to therapy, and valproate seems to be most efficacious. Tonic and atonic seizures may be secondarily generalized, and phenytoin and carbamazepine can be helpful.

Mattson RH, Cramer JA, Smith DB, et al: Comparison of carbamazepine, phenobarbital, phenytoin, and primidone in partial and secondarily generalized seizures. N Engl J Med 313:145–151, 1985.

Mattson RH, Cramer JA, Collins JF, et al: A comparison of valproate with carbamazepine for the treatment of complex partial seizures and secondarily generalized tonic-clonic seizures in adults. N Engl J Med 327:765–771, 1992.

32. What are the mechanisms of action of antiepileptic drugs?

Phenytoin, carbamazepine, and valproate block sodium channels and impair high-frequency action-potential generation. At higher than therapeutic concentrations, phenobarbital may also decrease repetitive firing. Some of these drugs may also reduce high-threshold calcium currents, although this often is in the supratherapeutic range. In the therapeutic range, the barbiturates and the diazepam derivatives enhance GABA responses. Diazepam derivatives increase the binding of GABA to the GABA receptor. The barbiturates appear to favor channel opening of the chloride ionophore associated with the GABA receptor. Lastly, ethosuximide appears to act by reducing the low-threshold calcium current that is responsible for burst behavior in thalamic neurons.

33. How often should antiepileptic medications be given?

Antiepileptic medications should be given at least every half-life. Some medications may need to be given more frequently because of peak dose side effects. This would be the case for ethosuximide, where patients tolerate twice daily or three times daily dosing rather than a single dose a day.

Half-life Frequencies for Antiepileptic Medications

DRUG	HALF-LIFE (HR)
Carbamazepine	12–18
Ethosuximide	48
Phenobarbital	96
Phenytoin	24
Primidone	8–12
Valproate	8–12

Values represent adult half-lives and may vary depending on whether the patient is on monotherapy or polytherapy. The half-life for phenytoin depends on the serum concentration; a higher concentration is associated with a longer half-life because of nonlinear kinetics.

34. What are the advantages of monotherapy?
1. In most situations, controls seizures as well as two drugs.
2. Prevents interactions between antiepileptic medications.
3. Is less expensive.
4. Improves compliance.

35. What are the main side effects of commonly used antiepileptic medications?
Side effects may be dose dependent or dose independent. In general, most anticonvulsants can have sedative properties and interfere with motor performance in a dose-dependent manner.

Side Effects of Anticonvulsants

DOSE DEPENDENT		DOSE INDEPENDENT	
Ataxia	Nausea, vomiting	Weight gain	Hirsutism
Phenytoin	Valproate	Valproate	Phenytoin
Carbamazepine	Carbamazepine	Carbamazepine	
Phenobarbital	Ethosuximide		Dupuytren's contrac-
Primidone	Phenytoin	Hair loss	tures
		Valproate	Phenobarbital
Diplopia, blurred vision	Headache		
Carbamazepine	Ethosuximide	Behavioral	Gingival hyperplasia
Phenytoin		Phenobarbital	Phenytoin
	Tremor	Primidone	
Sedation	Valproate	Ethosuximide	
Phenobarbital			
Phenytoin			
Carbamazepine			
Valproate			

36. What are the main drug interactions among antiepileptic medications?
Most antiepileptic medications influence the metabolism of other antiepileptic medications. This is seen most often with phenytoin, primidone, carbamazepine, and phenobarbital, which induce liver microsomal enzyme systems. Another mechanism of drug interaction is displacement of protein binding. Such an interaction often occurs with phenytoin and valproate, which are highly protein-bound in the serum. In some situations, antiepileptic medications will inhibit the metabolism of another antiepileptic medication.

Effects of Add-on Drugs on Original Drug Levels

	ADD-ON DRUG				
ORIGINAL DRUG	Carb	Pb	Pht	Prim	Val
Carbamazepine		↓	↓	↓	↑ *
Phenobarbital	↔		↑ ↓		↑
Phenytoin	↑ ↓	↑ ↓		↑ ↓	↓ *
Primidone	↑ pb		↑ pb		↑
Valproate	↓	↓	↓	↓	

* Valproate increases the epoxide metabolite of carbamazepine and may increase toxic side effects. Valproate increases the free level of phenytoin, although the total level may decrease.
Carb = carbamazepine, Pb = phenobarbital, Pht = phenytoin, Prim = primidone, Val = valproate, ↑ pb = increased phenobarbital level.

37. What are the main drug interactions between antiepileptic medications and other commonly used medications?

Whenever there is a change in seizure control or occurrence of toxic symptoms without a change in dosage of antiepileptic medication, drug interaction should be considered.

Effects of Drugs on Antiepileptic Drug Actions or Levels

INCREASE EFFECTS OF ANTIEPILEPTIC DRUG				DECREASE EFFECTS OF ANTIEPILEPTIC DRUG	
Phenytoin	Carbamazepine	Phenobarbital	Valproate	Phenytoin	Phenobarbital
Cimetidine	Cimetidine	Antihistamines	Chlorpromazine	Antacids	Dicumarol
Chloramphenicol	Diltiazem	Corticosteroids	Dicumarol	Carafate	Folate
Clofibrate	Danazol	Isoniazid	Phenylbutazone	Bleomycin	Phenylbutazone
Dicumarol	Erythromycin	Propoxyphene	Salicylates	Cisplatinum	
Disulfiram	Isoniazid	Tricyclic anti-		Diazoxide	
Imipramine	Lithium	depressants		Folate	
Isoniazid	Propoxyphene			Pyridoxine	
Phenylbutazone	Verapamil			Reserpine	
Propoxyphene				Vinblastine	
Salicylates					
Sulfonamides					
Trazodone					
Tolbutamide					

38. What are the idiosyncratic reactions to antiepileptic medications?

The most common is skin rashes, which may be relatively severe, leading to exfoliative dermatitis or Stevens-Johnson syndrome. Skin rashes are most common with phenytoin, carbamazepine, and barbiturates. Most antiepileptic medications can also suppress the bone marrow and cause aplastic anemia, agranulocytosis, or thrombocytopenia. These problems have been seen with all antiepileptic medications. Another idiosyncratic reaction consists of drug-induced hepatitis and, at times, a full-blown serum sickness picture. Valproate hepatic toxicity is most common in patients under the age of 2, who are retarded and are taking other medications. Phenytoin, phenobarbital, ethosuximide, and carbamazepine may produce vasculitis. Valproate has also been implicated as a cause of pancreatitis.

39. When and how often should blood levels of antiepileptic drugs be checked?

Monitoring of antiepileptic drug levels is indicated when the patient is initially loaded with the medication and when the drug reaches a steady-state concentration, usually after approximately 5 half-lives. Monitoring of drug levels is helpful in determining patient compliance and in documenting high levels when the patient has toxic symptomatology.

40. Which screening blood tests should be performed on patients taking antiepileptic medications? How often should they be done?

Many antiepileptic medications may affect the bone marrow's ability to produce blood cells or may cause liver dysfunction. It is reasonable to use a CBC and liver function tests as baseline studies to identify predisposing problems. After this initial screening, it is usually not necessary to perform these studies routinely unless the patient is symptomatic. The exceptions are young children or mentally retarded patients who cannot communicate their toxic syndromes.

Pellock JM, Willmore LJ: A rational guide to routine blood monitoring in patients receiving antiepileptic drugs. Neurology 41:961–964, 1991.

41. Should antiepileptic drugs be used following head trauma to prevent the development of epilepsy?
A definitive answer to this question does not exist. The most recent study assessing phenytoin concluded that therapy was useful only during the first week following head trauma. At later dates, the side effects produced by phenytoin appeared to be detrimental to patients with severe neurologic damage following the head trauma. At present, no drug clearly has been shown to be effective prophylaxis for posttraumatic epilepsy.

Tempkin NR, Dikmen SS, Wilensky AJ, et al: A randomized, double-blind study of phenytoin for the prevention of posttraumatic seizures. N Engl J Med 323:497–502, 1990.

42. What are the teratogenic risks of antiepileptic medications?
All antiepileptic medications have teratogenic features. In general, a pregnant patient taking a single antiepileptic medication has a three-fold increased risk of birth defects. The teratogenic effects of antiepileptic medication are more likely when more than one medication is used. The physician should try to treat the patient with only one antiepileptic medication during pregnancy. A patient and her family should be counseled about these potential effects, but rarely is pregnancy contraindicated because of antiepileptic therapy.

43. What are the primary teratogenic effects of antiepileptic medications?
Most of these are relatively minor and consist of cleft lip/cleft palate abnormalities, hypertelorism, hypoplastic fingernails, or distal phalanges. Major defects include congenital heart abnormalities, urogenital malformations, and neural tube defects. Valproate has been associated with approximately a 1% risk of a neural tube defect. Recent information suggests that carbamazepine may increase the risk of neural tube defects.

Rosa FW: Spina bifida in infants of women treated with carbamazepine during pregnancy. N Engl J Med 324:674–677, 1991.

44. What is status epilepticus? How is it classified?
Status epilepticus is a state of continuous seizures without return of normal neurologic function between them. Any of the classified seizure types may progress to status epilepticus. Another way to classify status epilepticus is convulsive or nonconvulsive. Convulsive status epilepticus is a medical emergency that can be produced by either primary generalized or secondarily generalized tonic-clonic seizures. Nonconvulsive status epilepticus refers to either absence or complex partial status epilepticus. In either case, the patient does not have major motor seizures, but is abnormal cognitively and may appear to be in a fugue state. Absence status appears to have no morbidity (unless injuries occur during the status), but complex partial status can lead to permanent cognitive deficits.

45. What are the most common causes of status epilepticus?

*1. Antiepileptic drug noncompliance or withdrawal	5. Cerebral infarction
2. Alcohol withdrawal	6. Cerebral hemorrhages
3. Metabolic abnormalities	7. Meningitis
4. Brain tumors	8. Undetermined (10–15% of patients)

* Most common.

Aminoff MJ, Simon RP: Status epilepticus: Causes, clinical features, and consequences in 98 patients. Am J Med 69:657–666, 1980.

46. How is absence status epilepticus treated?
Absence status is treated with intravenous diazepam or derivatives—not with phenytoin or the barbiturates.

47. How is complex partial status epilepticus treated?

Complex partial status is usually not associated with life-threatening systemic complications but may result in loss of memory function and should be treated aggressively, similar to generalized tonic-clonic status.

48. How is convulsive status epilepticus treated?

Generalized tonic-clonic or convulsive status epilepticus is a medical emergency and every effort should be made to stop the seizures within an hour. The mainstay of therapy is intravenous phenytoin, which should be given at a rate of 50 mg/min. During the time that phenytoin is being administered, either diazepam or lorazepam may be given acutely to suppress seizures. Following the phenytoin load, if the patient continues to have seizures, then phenobarbital should be given. If the patient has had benzodiazepines, addition of intravenous phenobarbital is more likely to cause respiratory arrest and the patient should be intubated. If a patient is resistant to phenytoin, phenobarbital, and diazepam, then anesthesia should be administered, preferably with pentobarbital. An outline for the treatment of status epilepticus is presented below.

Protocol for Treatment of Generalized Tonic-Clonic Status Epilepticus

0–5 min	Provide for maintenance of vital signs. Maintain airway. Give oxygen. Observe and examine patient.
6–10 min	Obtain 50 ml of blood for glucose, calcium, magnesium, electrolytes, BUN, liver functions, anticonvulsant levels, CBC, and toxicology screen. Begin normal saline IV and give 50 ml of 50% glucose and 100 mg of thiamine. Monitor EKG, blood pressure, and, if possible, EEG.
11–30 min	Use intravenous diazepam to stop seizures, 5 mg in 1–2 minutes; may repeat every 5–10 minutes if seizures recur, up to a total dose of 30 mg. An alternative approach is to use lorazepam, 2–4 mg IV every 5 minutes, up to a total dose of 10 mg.
11–30 min	Give phenytoin 18 mg/kg IV at a rate of 50 mg/min or less. If cardiac arrhythmias occur, then slow infusion rate.
31–60 min	If seizures persist 10–20 minutes after administration of phenytoin, intubate patient and give phenobarbital at a rate of 50–100 mg/min until seizures stop or 20 mg/kg is given.
After 60 minutes of status	Review laboratory results and correct abnormalities. Arrange for anesthesia, neuromuscular blockade, and EEG monitoring. Either inhalation anesthesia (isoflurane) or barbiturate anesthesia (pentobarbital, 6–15 mg/kg loading dose then 0.5–5 mg/kg/hr) should be used. Pentobarbital often causes circulatory collapse, so be prepared to administer a pressor agent such as dopamine.

Delgado-Escueta AV, Wasterlain C, Treiman DM, Porter RJ: Management of status epilepticus. N Engl J Med 306:1337–1340, 1982.

Lowenstein DH, Aminoff MJ, Simon RP: Barbiturate anesthesia in the treatment of status epilepticus: Clinical experience with 14 patients. Neurology 1988; 38:395–400.

49. What is epilepsia partialis continua? How is it treated?

Epilepsia partialis continua is simple partial motor status epilepticus, which consists of rhythmic contractions of a restricted region of the body, usually the face and the hand or fingers. These brief jerks are intermittent but occur at least every few seconds and may intensify or secondarily generalize. The patient is usually fully conscious during these seizures but there may be associated weakness in the affected limbs. The most common causes include nonketotic hyperglycemic states, cerebral infarction, encephalitis, and cerebral neoplasms. Treatment is directed at correcting metabolic abnormalities. Antiepileptic medications are used, but epilepsia partialis continua may be resistant to drug therapy short of anesthesia.

Thomas JE, Reagan TJ, Klass DW: Epilepsia partialis continua: A review of 32 cases. Arch Neurol 34:266–275, 1977.

50. Does continuous seizure activity cause nervous system damage?

Certain seizure types are not known to have any significant sequela, such as absence seizures. In other settings, after a certain duration of epileptiform activity, there is irreversible neuronal loss. A number of mechanisms probably mediate this neuronal death, including calcium loading of neurons and excitotoxicity produced by excessive glutamate release. Because continuous seizure activity can cause neuronal death, it is important to monitor the patient's EEG during the treatment of status, particularly if the patient is paralyzed by neuromuscular blockade. It is also important to try to prevent any neuronal death by controlling the patient's status within the first 60 minutes.

Meldrum BS, Vigouroux RA, Brierly JB: Systemic factors and epileptic brain damage. Arch Neurol 29:82–87, 1973.

Sloviter RS: Decreased hippocampal inhibition and a selective loss of interneurons in experimental epilepsy. Science 235:73–76, 1987.

51. What recommendations about driving should a physician make to a patient with epilepsy?

This depends upon the state where the physician is practicing medicine. Basically, states either require the physician to report any patient with a seizure, or require the patient to report any medical condition that may interfere with the ability to operate a motor vehicle. In general, physicians should caution against driving, especially if the patient's seizures are not controlled. It is usually most appropriate to have the patient's case evaluated by the state's driver-licensing authorities. Interestingly, drivers with epilepsy have only a slightly increased risk of an accident.

Krumholz A, Fisher RS, Lesser RP, Hauser WA: Driving and epilepsy: A review and reappraisal. JAMA 265:622–626, 1991.

52. When should patients be considered for epilepsy surgery?

Approximately 20% of patients with epilepsy have seizures that are not completely controlled despite adequate antiepileptic therapy and good patient compliance. These patients should be considered for epilepsy surgery.

53. What types of epilepsy surgery are available?

There are basically two types of epilepsy surgery: (1) focal resection of areas of epileptogenesis, and (2) disconnecting procedures, usually corpus callosotomy. Corpus callosotomy may be indicated in severe generalized seizures, usually associated with atonic or tonic seizures that produce falling. Resective surgeries should be considered in partial seizures, particularly those that seem to begin exclusively from one circumscribed area of the brain.

54. Which patients are good candidates for epilepsy surgery?

The actual criteria for choosing patients depends on a number of variables. First and foremost, the patient has seizures that are intractable to medical therapy. Second, the patient will have significant benefit from becoming seizure feee. Third, seizure onset can be localized. Fourth, the potential morbidity of the surgery is acceptable and less than the morbidity of the seizures. The recent NIH Consensus Statement estimates that there are 2000–5000 patients per year in the U.S. who develop epilepsy and could benefit from epilepsy surgery.

NIH Consensus Conference: Surgery for epilepsy. JAMA 264:729–733, 1990.

ACKNOWLEDGMENT

I would like to thank Dr. Richard Hrachovy for helpful comments on a draft of this chapter.

BIBLIOGRAPHY

1. Engel J: Seizures and Epilepsy. Philadelphia, F.A. Davis, 1989.
2. Hauser WA, Hesdorffer DC (eds): Epilepsy: Frequency, Causes, and Consequences. New York, Churchill Livingstone, 1988.
3. Laidlaw J, Richens A, Oxley J (eds): A Textbook of Epilepsy. New York, Churchill Livingstone, 1988.
4. Levy RH, Dreifuss FE, Mattson RH, et al (eds): Antiepileptic Drugs, 3rd ed. New York, Raven Press, 1989.
5. Porter RJ: Epilepsy: 100 Elementary Principles. Philadelphia, W.B. Saunders, 1989.

21. SLEEP DISORDERS

James D. Frost, Jr., M.D.

1. What is sleep?

Sleep is a complex physiologic state that occurs periodically in most vertebrate species, and similar states are often observed in invertebrate organisms. It is characterized by relative quiescence, immobility, and greatly decreased responsiveness to external stimuli. In mammals, two distinct sleep states are recognized: rapid-eye-movement sleep (REM) and non-REM sleep. REM sleep is characterized by pronounced muscular atonia, phasic twitches, and bursts of rapid eye movements. During this state the EEG is relatively low in amplitude and is often similar to that seen during drowsiness, although individuals in REM sleep appear deeply asleep by behavioral criteria. Most dreaming apparently occurs during the REM stage. Non-REM sleep is further subdivided into stages, 1, 2, 3 and 4, which are characterized by progressively increasing amplitude and decreasing frequency on EEG. Muscle tone tends to be higher than that seen during REM, and phasic movements are not typical. Individuals normally exhibit a fairly regular alternation of non-REM and REM sleep during the sleep period, with cycle times of approximately 90 minutes. There are relatively few awakenings (typically fewer than 10 per night), and the various stages of sleep are present in consistent amounts. In the typical adult, the total sleep time is divided as follows: stage 1, less than 5%; stage 2, 40–60%, stages 3 and 4, 10–20%; and stage REM, 18–25%.

2. How is normal sleep regulated by the brain?

Essentially every area of the brain is involved in sleep, as has been demonstrated by a variety of experimental manipulations. While no discrete "sleep center" exists, several regions appear to subserve crucial roles that govern the timing and sequencing of the sleep process. The suprachiasmatic area of the hypothalamus is directly involved in the regulation of circadian cycles that determine when sleep occurs within the 24-hour day. On the other hand, a group of nuclei in the pontomesencephalic region (including locus ceruleus, dorsal raphe, and several cholinergic areas) are critical for the alternating sequence of REM and non-REM cycles normally observed during sleep. Neurons of the basal forebrain and anterior hypothalamus also appear to play a primary role in control of sleep onset.

3. What are sleep disorders?

Currently, more than 50 individual entities are classified as sleep disorders. In addition, many other medical and psychiatric conditions can produce disturbed sleep as a secondary manifestation. Disordered sleep can be manifested in several ways: insomnia (difficulty initiating and/or maintaining sleep), excessive sleepiness ("hypersomnia"), and atypical motor or behavioral events occurring in a particular relationship to sleep states or sleep-wake transitions.

4. How are sleep disorders classified?

Three major categories are recognized:

1. **Dyssomnias** are conditions associated with difficulty initiating/maintaining sleep or excessive sleepiness. This group is further subdivided into intrinsic disorders, extrinsic disorders, and circadian disorders.

2. **Parasomnias** are conditions that occur with a particular relationship to the sleep process, but are not necessarily associated with disrupted sleep or excessive sleepiness. These include arousal disorders, sleep-wake transition disorders, REM-associated disorders, and a miscellaneous group.

3. **Disorders associated with medical or psychiatric conditions** are essentially secondary sleep disorders that accompany other recognized medical entities.

5. What specific conditions are included within the dyssomnia category?

Dyssomnias

INTRINSIC DISORDERS	EXTRINSIC DISORDERS	CIRCADIAN DISORDERS
Obstructive sleep apnea syndrome	Drug/alcohol-dependent insomnia	Time zone change syndrome
Central sleep apnea syndrome	Limit-setting sleep disorder	Delayed sleep phase syndrome
Psychophysiological insomnia	Insufficient sleep syndrome	Advanced sleep phase syndrome
Idiopathic insomnia	Inadequate sleep hygiene	Shift work sleep disorder
Narcolepsy	Environmental sleep disorder	Irregular sleep wake pattern
Idiopathic hypersomnia	Altitude insomnia	Non-24-hr sleep-wake disorder
Periodic limb movements	Adjustment sleep disorder	
Restless legs syndrome	Food-allergy insomnia	
Central aveolar hypoventilation	Nocturnal eating syndrome	
Posttraumatic hypersomnia	Toxin-dependent sleep disorder	
Recurrent hypersomnia		
Sleep state misperception		

6. What conditions are classified as parasomnias?

Parasomnias

Arousal Disorders	Sleep-Wake Transition Disorders
Confusional arousals	Rhythmic movement disorder
Sleepwalking	Sleep starts
Sleep terrors	Sleep talking
	Nocturnal leg cramps
REM-Associated Parasomnias	Other Parasomnias
Nightmares	Bruxism
Sleep paralysis	Enuresis
REM sleep behavior disorder	Primary snoring
REM sleep-related sinus arrest	Infant sleep apnea
Sleep-related painful erection	Nocturnal paroxysmal dystonia
Impaired sleep-related penile erection	Sudden unexplained nocturnal death
	Congenital central hypoventilation syndrome
	Sudden infant death syndrome
	Benign neonatal sleep myoclonus
	Sleep-related abnormal swallowing syndrome

7. How reliable are patients' reports of sleeping difficulties?
Subjective reports of sleep quality and quantity are often grossly incorrect. For example, individuals with significant hypersomnic conditions are sometimes unaware of the fact that they fall asleep at inappropriate times. Motor vehicle accidents may be attributed to "blackouts" or seizures. Impaired job performance may be related solely to poor memory function. Patients with certain conditions (such as sleep apnea or nocturnal myoclonus) may awaken literally dozens of times throughout the night, and may have both a low total sleep time and atypical sleep-stage distribution, and yet report to the physician that they fall asleep quickly every night and sleep soundly with few or no arousals. The opposite is also common, and many individuals who report the presence of severe insomnia later prove

(during sleep laboratory testing) to have normal sleep times and few awakenings. Because this phenomenon is common, the physician must be wary of all subjective reports of sleep characteristics and seek independent verification whenever there is evidence that a clinically significant condition may be present.

8. How much sleep is required for normal daytime function?
Most normal individuals average between 6 and 8 hours of sleep per night, but there is a great deal of individual variability in this requirement. As a general rule, if an individual's daytime performance is significantly impaired by excessive sleepiness, and this condition persists in spite of adherence to a regularly scheduled nocturnal sleep period of at least 8 hours, more definitive diagnostic tests are indicated. A significant change of an individual's apparent sleep requirements is also often an indication of an underlying sleep disorder.

9. Is total sleep time the only determinant of the ability to maintain a normal level of daytime alertness?
No. The structure, or architecture, of the sleep pattern is also crucial for normal waking function. When sleep is fragmented by frequent brief arousals, or if other factors disturb the normal stage distribution, excessive daytime sleepiness can sometimes result even if actual sleep time is not significantly reduced.

10. How can the physician objectively assess nocturnal sleep quality and quantity?
The most important diagnostic tool available to the physician dealing with sleep disorders is the sleep study or polysomnogram. By monitoring sleep/wake state throughout the night, concurrently observing multiple physiologic parameters, and continuously documenting behavioral status (video recording), it is possible to obtain diagnostic information that is highly reliable and objective. This test provides quantitative measures of total sleep time, number of awakenings, sleep-stage distribution, respiratory dysfunction, cardiac arrhythmias, atypical movements, nocturnal seizures, and character of parasomnias.

11. What variables are recorded during polysomnography?
1. Electroencephalogram (EEG)   5. Respiratory effort
2. Electro-oculogram (EOG)   6. Nasal/oral airflow
3. Electromyogram (EMG)   7. Oxygen saturation
   from submental area   8. End tidal PCO_2
4. Electrocardiogram (EKG)   9. Leg movement (EMG or accelerometer)

12. Can daytime sleepiness also be measured objectively?
Yes. The multiple sleep latency test (MSLT) evaluates the presence and degree of daytime sleepiness. This procedure makes use of polygraphic monitoring (EEG, EOG, EMG, and EKG) during a series of 4 or 5 nap sessions spaced at 2-hour intervals throughout the day. Quantitative information is provided about both average sleep latency and abnormalities of sleep-onset transition. The MSLT must be performed the day following an overnight sleep study in order to permit meaningful analysis of the results.

13. What is the normal sleep latency during the MSLT?
Normal individuals have an average sleep latency (time from onset of the nap until the first appearance of any stage of sleep) of 10 minutes or longer.

14. Will medications alter the results of polysomnography and multiple sleep latency testing?
Many drugs (e.g., hypnotics, sedatives, tranquilizers, and stimulants) can significantly alter the results of polysomnographic and MSLT examinations. In particular, both periods of

drug initiation and acute withdrawal are often associated with major alterations of sleep characteristics, and the findings may mimic other sleep disorders, including narcolepsy. Consequently, whenever possible, CNS active drugs should be discontinued for a period of 2 weeks or longer prior to diagnostic studies. When this is not possible, such drugs should be administered at constant and stable levels for at least 2 weeks prior to polysomnography and MSLT studies. *Patients should never be told to simply refrain from taking a medication on the night of a study, or for several nights prior to the examination, since this could invalidate the results.*

15. What is the most common condition associated with excessive daytime sleepiness and sleep at inappropriate times?
The obstructive sleep apnea syndrome. In this disorder sleep onset is typically associated with increased upper airway resistance, and partial or complete airway obstruction often occurs. The patient is usually aroused within a short period of time by ensuing hypoxia or hypercarbia as well as by the increased effort associated with attempts to breathe. Resultant sleep deprivation or fragmentation is presumably the basis for the daytime sleepiness. Pronounced oxygen desaturation can occur and may cause potentially life-threatening cardiac arrhythmias. The polygraphic characteristics are conclusive.

16. What is the treatment for obstructive sleep apnea?
Therapy must be directed toward correction of the airway obstruction (which may result from anatomic factors causing increased upper airway resistance to air flow, or abnormal relaxation of musculature in the oropharynx). Administration of continuous positive airway pressure (CPAP) by means of a nasal mask is currently the most frequently used therapeutic modality. Surgical procedures are effective in some cases, particularly when a discrete anatomic factor producing airway obstruction can be demonstrated. In some individuals significant improvement is achieved by preventing assumption of the supine position during sleep. Tongue-retaining devices are beneficial in a small number of instances, particularly when the respiratory disturbance is mild.

17. What is the classic narcoleptic tetrad?
Narcolepsy is the most familiar condition associated with episodes of sleep at inappropriate times, although it is clear that many individuals diagnosed with this condition in the past actually had sleep apnea (or one of the other conditions associated with disturbed nocturnal sleep). The classic narcoleptic tetrad is:
1. Excessive sleepiness
2. Cataplexy
3. Sleep paralysis
4. Hypnagogic hallucinations

The tetrad is observed in no more than 50% of patients meeting current criteria for the diagnosis of narcolepsy, and 90% lack at least one of the primary symptoms.

18. What is cataplexy?
Cataplexy is a condition characterized by episodes of weakness or paralysis, without loss of consciousness, typically precipitated by emotional changes such as laughter, excitement, or anger. Episodes typically do not last more than a few seconds and may be terminated by a direct transition to stage REM sleep.

19. What is sleep paralysis?
This condition is characterized by a transient inability to move during onset of sleep, or during arousal from sleep. Episodes usually last no more than several minutes and may be associated with hallucinations.

20. What are hypnagogic hallucinations?

Hallucinations involving various sensory modalities (most commonly visual) that occur during sleep/wake transitions. Although this entity is typically observed in association with narcolepsy, it does occasionally occur in normal individuals.

21. How is narcolepsy diagnosed?

An unambiguous diagnosis of narcolepsy requires that all of the following criteria be met during polysomnographic and MSLT testing:

1. A total nocturnal sleep time of at least 80% of the total monitoring time (the monitoring time should approximate the patient's typical time in bed at night).

2. Stage REM should occupy more than 17% of the total nocturnal sleep time.

3. An excessive degree of daytime sleepiness should be demonstrated during a MSLT (average sleep latency less than 10 minutes).

4. Stage REM should occur within 10–15 minutes of onset of sleep on at least two occasions during the MSLT.

22. How is narcolepsy treated?

Excessive daytime sleepiness is usually managed with stimulant medications (e.g., methylphenidate or dextroamphetamine). The requirement for stimulants can sometimes be reduced by prescribing several (typically 2 or 3) regularly scheduled short (1 hour or less) naps during the day. Cataplexy and sleep paralysis are often treated successfully with tricyclic antidepressants.

23. What other disorders, in addition to narcolepsy and obstructive sleep apnea, may present as excessive daytime somnolence?

1. Periodic limb movements (nocturnal myoclonus)
2. Insufficient nocturnal sleep syndrome
3. Circadian rhythm disorders (e.g., jet lag)
4. Drug or alcohol dependency
5. Central sleep apnea
6. Toxin-induced sleep disorder
7. Mood disorders (depression)
8. Cerebral degenerative disorders
9. Dementia
10. Trypanosomiasis
11. Idiopathic hypersomnia
12. Periodic hypersomnia (e.g., Kleine-Levin syndrome)
13. Posttraumatic hypersomnia

24. Is the occurrence of sleep paralysis pathognomonic of narcolepsy?

No. Although sleep paralysis is most commonly encountered as one of the ancillary manifestations of narcolepsy, it is sometimes seen as an independent entity in the absence of other signs of narcolepsy. It may occur independently or in a familial form. It is characterized by a transient (usually from less than 1 minute to several minutes) inability to move voluntarily either at the time of onset of sleep or during an arousal from sleep. Consciousness is maintained and the individual may experience severe anxiety and fear. Eye and respiratory movements are not impaired. The condition disappears spontaneously but may be terminated immediately if the individual is stimulated externally. In some individuals this phenomenon may occur more frequently in the presence of sleep deprivation or other sleep disturbance. Although this condition is typically identified by its symptomatology, a sleep study may be required to rule out narcolepsy or the presence of another sleep disorder that could be triggering the sleep paralysis through sleep disruption. Treatment is usually not required, although if the condition is frequent and/or results in a high degree of anxiety, treatment may be indicated. Tricyclic antidepressant medications are often effective.

25. Is HLA typing useful in the diagnosis of narcolepsy?

Although nearly 100% of narcoleptic patients have been found to be HLA-DR2 and DQw1 positive in several studies, this test is of limited value because 10 to 35% of the general population is also DR2 positive. DR2 negativity, although rare, does not exclude the presence of narcolepsy.

26. What is the most significant risk factor common to all conditions associated with excessive daytime sleepiness?
Individuals with hypersomnic conditions are at a significantly increased risk for death or serious injury as a result of motor-vehicle and job-related accidents.

27. How is insomnia defined?
Insomnia is a subjective symptom characterized by the perception that sleep is inadequate or otherwise abnormal. It includes complaints of a low total sleep time, difficulty falling asleep, frequent awakenings, or unrefreshing sleep. It is a common symptom and is associated with a wide spectrum of underlying medical conditions as well as with specific sleep disorders.

28. What are the commonest causes of insomnia?
1. Circadian rhythm disturbances
2. Primary or idiopathic insomnia
3. Underlying medical or psychiatric disorders
4. Periodic limb movements (nocturnal myoclonus)
5. Drug or alcohol dependency
6. Irregular or improper sleep habits (poor sleep hygiene)
7. Sleep apnea

29. What is the appropriate treatment for idiopathic or primary insomnia?
The individual with chronic insomnia should be encouraged to:
1. Establish a regular and fixed sleep period, with a consistent bedtime and time of arousal. The sleep period should be long enough to permit adequate sleep time (typically 8 hours for an adult), but no longer.
2. Avoid daytime napping.
3. Minimize concern about inability to sleep.
4. Establish a regular, daily program of exercise, but do not exercise immediately prior to bedtime.
5. Avoid excessive consumption of caffeine and alcohol, and exclude these substances entirely during the evening prior to bedtime.
6. Ensure that the sleeping environment is optimal with respect to noise and temperature.
7. Avoid use of medication to induce sleep.
8. Obtain behavioral treatment (e.g., relaxation therapy) if indicated.

30. What is the time zone change syndrome?
This condition, also known as jet lag, consists of symptoms of insomnia that begin immediately following rapid travel across several time zones. It results from a loss of proper synchronization between the endogenous circadian timing system of the brain and external environmental cues (primarily day/night cycles).

31. What is the best way to manage insomnia resulting from a time zone change?
Some individuals adapt without difficulty, whereas others (particularly those over 50 years of age) experience a prolonged period of disturbed sleep. These symptoms can be minimized by:
1. Immediately adopting a sleep/wake schedule appropriate for the new environment.
2. Avoiding prolonged napping immediately after arrival in a new location. A mild degree of sleep deprivation the first day will facilitate adaptation to the new environment.

3. Spending some time outdoors during the daytime on the first few days after arrival. This facilitates resetting of the circadian clock.
4. Avoiding excessive use of caffeine and alcohol.
5. Avoiding use of sleep medications.

32. What are sleep terrors (parvor nocturnus)?
Sleep terrors are episodes of apparent intense fear, often associated with crying and/or screaming, that occur during arousal from non-REM (typically stages 3 or 4) sleep. These events are characteristically accompanied by elevated heart and respiratory rates, and the patient may exhibit confusion and disorientation. Amnesia is most common, although some individuals report brief dream-like images. This condition is most common in children between 4 and 12 years of age but may persist into the adult years. Drug treatment is usually unnecessary, but benzodiazepines may be effective for short-term use, especially when episodes become frequent.

33. What are the major characteristics of the periodic limb movement disorder?
Periodic limb movement disorder, or nocturnal myoclonus, is characterized by the frequent occurrence of clusters of extremity movements (typically the legs, but occasionally the arms) that tend to recur periodically at intervals of 10 to 90 seconds for an extended time. When these events produce arousal, as they often do, sleep may be disrupted. This condition is readily apparent during sleep laboratory evaluation, and its severity can be quantitatively assessed. This condition is typically resistant to therapy, but daytime symptoms are often relieved by medications (e.g., clonazepam) that reduce the number of nocturnal arousals associated with the limb movements.

34. Which conditions other than epilepsy may be associated with paroxysmal episodes of atypical, often complex, motor activity during the sleep period in adult patients?
1. Sleepwalking
2. Paroxysmal nocturnal dystonia
3. REM sleep behavior disorder

35. What are the key clinical and polysomnographic features of sleepwalking?
Sleepwalking consists of complex and usually inappropriate behavior beginning during non-REM (typically stages 3 and 4) sleep. It occurs most frequently early in the night, but may occur at other times on occasion. Although walking is common, other behavior such as sitting up in bed, talking, etc. is also frequent. The patient is difficult to awaken, may be confused, and usually is amnesic for the event. It occurs most commonly in children (3 to 10 years) but may occur in older individuals. Some medications and other medical conditions can induce or potentiate sleepwalking. Because serious accidental injury may result during these episodes, patients of all ages should be protected by appropriate safety precautions. Although drug treatment is usually not necessary, benzodiazepines (e.g., diazepam) are often effective, especially for short-term use.

36. What are the characteristics of paroxysmal nocturnal dystonia?
Paroxysmal nocturnal dystonia is a disorder of unknown etiology characterized by repeated dystonic or dyskinetic episodes that occur during or immediately following arousal from non-REM sleep, or, more rarely, during wakefulness. Episodes typically last less than 1 minute, but in some cases are much more prolonged (reportedly up to 1 hour), and often occur several times per night. Movements are often relatively violent and can result in injury to the patient or bed partner. Patients typically do not recall these events following arousal. This condition has been reported in both children and adults, and can be isolated or familial. Episodes are not associated with epileptiform EEG activity or other abnormal

EEG findings. This condition is apparently long-lasting. Carbamezapine is efficacious in many instances, suggesting the possibility of an epileptogenic origin.

37. Which features distinguish the REM sleep behavior disorder from other conditions associated with atypical nocturnal events?
The REM sleep behavior disorder is typified by repeated episodes of complex, often violent, motor activity during periods of REM sleep. These episodes appear to represent enactment of dream mental activity as a result of loss of normal inhibitory mechanisms originating in the brainstem (specifically, in the peri-locus ceruleus region of the pons). Patients with this condition often kick or punch repeatedly and may jump from the bed and run through the bedroom, frequently colliding with furniture or walls. Injuries to the patient and bed partner are common. Although full-blown episodes may occur infrequently, atypical movements and abnormally increased EMG tonic activity are typically present during all REM periods, as demonstrated during polysomnographic testing. Patients often recall the dream content after the event is over. The majority of cases are idiopathic, but a significant number are associated with specific neurologic disorders (e.g., ischemic cerebrovascular disease, olivopontocerebellar degeneration, multiple sclerosis, brainstem neoplasm, etc.). Clonazepam is often efficacious. Patients should be advised to take safety precautions to minimize injury if an occasional episode does occur.

38. What is the restless legs syndrome?
The restless legs syndrome is characterized by unpleasant sensations in the lower legs prior to sleep onset (and sometimes at other times as well) that produce a strong urge to move the legs. This sensation is typically described as a "crawling" or "creeping" feeling, and it disappears temporarily when the lower extremities are moved, only to recur again within a few seconds. The symptoms last from minutes to several hours and can significantly delay sleep onset, with resultant sleep deprivation. Many individuals with this condition also experience periodic limb movements (noctural myoclonus) during sleep. The cause is unknown and the condition is typically long term, although gradual improvement is sometimes observed. Medications reported to be beneficial in this disorder include benzodiazepines (clonazepam, temazepam, and nitrazepam), L-dopa, and opioids.

BIBLIOGRAPHY

1. Culebras A (ed): The neurology of sleep. Neurology 42(Suppl 6):1–94, 1992.
2. Diagnostic Classification Steering Committee, Thorpy MJ, Chairman. International Classification of Sleep Disorders: Diagnostic and Coding Manual. Rochester, MN, American Sleep Disorders Association, 1990.
3. Kryger MH, Roth TR, Dement WC: Principles and Practice of Sleep Medicine. Philadelphia, W.B. Saunders, 1989.

22. NEUROLOGIC COMPLICATIONS OF SYSTEMIC DISEASE

R. Glenn Smith, M.D., Ph.D.

CARDIAC DISEASE

1. What is the major neurologic complication of cardiac disease?
By far, stroke is the most common neurologic sequela of cardiac disease. The risks for embolic, thrombotic, and hemorrhagic stroke are all elevated in the presence of cardiac disease. Nonvalvular atrial fibrillation, followed by ischemic heart disease and valvular heart disease are the most common types of cardiac abnormalities causing embolic ischemic strokes. Infective endocarditis is most frequently associated with hemorrhagic strokes.

Tegeler CH, et al: Thrombosis and the heart. Semin Neurol 11:339–352, 1991.
Davis WD, et al: Cardiogenic stroke in the elderly. Clin Geriatr Med 7:429–442, 1991.

2. What is the risk of stroke secondary to atrial fibrillation?
There is at least a five-fold increased risk of stroke in patients with atrial fibrillation relative to control patient populations. Atrial fibrillation secondary to rheumatic mitral valve disease has the highest stroke risk, with a 17-fold increase over unaffected controls. Atrial fibrillation causes 10–20% of all ischemic strokes.

Wipf JE, et al: Atrial fibrillation: Thromboembolic risk and indications for anticoagulation. Arch Intern Med 150:1598–1603, 1990.
Alpert JS, et al: Atrial fibrillation: Natural history, complications, and management. Annu Rev Med 39:41–52, 1988.

3. What other atrial abnormalities predispose to stroke?
Even in the absence of atrial fibrillation, isolated enlargement of the atria may result in thrombus formation and subsequent stroke. Atrial infarction leads to decreased myocardial motility or aneurysm formation, and also increases the incidence of embolic stroke. Tumors of the atria, like atrial myxoma, reduce atrial blood flow and thus predispose the patient to thrombus formation and stroke.

Cerebral Embolism Task Force: Cardiogenic brain embolism. Arch Neurol 46:727–743, 1989.

4. What is the relationship between myocardial infarction (MI) and stroke?
One in 40 patients will suffer a stroke within 1 month of MI. Persons who have had an anterior wall MI are at greatest risk, with up to a 10% chance for a subsequent cerebrovascular accident. This risk for embolic stroke is directly related to the propensity for left ventricular thrombus formation, with the highest risk being found after anterior wall MI. Anticoagulation reduces post-MI embolic stroke risk by about 60%, if maintained for 3 to 6 months. The risk for thrombotic stroke is likewise greater in patients with MI. This reflects the similar risk factors and mechanisms for atherogenic plaque formation in cardiac and cerebral vessels.

Haugland JM, et al: Embolic potential of left ventricular thrombi detected by two-dimensional echocardiography. Circulation 70:588–593, 1984.
Johannessen KA, et al: Risk factors for embolization in patients with left ventricular thrombi and acute myocardial infarction. Br Heart J 60:104–111, 1988.

5. What is the association between transient ischemic attack (TIA) and MI?
Patients who suffer a TIA are more likely to have an MI than a stroke in the subsequent 5 years. All patients who have suffered a mild stroke or TIA should undergo careful cardiac assessment as soon as possible.

Scheinberg P: Transient ischemic attacks: An update. J Neurol Sci 101:133–140, 1991.

6. What is the association between sleep, MI, and stroke?

In the stage of sleep associated with rapid eye movements (REM sleep), profound changes in centrally mediated sympathetic activity occur. These large changes in autonomic output are manifest by smaller increases in blood pressure and heart rate, skin conductance changes, momentary restorations in muscle tone, mesenteric and renal vasodilation, and skeletal muscle vasoconstriction. In the elderly, it is hypothesized that large fluctuations in sympathetic activity associated with REM sleep also cause increased rates of arrhythmias and increased risk for cardiac vasospasm. This, in turn, may increase the risk for embolic stroke and MI, respectively.

Somers VK, et al: Sympathetic nerve activity during sleep in normal subjects. N Engl J Med 328:303–307, 1993.

7. When is stroke likely to be a late complication of MI?

Conditions that lead to the persistent presence of mural thrombi may predispose patients to stroke. Ventricular aneurysm formation with intraventricular thrombi (especially when thrombi are mobile or protruding) may provide the greatest long-term risk for embolic stroke. Atrial septal aneurysms may also form after MI and predispose the patient to delayed embolic stroke.

Weinreich DJ, et al: Left ventricular mural thrombi complicating acute myocardial infarction: Long-term follow-up with serial echocardiography. Ann Intern Med 100:789–795, 1984.

8. How is myocardial hypokinesis associated with stroke?

Areas of focal myocardial hypokinesis, even in the absence of aneurysms or reduced cardiac output, serve as sites for thrombus formation and increase the risk of embolic stroke. Impaired myocardial contractility provides relative stasis of cardiac blood flow and increases the risk for mural thrombus formation. The risk for embolic stroke usually worsens with the severity of the underlying cardiomyopathy, but this risk is modified by the patient's coagulation state. Hypercoagulable states, such as can occur in patients with paraneoplastic cardiomyopathy, further heighten the risk for embolic stroke, whereas chronic anticoagulation reduces this risk.

Leier CV: The cardiomyopathies: Mortality, sudden death, and ventricular arrhythmias. Cardiovasc Clin 22:275–306, 1992.

9. How is valvular cardiac disease associated with stroke?

Left-sided valvular cardiac disease carries a great danger of embolic stroke. Mitral valve annulus calcification, calcific aortic stenosis, rheumatic mitral valve stenosis, mitral valve prolapse, and infective or noninfective endocarditis all predispose to stroke.

Prosthetic valves account for the greatest number of embolic strokes. Even with appropriate anticoagulation, the risk for stroke is 2–4%/year for mitral prostheses, and half that for aortic prostheses.

In rheumatic valvular disease, the prevalence of CNS embolism is 20%, while 33% of patients with both mitral disease and atrial fibrillation will experience an embolic stroke.

Septic emboli to the brain complicate the course of infective endocarditis in 20% of patients. Hemorrhagic sequelae from focal arteritis or from mycotic aneurysmal rupture are the most serious complications of such embolization. In the presence of immunocompromised or hypercoagulable states, nonbacterial thrombotic endocarditis assumes greater importance. This form of valvular disease accounts for 25% of strokes in patients with malignancies.

Paradoxical embolism can also occur from tricuspid or pulmonary valves in the presence of pulmonary or intracardiac right-to-left shunts. Because approximately 15% of otherwise normal individuals will have intermittent right-to-left shunting through a patent foramen ovale, right-sided valvular disease must be considered a source for brain emboli.

Aronow WS: Etiology and pathogenesis of thromboembolism. Herz 16:395–404, 1991.

10. What are the non-stroke-related neurologic complications of cardiac disease?

Cardiac arrhythmias (especially sick sinus syndrome) may produce decreased cardiac output, causing syncope, and, rarely, encephalopathy. Cardiac failure may likewise impair cardiac output and produce encephalopathy. Cerebral blood flow is not directly altered in patients with cardiac failure or arrhythmias, except with major reductions in cardiac function. Instead, there appears to be a change in cerebral autoregulation caused by abnormal autonomic vagal activity. Persistent decreased brain perfusion may lead to laminar necrosis of the cerebral cortex or hippocampus, even in the absence of stroke. Delayed demyelination leading to coma and death may also occur after apparent recovery from hypotension or cardiac failure.

Leier CV: The cardiomyopathies: Mortality, sudden death, and ventricular arrhythmias. Cardiovasc Clin 22:275–306, 1992.

Helgason CM, et al: Neurologic manifestations of cardiac disease. Neurol Clin 7:469–488, 1989.

11. Is dementia associated with cardiac disease?

Multi-infarct dementia most commonly results from hypertensive vascular disease that affects the thalamus, hippocampus, and/or amygdala, manifesting as a lacunar state. Isolated cardioembolic multi-infarct dementia is much less common, due in part to the relatively small chance that emboli will occlude the small caliber vessels that arise directly from major cerebral arteries to feed these regions. Although dementia may arise secondary to multiple bilateral large embolic branch occlusions affecting the central thalamic nuclear group or hippocampus, it is often difficult to distinguish as an entity separate from many other defects caused by such focal lesions. Prolonged hypotension in the absence of stroke may lead to hippocampal laminar necrosis and also result in dementia.

Liston EH, et al: Clinical differentiation of primary degenerative and multi-infarct dementia: A critical review of the evidence. II. Pathological studies. Biol Psychol 18:1467–1483, 1983.

GASTROINTESTINAL DISEASE

12. What is the major cause of neurologic symptoms associated with gastrointestinal (GI) disease?

Most known neurologic complications of GI disease are the consequence of malabsorption. This is likewise true of neurologic problems arising after GI trauma or surgical resection. Although in many cases the specific absorptive deficiencies are unclear, the consequences of some nutrient deficiencies have been well described, including those involving thiamine, folate, cyanocobalamin, niacin, vitamin D, and vitamin E.

13. What are the neurologic manifestations of celiac disease?

Celiac disease, or gluten enteropathy, produces chronic small bowel malabsorption, often with iron deficiency anemia, osteoporosis and osteomalacia, and hypoalbuminemia. At least 10% of affected patients also have neurologic complaints, the most notable being cerebellar dysfunction secondary to chronic fat malabsorption. Patients may also have tremor, intranuclear ophthalmoplegia, symptoms suggesting Wernicke's encephalopathy or subacute combined degeneration, seizures, or myopathy. The observed myopathy is often treatable by vitamin D replacement.

Cooke WT, et al: Neurologic disorders associated with adult coeliac disease. Brain 89:683–722, 1966.

Falchuk ZM: Gluten-sensitive enteropathy. Clin Gastroenterol 12:475–494, 1983.

14. What is the triad of neurologic complaints commonly ascribed to Whipple's disease?

In Whipple's disease, a multisystem granulomatous infection, neurologic complaints develop in 10% of afflicted patients. The common triad of findings associated with this disease includes ocular disturbance (often ophthalmoparesis), gait ataxia, and dementia.

Other abnormalities sometimes associated with this disease include seizures, myelopathy, meningoencephalitis, autonomic dysfunction, and steroid-unresponsive myopathy. Untreated, most patients die within 1 year of the onset of neurologic symptoms.

Fleming JL, et al: Whipple's disease: Clinical, biochemical, and histopathological features and assessment of treatment in 29 patients. Mayo Clin Proc 63:539–551, 1988.

15. What is the triad of neurologic complaints commonly ascribed to Wernicke's encephalopathy?

Thiamine deficiency may manifest as Wernicke's encephalopathy, whose clinical symptoms include the triad of ocular disturbance (with nystagmus), gait ataxia, and disturbances of mental function. The similarity of this triad to that found in Whipple's disease has suggested to some that thiamine uptake or utilization is altered in that disease. An axonal sensorimotor neuropathy appears in half of patients with this deficiency state, and Korsakoff's psychosis (dementia associated with profound amnesia and confabulation) is also variably present. The mortality associated with Wernicke's encephalopathy is still greater than 10%, although this is more due to concomitant infections and malnutrition than to the neurologic disorders.

Reuler JB, et al: Wernicke's encephalopathy. N Engl J Med 312:1035–1039, 1989.

16. What is Strachan's syndrome?

Strachan described a triad of sensory spinal ataxia, optic nerve atrophy, and sensorineural deafness that is partially responsive to high-dose thiamine therapy.

Strachan RW, et al: Psychiatric syndromes due to avitaminosis B12 with normal blood and marrow. Q J Med 34:303–310, 1965.

17. What is known about the etiology of nervous system impairment associated with B12 malabsorption?

The deficiency of methionine synthetase activity secondary to absence of its cofactor (B12) leads to accumulation of homocysteine. The resulting impairment in DNA synthesis is responsible for the megaloblastic anemia associated with B12 deficiency, while neurologic abnormalities are the result of failure to maintain methionine biosynthesis.

Scott JM, et al: Pathogenesis of subacute combined degeneration: A result of methyl group deficiency. Lancet 2:334–340, 1981.

18. What are the neurologic manifestations of vitamin B12 deficiency?

Psychiatric symptoms fall into several clinical categories. Many patients manifest slowed cerebration, dementia, or delirium (with or without delusions), while others exhibit depression, amnesia, or acute psychotic states. Rarer are those patients whose B12 deficiency results in reversible manic or schizophreniform states. Nonbehavioral findings in B12 deficiency include myelopathy that affects the dorsal and lateral columns, and sensorimotor neuropathy.

Hector HM, et al: What are the psychiatric manifestations of B12 deficiency? J Am Geriatr Soc 36:1105–1132, 1988.

19. Which vitamin deficiencies cause different neurologic syndromes in children than in adults?

Lack of absorption of vitamin D from the intestinal tract leads to rickets in children and osteomalacia in adults. In children with rickets, neurologic sequelae include head shaking, nystagmus, and increased irritability that may evolve into tetany with a sufficient fall in serum calcium concentrations. **Malabsorption of folate** in infants leads to mental retardation, seizures, and athetotic movements, whereas in adults, polyneuropathy and depression are the primary complications. **Pyridoxine deficiency** leads to seizures in infants, but a sensory polyneuropathy in adults.

Albers JW, et al: Neurologic manifestations of gastrointestinal disease. Neurol Clin 7:525–548, 1989.

20. Malabsorption of which vitamins will lead to an increased risk for subdural hematoma?
Malabsorption of vitamin C or vitamin K results in an increased tendency for hemorrhage, especially following trauma. Lack of thiamine, vitamin B12, or vitamin E all can result in ataxia, with an increased tendency for falls and head trauma.

21. Besides thiamine, malabsorption or dietary lack of which vitamin may produce a syndrome resembling Korsakoff's dementia?
Nicotinic acid deficiency results in pellagra, whose major and often sole manifestation is psychiatric disturbance, sometimes mimicking Korsakoff's psychosis. Although vitamin B12 deficiency can also produce disturbances of cognitive function, the concomitant presence of other neurologic deficits usually serves to separate pernicious anemia from Korsakoff's psychosis.

Spivak JL, et al: Pellagra: An analysis of 18 patients and a review of the literature. Johns Hopkins Med J 140:295–308, 1977.

HEPATIC DISEASE

22. What are the six major neurologic syndromes associated with hepatic dysfunction?

1. Encephalopathy
2. Acquired hepatocerebral degeneration
3. Wilson's disease
4. Reye syndrome
5. Intracranial hemorrhage
6. Hemochromatosis

23. What causes hepatic encephalopathy?
This complication may occur with hepatic failure or with portal or hepatic circulatory dysfunction, as caused by acute or chronic hepatitis, hepatic necrosis, cirrhosis, or portocaval anastomosis. No single cause has been identified for the production of neuropsychiatric manifestations associated with this syndrome. Ammonia is considered an important toxin, precipitating encephalopathy by increasing glutamine and gamma-aminobutyric acid (GABA) synthesis and by altering reductive amination of alpha-ketoglutarate. Also, endogenous GABA neurotransmitter agonists (like diazepine-binding inhibitor) are elevated in both the serum and cerebrospinal fluid (CSF) of patients with hepatic encephalopathy, and their concentrations correlate with the degree of encephalopathy. Both these agents, as well as other undefined endogenous toxins appear to affect central neurotransmission, especially of the dopaminergic and GABA-nergic systems. Reduction in the serum concentration of ammonia, or addition of centrally acting GABA antagonists may temporarily improve hepatic encephalopathy, although correction of the precipitating causes of hepatic dysfunction are necessary for ultimate recovery.

Ferenci P: Pathophysiology of hepatic encephalopathy. Hepatogastroenterology 38:371–376, 1991.
Butterworth RF: Pathogenesis and treatment of portal-systemic encephalopathy: An update. Dig Dis Sci 37:321–327, 1992.

24. What are the clinical stages of hepatic encephalopathy?
Stage 1: Subtle changes in sleep patterns, mentation, and behavior may be accompanied by slight motor incoordination and postural tremor.

Stage 2: Lethargy, increasing disorientation to time, and forgetfulness are associated with ataxia, signs of frontal release, asterixis, and paratonia.

Stage 3: Delirium and somnolence are apparent, as are signs of autonomic changes (hyperventilation, hypothermia, incontinence), hyperreflexia, myoclonus, worsened asterixis, and seizures.

Stage 4: Coma develops, with decorticate or decerebrate posturing.

Zieve L: Hepatic encephalopathy. In Schiff L, Schiff ER (eds): Diseases of the Liver, 6th ed. Philadelphia, J.B. Lippincott, 1987, pp 925–948.

25. In patients with chronic hepatic disease, what acute changes may lead to the development of hepatic encephalopathy?

Patients with acute hepatic encephalopathy must be assessed for an intercurrent source of infection. Excessive dietary protein intake or GI hemorrhage may be the source of increased ammonia production in the gut, with resultant increased absorption of ammonia. Electrolyte abnormalities, such as hypokalemia, also produce elevated renal ammonia production.

26. How is hepatic encephalopathy treated?

Acute therapy for hepatic encephalopathy requires removal or blockade of neurologically-acting toxins produced in the gut. Reduction of protein intake, associated with lactulose therapy to enhance ammonia excretion and reduce ammonia absorption, is the mainstay of therapy. Oral antibiotics that are poorly absorbed from the gut, such as neomycin, are used as second-line agents to reduce gut bacterial levels and ammonia formation. Benzodiazepine antagonists, such as flumazenil, may be useful in blocking the central effects of gut-produced CNS-acting toxins, although human studies are still ongoing. Long-term treatment of hepatic encephalopathy by medical therapies has only limited success, depending in part upon whether the hepatic damage is reversible, static, or progressive. "Cure" of hepatic encephalopathy requires reversal of hepatic failure, and surgical shunting procedures and liver transplantation have been successful treatments for selected individuals.

Morgan MY: The treatment of chronic hepatic encephalopathy. Hepatogastroenterology 38:377–387, 1991.

Gyr K, et al: Flumazenil in the treatment of portal systemic encephalopathy—an overview. Intens Care Med 17(Suppl 1):S39–S42, 1991.

27. What is Reye syndrome?

Reye syndrome is a rare acute noninflammatory encephalopathy that primarily affects children and adolescents. An epidemiologic correlation has been found between this disease and immediately preceding viral infection (especially influenza and varicella) treated with salicylates, although apparently it may be precipitated by other toxic, metabolic, or hypoxic insults. Hyperammonemia, hypoglycemia, coagulopathy, and cerebral edema with hypoxia may be present. The biochemical changes found in this disease suggest mitochondrial dysfunction, as substantiated on electron microscopy. Toxic metabolites suggested to accumulate in this disease are similar to those incriminated in hepatic encephalopathy, and can produce their damage by direct neuronal destruction, neurotransmitter blockade, demyelination, and cerebral edema, with concomitant vascular/ischemic damage. Treatment is supportive, including administration of intravenous glucose to prevent hypoglycemia, and in severe cases, hyperventilation, mannitol, etc. to reduce intracranial pressure.

DeVivio DC: Reye syndrome. Neurol Clin 3:95–115, 1985.

Brown JK, et al: Interrelationships of liver and brain with special reference to Reye syndrome. J Inherit Metab Dis 14:436–458, 1991.

28. In addition to hepatic encephalopathy, what other diseases cause asterixis?

Asterixis, or flapping tremor, is best elicited by the extension of outstretched, opened hands. This sign is encountered in many metabolic encephalopathies, including uremia, malnutrition, severe pulmonary disease, and polycythemia rubra vera.

29. In addition to hepatic encephalopathy, what other diseases cause the electroencephalographic (EEG) abnormality of slow triphasic waves?

This abnormal EEG pattern, although commonly used to diagnose hepatic encephalopathy, may also accompany head trauma (especially with subdural hematoma), acute cerebral anoxia, uremia, or electrolyte imbalance.

30. How much is the risk for intracranial hemorrhage (ICH) increased in patients with hepatic disease?
When compared to individuals without liver disease, persons with hepatic dysfunction due to cirrhosis, neoplasm, viral hepatitis, or chemical hepatitis have a five-fold higher incidence of spontaneous ICH. This accounts for an association with hepatic disease in 10 to 20% of all ICH presentations, and in even a higher percentage of cases when ICH from arteriovenous malformation or aneurysm are excluded.

Calandare A, et al: Risk factors for spontaneous cerebral hematoma. Stroke 16:1126–1128, 1986.

31. What are the neurologic manifestations of Wilson's disease?
In almost half of patients with Wilson's disease, neurologic sequelae predominate. Signs include gait instability and clumsiness, chorea, rigidity, tremor, dystonia, and seizures. The cerebellar manifestations tend to involve the upper extremities earlier and more severely than the lower extremities, unlike those seen with Wernicke's syndrome and alcoholism. Psychiatric symptoms, including those of dementia, mania, depression, or schizophrenia, may dominate the presentation in up to 20% of patients.

Walshe JM: Wilson's disease. In Vinken PJ, et al (eds): Handbook of Clinical Neurology, Vol. 49. New York, Elsevier, 1986, pp 223–238.

32. What is the treatment for Wilson's disease?
Early diagnosis and copper chelation therapy are the mainstays of therapy. The chelation therapy of choice is 250 mg of penicillamine given PO QID between meals. Penicillamine should be administered concomitantly with pyridoxine to prevent vitamin B6 deficiency. Side effects of this treatment include rash, fever, thrombocytopenia, relative eosinophilia with total leukopenia, and reversible lupus-like and myasthenia-gravis-like syndromes. Alternative therapies include oral administration of zinc sulfate or triethylenetetraamine.

Walshe JM: Wilson's disease. In Vinken PJ, et al (eds): Handbook of Clinical Neurology, Vol. 49. New York, Elsevier, 1986, pp 223–238.

Brewer GJ, et al: Treatment of Wilson's disease with zinc. III. Prevention of reaccumulation of hepatic copper. J Clin Lab Med 109:526–531, 1987.

33. How does acquired hepatocerebral degeneration differ from Wilson's disease?
Symptoms for acquired hepatocerebral degeneration (or hepatic dementia) and Wilson's disease are very similar, making differentiation difficult on this basis. MRI findings are likewise similar. However, acquired hepatocerebral degeneration occurs later in life than does Wilson's disease, primarily in patients who have received portal-systemic or splenorenal shunting. These diseases can also be differentiated based on family history and slit-lamp examination.

Mendez MF: Hepatic dementia or acquired hepatocerebral degeneration. J Am Geriatr Soc 37:259–260, 1989.

Hanner JS, et al: Acquired hepatocerebral degeneration: MR similarity with Wilson disease. J Comp Assist Tomogr 12:1076–1077, 1988.

34. What are the neurologic complications of hemochromatosis?
Encephalopathy, truncal ataxia, neuritis, and rigidity may all complicate hemochromatosis. Hepatomegaly and liver failure in these patients are due to cirrhosis, resulting from massive iron deposition in the liver. CNS abnormalities, including demyelination, are caused by the liver disease. Neuritis is either a complication of the diabetes mellitus that accompanies most cases of hemochromatosis, or is a result of local iron deposition.

Differentiation of this disease from other secondary causes of hepatic dysfunction, such as Wilson's disease and acquired hepatocerebral syndrome, is important, due to its improvement with appropriate therapy. One screening device that may be helpful for hemochromatosis is HLA typing, since the gene defect in this disease is closely linked on chromosome 6 to HLA loci. However, due to the insensitivity of this method, HLA typing can be used only within a family to screen for heterozygotes and preclinically affected individuals, once an index case has been identified.

Treatment requires serial phlebotomies four to six times per year. Lifetime treatment with phlebotomies is currently the treatment of choice, although newer therapies using growth factor control over red blood cell production may soon be tested.

Flexner JM: Hemochromatosis: An update. Compr Ther 17:7–9, 1991.

35. Which porphyrias are associated with primarily neurologic manifestations?

So-called hepatic porphyrias, such as acute intermittent porphyria (AIP) and variegate (South African) porphyria, can be distinguished from the rare "erythropoietic" forms that produce dermatologic symptoms without neurologic disease. In AIP, clinical symptoms develop during crises, most often precipitated by ingestion or administration of drugs that adversely affect porphyrin metabolism. Manifestations of AIP during crisis may include (1) abdominal pain with vomiting, constipation or diarrhea, and often a previous history of exploratory abdominal surgery; (2) psychiatric disorder, with symptoms suggesting conversion reactions, delirium, or psychosis; (3) peripheral neuropathy, primarily motor, often with autonomic abnormalities, that may be severe or fatal and mimic Guillain-Barré syndrome; and (4) central abnormalities, such as SIADH or convulsions.

Straka JG, et al: Porphyria and porphyrin metabolism. Annu Rev Med 41:457–469, 1990.

36. Chronic ingestion of what substance may produce a condition similar to AIP?

Lead poisoning produces a condition (termed saturnism) that closely resembles AIP clinically, and also appears to share heme synthetic dysfunction with accumulation of delta-aminolevulinic acid. Increased levels of superoxide dismutase and glutathione reductase are also reported, presumably in response to the toxic effects of free radical–associated cellular damage.

Montiero HP, et al: Free radical involvement in neurological porphyrias and lead poisoning. Mol Cell Biochem 103:73–83, 1991.

37. What is the treatment for neurologic crises in acute intermittant porphyria (AIP)?

Therapy is directed at modifying the biochemical abnormalities found in the disease, including overproduction of the neurotoxin delta-aminolevulinic acid (which has been proposed as a source for free radical formation) and heme deficiency. Intravenous administration of hematin increases available heme and downregulates the patient's abnormal heme biosynthetic pathway, thus reducing delta-aminolevulinic acid levels. Prevention of crises is the primary goal in treating patients with AIP. Education of the patient to the many precipitants of acute attacks is necessary for their survival.

Karcz A, et al: Acute porphyria in the emergency department. J Emerg Med 73:279–285, 1989.

RENAL DISEASE

38. What are the most common neurologic complications of renal disease?

Typical neurologic complications of renal disease are peripheral neuropathy and metabolic encephalopathy.

39. What are the characteristics of uremic neuropathy?

Uremic neuropathy appears as a symmetric distal sensorimotor axonal neuropathy and is almost invariably present in patients by the time they require dialysis. Because conditions that predispose to renal failure (e.g., diabetes and vasculitis) may also produce neuropathy, symptoms can result from several different etiologies. The presence of mononeuritis multiplex or of autonomic dysfunction suggests nonuremic pathology, whereas a pattern of stocking-and-glove numbness without severe parasthesias is consistent with uremic neuropathy. Uremic neuropathy is at least partially reversible by repeated dialysis or by kidney transplantation.

Fraser CL, et al: Nervous system complications in uremia. Ann Intern Med 109:143–153, 1988.

40. What are the characteristics of uremic encephalopathy?

Patients with uremia often develop a metabolic encephalopathy. The mechanisms responsible for this encephalopathy remain unclear, but presumably involve the retention of inorganic and organic acids, fluid alterations among cerebral cellular compartments, and abnormalities caused by hypertension, hypocalcemia, hyperkalemia, hypernatremia, hyperphosphatemia, and hypochloremia. Uremic encephalopathy is unusual because of the coexistence of signs of neuronal depression (lethargy, coma) with those of neuronal excitation (agitation, muscle cramps, myoclonus, tetany, asterixis, and seizures).

Raskin NH, et al: Neurologic disorders in renal failure. N Engl J Med 294:143–148, 1976.

De Deyn PP, et al: Clinical and pathophysiological aspects of neurological complications in renal failure. Acta Neurol Belg 92:191–206, 1992.

41. Name three neurologic complications associated with dialysis.

Dialysis disequilibrium, dialysis dementia, and intracranial hemorrhage.

Alter MJ, et al: National surveillance of dialysis-associated diseases in the United States, 1988. ASAIO Trans 36:107–118, 1990.

42. What is the dialysis disequilibrium syndrome?

Dialysis disequilibrium is the name given to the cerebral edema produced by too-rapid removal of urea and other osmoles, with resultant fluid and electrolyte shifts. Symptoms of dialysis disequilibrium may be mild, such as persistent headache or fatigue, or may be sufficiently severe to produce seizures, coma, and death. Recognition of this problem has led to newer protocols using more frequent, but less vigorous dialysis.

DeDeyn PP, et al: Clinical and pathophysiological aspects of neurological complications in renal failure. Acta Neurol Belg 92:191–206, 1992.

43. What is dialysis dementia?

Dialysis dementia refers to a rarer but much more serious syndrome of irreversible progressive dementia with apraxias, dysarthria, hyperreflexia, myoclonus, and multifocal seizures. Aluminum present in the dialysate is thought to be the primary agent causing CNS toxicity, and removal of aluminum with ion exchange resins prior to dialysis has significantly reduced the problem.

Mach JR, et al: Dialysis dementia. Clin Geriatr Med 4:853–867, 1988.

44. What causes intracranial hemorrhage in patients undergoing dialysis?

Because of the need for anticoagulation during dialysis, the incidence of trauma-related hemorrhage is elevated. Chronic hypertension is also associated with renal failure, further increasing the incidence of intracranial hemorrhage.

45. What neurologic complications are associated with renal transplantation?

Neurologic sequelae of renal transplantation are primarily the result of immunosuppression. *Listeria monocytogenes* and Cryptococcus and Aspergillus species account for 90% of the nonviral CNS infections in these patients. Cytomegalovirus, varicella zoster, and herpes simplex are more common viral infective agents that cause clinical nervous system involvement following renal transplantation. Malignancies, such as primary lymphomas, are also seen. The overall risk of developing cancer following renal transplantation is approximately 6%, or about 100-fold greater than that expected for the general nonimmunosuppressed population.

Bruno A, et al: Neurologic problems in renal transplant recipients. Neurol Clin 6:305–316, 1988.

Lockwood AH: Neurologic complications of renal disease. Neurol Clin 7:617–627, 1989.

PULMONARY DISEASE

46. What are the neurologic signs and symptoms of respiratory insufficiency?
Neurologic features of this medical emergency result from hypoxemia and acute hypercapnia. Initial symptoms may be those of a nocturnal or early morning headache, associated with lethargy, drowsiness, inattentiveness, and irritability. Motor signs at this stage include tremor and twitching, caused by hypercapnia-induced stimulation of sympathetic nervous system output. More severe levels of hypoxia result in somnolence, confusion, and asterixis. Prolonged severe hypoxia results in coma and generalized seizures. Ocular findings include papilledema in 10% of patients, probably from hypercapnia-induced increases in intracranial pressure. However, isolated chronic hypercapnia with PCO_2 measurements of up to 110 mm Hg may exist without apparent neurologic symptoms or signs.

Jozefowicz RF: Neurologic manifestations of pulmonary disease. Neurol Clin 7:605–617, 1989.

47. What neurologic diseases may result in respiratory insufficiency?
Various neuromuscular diseases may either acutely or insidiously result in respiratory insufficiency or failure:

1. Myotonic dystrophy
2. Limb-girdle muscular dystrophy
3. Nemaline myopathy
4. Centronuclear myopathy
5. Inclusion body myositis
6. Acid maltase deficiency
7. Hexosaminidase A deficiency
8. Myasthenia gravis
9. Congenital myasthenic syndromes
10. Postpolio syndrome
11. Spinal muscular atrophy
12. Amyotrophic lateral sclerosis
13. Duchenne muscular dystrophy
14. Guillain-Barré syndrome
15. Polymyositis

Bennett DA, et al: Diagnosis and treatment of neuromuscular causes of acute respiratory failure. Clin Neuropharmacol 11:303–347, 1988.

48. What is sleep apnea?
Sleep apnea refers to a group of syndromes of hypersomnia, snoring, and frequent nocturnal apnea during sleep, resulting in hypercapnia and alveolar hypoxemia. These syndromes may lead to systemic hypertension, cardiac arrhythmias and infarction, polycythemia, pulmonary hypertension, cardiac hypertrophy, and cerebrovascular accidents.

Nasser S, et al: Sleep apnoea: Causes, consequences, and treatment. Br J Clin Pract 46:39–43, 1992.

49. What are the different types of sleep apnea?
Sleep apnea can be separated into an obstructive form, in which upper airway obstruction prevents normal air flow despite persistent respiratory movements, and a central type, in which medullary respiratory centers are damaged or altered. Central sleep apnea may be the result of congenital primary alveolar hypoventilation (Ondine's curse), bilateral cervical cordotomy, brainstem infarction, bulbar poliomyelitis, or a neurodegenerative process.

Guilleminault C, et al: The sleep apnea syndromes. Annu Rev Med 27:465–481, 1976.

50. How is sleep apnea treated?
Treatment of obstructive sleep apnea may require only weight loss, or may necessitate use of oxygen, continuous positive airway pressure (CPAP), or surgical intervention. Central apnea may improve with acetazolamide therapy, pharmacologic respiratory stimulants, or diaphragmatic pacing.

Series F, et al: Mechanisms of the effectiveness of continuous positive pressure airway pressure in obstructive sleep apnea. Sleep 15(Suppl):S47–S49, 1992.

Nasser S, et al: Sleep apnoea: Causes, consequences, and treatment. Br J Clin Pract 46:39–43, 1992.

51. Describe the clinical features of prolonged hyperventilation.
Anxious patients with acute psychogenic hyperventilation usually complain of lightheadedness, dyspnea, circumoral and acral parasthesias, and the presence of visual phosphenes. Visual blurring, tremor, muscle cramps, carpopedal spasm, and chest pain are found with prolonged hyperventilation. In addition to psychogenic etiologies, prolonged hyperventilation may be the result of drug effects, metabolic acidosis, CNS damage or edema, or response to heat stroke or overexercise.

52. What causes high-altitude sickness? How is it treated?
Cerebral hypoxia results from the lower partial pressure of oxygen at high altitudes. A shift of water and sodium into neurons may also occur as the result of the failure of glycolysis-dependent cellular enzymes and transporters, such as the Na/K pump. Exercise in the cold temperatures encountered at high altitude worsens cerebral edema by further increasing cerebral blood flow. Treatment prophylactically with dexamethasone will prevent most cases of acute mountain sickness. The use of high pressure oxygen, removal to lower altitudes, and acetazolamide therapy may reduce symptoms in patients with preexisting high-altitude sickness.

Sutton JR: Mountain sickness. Neurol Clin 10:1015–1030, 1992.

HEMATOLOGIC DISEASE

53. Name the most common symptoms associated with anemia.
Regardless of cause, headache, lightheadedness, and fatigue are the most commonly reported neurologic complaints of the anemic patient.

54. What is the most serious neurologic complication of sickle cell anemia?
Ischemic stroke, often affecting patients in childhood or adolescence, is the most frequent serious sequela of a vascular crisis in sickle cell disease. Intimal hyperplasia and stenosis of proximal cerebral vessels have been described in the pathogenesis for medium- and large-vessel stroke in these patients. Hyperventilation (with associated vasoconstriction) is thus a common precipitating event for stroke in the young patient with sickle cell disease. Recurrence rates for stroke in patients with sickle cell disease exceed 67%. Intracranial hemorrhage (ICH) may also be seen in patients with sickle cell disease. Rupture of intracranial aneurysms is the usual cause for ICH in affected individuals.

Powers D, et al: Cerebrovascular accidents in sickle cell anemia. Texas Rep Biol Med 40:293–303, 1980.

Overby MC, et al: Multiple intracranial aneurysms in sickle cell anemia. J Neurosurg 62:430–434, 1985.

55. What forms of anemia affect muscle?
Iron deficiency anemia may produce muscle dysfunction independent of the degree of anemia, secondary to the importance of iron as a cofactor for myoglobin and cytochrome C. Sickle cell anemia and hemoglobin C or SC diseases may cause muscle ischemia and necrosis during crises.

Rector WG, et al: Non-hematologic effects of chronic iron deficiency. Medicine 61:382–389, 1982.

Dorwart BB, et al: Symmetric myositis and fascitis: A complication of sickle cell anemia during vasoocclusion. J Rheumatol 12:590–595, 1985.

56. What are the primary neurologic manifestations of hyperviscosity states?
Hyperviscosity states are conditions in which red blood cells, white blood cells, or serum proteins are increased to a sufficient degree that impedance of blood flow and/or oxygen delivery results. Neurologic manifestations include symptoms of chronic or acute vertebrobasilar

insufficiency (tinnitus, lightheadedness, and headache), paresthesias, problems with mentation, visual/auditory disturbances, seizures, stroke, stupor, or coma.

Massey WE, et al:Neurologic manifestations of hematologic disease. Neurol Clin 7:549–561, 1989.

57. What red cell diseases can produce a hyperviscosity state?

Polycythemia rubra vera and "secondary" or "relative" polycythemia increase the hematocrit or the red cell volume/plasma volume ratio, respectively. This increases blood viscosity, producing symptoms. Chronic reduction in hematocrit by phlebotomy or acute expansion of the plasma volume both reduce symptoms and may decrease the risk for serious sequelae.

Burge PS, et al: Morbidity and mortality in pseudopolycythemia. Lancet 1:1266, 1975.

Toghi H, et al: Importance of the hematocrit as a risk factor in cerebral infarction. Stroke 9:369–373, 1978.

58. What diseases produce elevated serum proteins and cause hyperviscosity states?

Paraproteinemias may be first detected by the onset of neurologic symptoms. Multiple myeloma and Waldenström's macroglobulinemia are the most common causes of increased serum viscosity, which appears to produce the complications of this state. Treatment usually requires plasmapheresis and therapy for the underlying condition.

59. What are the neurologic complications of hemophilia?

Intracranial hemorrhage is the most serious consequence of factor VIII deficiency. A history of head trauma is often obtained, preceding symptoms of a subdural hemorrhage by days. Subarachnoid and intraparenchymal hemorrhages cause more rapid progression of symptoms, and carry increased mortality. Intraspinal hemorrhage, while rare, rapidly produces cord compression and paralysis, while soft-tissue hematomas may cause focal compressive neuropathies.

Eyster ME, et al: Central nervous system bleeding in hemophiliacs. Blood 51:1179–1188, 1978.

Massey WE, et al: Neurologic manifestations of hematologic disease. Neurol Clin 7:549–561, 1989.

60. How does hemochromatosis cause neurologic symptoms?

Excessive iron deposition in the liver produces cirrhotic and noncirrhotic hepatic changes and may lead to hepatic encephalopathy from liver failure. Thus, hemochromatosis is not considered to be a cause of focal neurologic deficits.

Neiderau C, et al: Survival and causes of death in cirrhotic and in non-cirrhotic patients with primary hemochromatosis. N Engl J Med 313:1256–1262, 1985.

61. Which platelet disorders produce neurologic disease?

Neurologic complications may arise from having too few or too many platelets, sometimes associated with platelet dysfunction. Thrombocytopenia-caused neurologic manifestations may be due to primary acute or chronic immune thrombocytopenia purpura (ITP), disseminated intravascular coagulation (DIC), thrombotic thrombocytopenic purpura (TTP), dysimmune thrombocytopenia (DIT) secondary to rheumatic disease (associated with anticardiolipin antibodies) or hyperviscosity states, and heparin-associated thrombocytopenia (HAT). TTP produces a microangiopathic hemolytic anemia with prominent neurologic symptoms of headache, encephalopathy, or seizures, whereas DIC and (less commonly) ITP may produce larger intracerebral hemorrhages. HAT and DIT more commonly cause stroke. Thrombocytosis usually results from essential thrombocythemia, which produces symptoms of a hyperviscosity state when platelet counts exceed $600,000–1,000,000/\mu l$. Cerebrovascular complications—TIAs and stroke—are the serious consequences of this disease.

Mueller-Eckhardt C: Idiopathic thrombocytopenic purpura (ITP): Clinical and immunologic considerations. Semin Thromb Hemost 3:125–159, 1977.

Ridolfi RL, et al: TTP: Report of 25 cases and review of the literature. Medicine 60:413–428, 1981.

Jabaily J, et al: Neurologic manifestations of essential thrombocythemia. Ann Intern Med 99:513–518, 1983.

ENDOCRINE DISEASE

62. Which endocrine diseases are commonly associated with neurologic complications?

1. Diabetes mellitus	4. Hyperparathyroidism	7. Adrenal insufficiency
2. Hyperthyroidism	5. Hypoparathyroidism	8. Glucocorticoid excess
3. Hypothyroidism	6. Acromegaly	9. Diabetes insipidus

63. Which endocrine diseases are complicated by seizures?

Seizures most commonly occur after an acute change in endocrine function and usually result from electrolyte imbalance. They occur in 50% or more of patients with hypoparathyroidism because of the hypocalcemia. Although seizures are usually generalized, partial or absence seizures may also complicate hypoparathyroidism. Seizures do not occur in hyperparathyroidism.

Seizures may be the presenting sign in 20% of all hypothyroid patients, and are nearly always generalized. In contrast, the incidence of seizures in thyrotoxicosis is only 5–10%.

In Addison's disease, seizures follow the rapid onset of serum hyponatremia (<115 mEq/L), and carry a subsequent mortality of greater than 50%. Seizures are seen in diabetes insipidus (DI) only with rapid elevation of serum sodium (usually to greater than 160 mEq/L). In DI, seizures are often partial and may occur as a result of brain shrinkage with focal hemorrhage, or during rehydration.

Seizures are observed with other endocrine causes of brain shrinkage, such as in non-ketotic hyperosmolar states from diabetes mellitus (DM). In this setting, up to 25% of patients develop partial or generalized motor seizures that may evolve into epilepsia partialis continua or generalized status epilepticus. Seizures may also be seen in DM as the result of hypoglycemia from insulin therapy, but are distinctly uncommon in diabetic keto-acidosis. Seizures are not typically associated with Cushing's disease or acromegaly.

Kaminski HJ, et al: Neurologic complications of endocrine disease. Neurol Clin 7:489–508, 1989.

64. Which endocrine diseases may cause coma?

Coma is a rare and life-threatening complication of both hypothyroidism and hyperthyroidism. In the latter case, coma is almost always associated with thyroid storm. Coma is also found in hyperparathyroidism when serum calcium is greater than 19 mg/dl, in adrenal hypofunction with severe hyponatremia, and in diabetes mellitus.

Berek K, et al: Neurologic symptoms within the scope of endocrine emergencies. Wein Klin Wochenschr 104:613–619, 1992.

65. What are the potential causes of coma in diabetes mellitus?

1. Nonketotic hyperglycemic coma	6. Hypotension
2. Lactic acidosis	7. Disseminated intravascular coagulation
3. SIADH	8. Uremia with hypertensive encephalopathy
4. Hypophosphatemia	9. Cerebral edema
5. Cerebral infarction	10. Hypoglycemia or acidosis as complications of therapy

Alberti KG: Diabetic emergencies. Br Med J 45:242–263, 1989.

66. What are the most common neurologic complications of hypothyroidism? What are several rare complications?

In more than 90% of tested patients, hypothyroidism causes headache, fatigue, slowness of speech and thought, apathy, and inattention. These symptoms are often mistaken for early dysthymia or depression. Reversible sensorineural hearing loss, with or without tinnitus, develops in 75% of hypothyroid patients, while 60% of patients have reversible ptosis as a result of diminished sympathetic tone. Sleep apnea occurs in up to half of hypothyroid patients and usually results from obstructive problems due to associated obesity and myxedema. Seizures may be found in 20% of patients, often as the presenting neurologic sign. Prolonged relaxation time for deep tendon reflexes can be elicited in many hypothyroid patients, but similar changes are noted in many other diseases.

More rare are findings of demonstrable muscle weakness, limb ataxia, nystagmus, carpal tunnel syndrome or demyelinating polyneuropathy, optic neuropathy, myxedematous constriction of extraocular movements, papilledema from pseudotumor cerebri, trigeminal neuralgia, Bell's palsy, reversible dementia, or overt psychosis (myxedema madness).

Kaminski HJ, et al: Neurologic complications of endocrine disease. Neurol Clin 7:489–508, 1989.

Klein K, et al: Unusual manifestations of hypothyroidism. Ann Intern Med 144:123–128, 1984.

67. What are the most dangerous neurologic complications of hypothyroidism? How are they treated?

Although myxedema coma develops in only 1% of hypothyroid patients, its often-rapid onset with associated bradycardia, ventricular arrhythmias, hypotension, hypopnea, hypothermia, hypoglycemia, electrolyte disturbance, and seizures make it life threatening. Treatment is supportive, with correction of metabolic abnormalities, rewarming, ventilatory and/or cardiovascular support, and adequate replacement of thyroxine and corticosteroids. In utero and in the newborn period, undiagnosed and untreated hypothyroidism leads to cretinism. Treatment requires early screening prior to the onset of symptoms and thyroid hormone replacement before permanent damage occurs.

Myers L, et al: Myxedema coma. Crit Care Clin 7:43–56, 1991.

Fisher DA, et al: Thyroid development and disorders of thyroid function in the newborn. N Engl J Med 304:702–712, 1981.

68. What is the spectrum of neurologic symptomatology in hyperthyroidism? Do symptoms resolve after correction of hyperthyroidism?

Thyrotoxicosis may manifest with reversible behavioral and cognitive changes, including emotional lability, euphoria, irritability, mania, and psychosis. Delirium may be observed as a manifestation of thyroid storm. Apathetic hyperthyroidism may appear as fatigue, with symptoms suggesting depression or dementia. Seizures are a feature of thyrotoxicosis, as are tremor of the hands, eyelids or tongue, chorea, spasticity (sometimes with clonus and Babinski signs), thyrotoxic periodic paralysis, and myopathy.

Neurologic problems usually resolve after treatment of the underlying thyrotoxicosis, but thyroid ophthalmopathy often requires surgical orbital decompression. Additionally, bulbar palsies and motor weakness may not recover following correction of hyperthyroidism secondary to autoimmune disease, and may result from coincident affliction with other associated diseases, such as acute myasthenia gravis or amyotrophic lateral sclerosis.

Bulens C: Neurologic complications of hyperthyroidism. Arch Neurol 38:669–670, 1981.

69. Which psychiatric diseases have been mistakenly diagnosed in cases of parathyroid dysfunction?

Up to 25% of patients with hyperparathyroidism have prominent psychiatric symptoms resembling mania, schizophrenia, or acute confusional state. An additional 50% of hyperparathyroid patients may have symptoms suggesting depression. Interestingly, 80% of patients with hypoparathyroidism also exhibit psychologic manifestations of their disease, including symptoms resembling depression, pseudodementia, mania, schizophrenia, and toxic delirium.

Cogan MG, et al: Central nervous system manifestations of hyperparathyroidism. Am J Med 65:563–630, 1978.

Houssain M: Neurologic and psychiatric manifestations in idiopathic hypoparathyroidism: Response to treatment. J Neurol Neurosurg Psychiatry 33:153–156, 1970.

70. Which neurologic sequelae of parathyroid disease pose serious health threats to afflicted patients?

In hyperparathyroidism, hypercalcemia-induced coma and spinal cord or root compression caused by collapse of decalcified vertebrae are the major nonpsychiatric symptoms that threaten a patient's health. Myopathy, which at times may be severe, is also a common finding in hyperparathyroidism. In contrast, hypocalcemia resulting from hypoparathyroidism is more closely associated with seizures and tetany. Seizures are often difficult to control without correction of the electrolyte imbalance. Latent tetany, which may become apparent as laryngeal spasm, can be evoked by mechanical stimulation of the facial nerve (Chvostek sign), by hyperventilation, or by occlusion of venous return from an arm, producing carpopedal spasm (Trousseau sign).

Fonesca OA, et al: Neurological manifestations of hypoparathyroidism. Arch Intern Med 120:202–206, 1967.

Cogan MG, et al: Central nervous system manifestations of hyperparathyroidism. Am J Med 65:563–630, 1978.

71. How may adrenal insufficiency lead to weakness?

Up to 50% of patients with Addison's disease have a glucocorticoid-sensitive myopathy with associated cramping. Adrenal insufficiency results in decreased blood flow to the muscle, reduced muscle carbohydrate metabolism, and altered Na/K pump function and potassium homeostasis with resulting reduced muscle intracellular potassium and altered muscle contractility. Decreased adrenergic sensitivity in patients with Addison's disease also results in reduced exercise tolerance and exercise-related hypotension. Abnormalities in potassium homeostasis may additionally result in the episodic appearance of extreme weakness, resembling hyperkalemic periodic paralysis.

Ruff RL, et al: Endocrine myopathies. Neurol Clin 6:575–586, 1988.

Van Dellen RG, et al: Hyperkalemic paralysis in Addison's disease. Mayo Clin Proc 44:904–914, 1969.

72. How does prolonged glucocorticoid excess lead to weakness?

Most patients with Cushing's disease have frank weakness with demonstrable myopathic findings on electromyography and selective type IIb atrophy on muscle biopsy. Chronic treatment with glucocorticoids, especially with the fluorinated steroids, will reproduce these effects of ectopic ACTH production in 10–20% of patients. Glucocorticoids produce an insulin-resistant state in myotubes, in which both glycolytic (nonoxidative) carbohydrate metabolism and protein synthesis are adversely affected. Type IIb fibers, which are least able to compensate for this reduction of glycolytic metabolism, are most affected.

Kakulas BA, et al: Metabolic, endocrine and miscellaneous diseases. In Kakulas BA, Adams RD (eds): Diseases of Muscle, 4th ed. Philadelphia, Harper and Row, 1985, pp 643–644.

73. Does acromegaly (excess growth hormone production) directly cause neurologic damage?

Sustained excessive growth hormone (GH) appears to directly produce myopathy. GH-induced changes in the myotube include impaired glycolytic carbohydrate metabolism, increased fatty acid oxidation, and increased protein synthesis with reduced protein degradation. The more highly oxidative type I and type IIa muscle fibers typically are most affected by GH. Myotube hypertrophy from abnormal protein synthesis produces weakness in the face of increased muscle size. Although central sleep apnea may also be caused directly by excessive GH production, the obstructive sleep apnea, basilar impression, myelopathy, and compressive neuropathies reported in this disease are all indirect effects of bony, ligamentous, and soft-tissue hyperplasia with secondary compression of neural tissue.

Pickett JBE, et al: Neuromuscular complications of acromegaly. Neurology 25:638, 1975.

Perks WH, et al: Sleep apnea in acromegaly. Br Med J I(36):894, 1980.

Woo CC: Neurologic features of acromegaly: A review and report of two cases. J Manip Physiol Ther 11:314–321, 1988.

74. How does diabetes mellitus affect the nervous system?
Damage to the peripheral nervous system accounts for the main neurologic manifestations of diabetes. Initially, a symmetric distal stocking-and-glove sensory neuropathy involving small, unmyelinated or thinly myelinated fibers appears and is often associated with painful, burning paresthesias. In more severe cases, larger proprioceptive fibers are also affected, leading to Charcot joints. Autonomic nerve damage causes atrophic skin changes, impotence, orthostatic hypotension, arrhythmias, gastroparesis, and sphincter incontinence. Motor fibers may also be damaged, leading to symmetric distal weakness, especially of the lower extremities. Focal destruction of nerves may cause cranial nerve palsies, diabetic amyotrophy, and thoracoabdominal neuropathy.

Kaminski HJ, et al: Neurologic complications of endocrine disease. Neurol Clin 7:489–508, 1989.

75. Which neurologic complications of diabetes mellitus result from vascular occlusive disease?
Most focal neurologic complications of diabetes result directly or indirectly from infarction. In diabetes, the risk of stroke is increased between two- and four-fold. This may be due to accelerated atherogenesis, as well as to autonomic dysfunction that leads to hypotension and infarction. Most CNS abnormalities observed with diabetes, including hemiparesis, aphasia, and dementia, are the result of such pathology. Mononeuropathies, including those affecting median, ulnar, peroneal, femoral, and cranial nerves, are also thought to be vascular in origin, as is the lumbosacral pathology observed in diabetic amyotrophy, and the thoracic root damage with severe visceral pain found in thoracoabdominal neuropathy. Focal infarction of the vasa nervorum may be responsible for these abnormalities.

FLUID AND ELECTROLYTE DISORDERS

76. How do changes in serum potassium affect the nervous system?
In vitro experimental alterations in neuronal intracellular potassium change both the cell resting potential and neuronal excitability. However, the presence of mechanisms for active potassium transport into neurons, combined with the local control of perineuronal extracellular potassium by glia, prevents significant fluctuations in neuronal potassium over wide ranges of serum potassium concentration. For these reasons, neurologic complications of hypokalemia or hyperkalemia are few and are typically nonneuronal.

77. Name the most common neurologic complications of hypokalemia.
Myalgias and weakness can be found with serum potassium concentrations of 2.5–3.0 mEq/L. Prolonged hypokalemia of less than 2.5 mEq/L will lead to rhabdomyolysis, myoglobinuria, and cardiac arrhythmias.

Corbett AJ: Electrolyte disorders affecting muscle. Semin Neurol 3:248–257, 1983.
Knochel JP: Neuromuscular manifestations of electrolyte disorders. Am J Med 72:521–535, 1982.

78. What are the most common neurologic complications of hyperkalemia?
Hyperkalemia (>6.0 mEq/L) likewise causes functional and structural muscle abnormalities, including weakness and cardiac arrhythmias. Ventricular asystole or fibrillation are life-threatening and occur long before neurologic symptoms are usually manifested. The few previous reports of drowsiness, lethargy, and coma in hypokalemia may actually be the result of acid-base disequilibrium.

DeFronzo RA: Hyperkalemic states. In Maxwell MH, et al (eds): Clinical Disorders of Fluid and Electrolyte Metabolism, 5th ed. New York, McGraw-Hill, 1987, pp 547–584.

79. What is familial periodic paralysis?
Familial periodic paralysis refers to a group of genetic diseases with recurrent attacks of limb weakness caused by failure of the muscle to contract to electrical stimulation. At least

two forms of this disease occur: one is associated with serum hypokalemia, and the other with normal or elevated serum potassium. In both forms, changing the serum potassium by oral or intravenous intervention alters clinical symptoms: potassium supplementation prevents or resolves the symptoms of hypokalemic periodic paralysis, but precipitates an episode of hyperkalemic periodic paralysis. Familial periodic paralysis must be differentiated from other causes of weakness associated with renal or GI dysregulation of serum potassium, including thyrotoxicosis, hyperaldosteronism, malabsorption syndromes, uremia, or Addison's disease.

Riggs JE: The periodic paralyses. Neurol Clin 6:485–498, 1988.

80. How do changes in serum sodium affect the nervous system?

Because extracellular fluid volume changes as a direct function of total body sodium, patients who are hyponatremic are usually hyposmolar, whereas hypernatremic patients are hyperosmolar. Neurologic manifestations of sodium dysregulation mainly result from shrinkage or swelling of the brain, and the degree to which these changes occur depend both on the amount and the rapidity of the sodium changes.

81. What are the most common neurologic complications of hyponatremia?

Alteration of mental status is the common neurologic alteration resulting from hyponatremia. This may occur after acute reduction of serum sodium to below 130 mEq/L, or with chronically depressed sodium concentrations of below 115 mEq/L. Seizures, seen in the presence of acute reduction of serum sodium to less than 125 mEq/L, are generalized in nature and prognostically signify mortality of greater than 50%.

Riggs JE: Neurologic manifestations of fluid and electrolyte disorders. Neurol Clin 7:509–523, 1989.

82. What are the neurologic complications of therapy for hyponatremia?

The most devastating complication of rapid sodium replacement is **central pontine myelinolysis.** This disease causes myelinolysis throughout the brain and can result from rapid osmotic shifts. Symptoms of corticospinal and corticobulbar destruction are prominent, and patients may develop a "locked in" syndrome. Rapid dehydration of persons who are hyponatremic may result in hyperviscosity syndrome from plasma volume depletion, despite the presence of persistent tissue edema. **Strokes** are the primary complication of this treatment and are especially numerous when fluid restriction is used as therapy for subarachnoid hemorrhage–induced hyponatremia.

Sterns RH, et al: Osmotic demyelination syndrome following correction of hyponatremia. N Engl J Med 314:1535–1542, 1986.

83. Describe the most common neurologic complications of hypernatremia.

Hypernatremia (serum sodium >160 mEq/L) may lead to an altered mental state, progressing to coma or to seizures. Focal cerebral hemorrhage resulting from the tearing of parenchymal vessels or bridging veins produces multiple neurologic symptoms, including hemiparesis, rigidity, tremor, myoclonus, cerebellar ataxia, and chorea, as well as signs of subarachnoid hemorrhage or subdural hematoma.

Arieff AI: Central nervous system manifestations of disordered sodium metabolism. Clin Endocrinol Metab 13:269–294, 1984.

Morris-Jones PH, et al: Prognosis of the neurological complications of acute hypernatremia. Lancet 2:1385–1389, 1967.

84. What are the neurologic complications of hypercalcemia?

Hypercalcemia (>12 mg/dl) leads commonly to symptoms of progressive encephalopathy and coma, and more rarely to seizures or signs of corticobulbar, corticospinal, or cerebellospinal tract dysfunction. Elevated serum calcium may also produce weakness with reduced membrane excitability at the level of the neuromuscular junction, and may possibly cause a reversible myopathy.

Mundy GR, et al: Primary hyperparathyroidism—changes in the pattern of clinical presentation. Lancet 1:1317–1320, 1980.

Patten BM, et al: Neuromuscular disease in primary hyperparathyroidism. Ann Intern Med 80:182–193, 1984.

85. Name common neurologic complications of hypocalcemia.

Hypocalcemia may present with seizures or with neurobehavioral changes and dementia. Some patients develop parkinsonism after prolonged hypocalcemia. Increased excitability at the neuromuscular junction with reduced serum calcium may manifest as tetany.

Fonesca OA, et al: Neurological manifestations of hypoparathyroidism. Arch Intern Med 120:202–206, 1967.

86. What are the most common neurologic complications of hypomagnesemia?

Because, like potassium, magnesium is an intracellular ion whose intracellular concentrations are tightly controlled, the presence of neurologic complications may not directly correlate with extracellular magnesium concentrations. Hypomagnesemia, however, appears to present in patients with essentially the same findings as hypocalcemia. Because serum ionized calcium concentrations are reduced in the presence of hypomagnesemia, some of these symptoms may in fact be the functional result of hypocalcemia.

Fishman RA: Neurologic aspects of magnesium metabolism. Arch Neurol 12:562–569, 1965.

Zimmet P, et al: Plasma ionized calcium in hypomagnesaemia. Br J Med I:622–623, 1968.

87. What are common neurologic complications of hypermagnesemia?

Hypermagnesemia results in CNS depression and muscle paralysis. While the mechanism of CNS depression is still being addressed, muscle paralysis occurs as a result of direct neuromuscular blockade.

Swift TR: Weakness from magnesium-containing cathartics: Electrophysiologic studies. Muscle Nerve 2:295–298, 1979.

RHEUMATOLOGIC DISEASE

88. What are the neurologic effects of systemic lupus erythematosus (SLE) on the CNS?

Symptoms of central dysfunction include neuropsychiatric and behavioral changes, such as dementia, psychosis, and confusional states (the most common central manifestation of SLE). Physical signs of this disease include such localizing neurologic findings as hemiparesis, chorea, tremor, cerebellar ataxia, cranial neuropathies and optic neuritis, and transverse myelitis. These signs and symptoms may be due to SLE vasculitis or to stroke and vascular dementia seen in patients with SLE and antiphospholipid antibodies. Aseptic meningitis, seizures, and signs of increased intracranial pressure may also develop in patients with SLE.

Brick JE: Neurologic manifestations of rheumatologic disease. Neurol Clin 7:629–639, 1989.

89. What are the neurologic effects of SLE on the peripheral nervous system?

Peripheral neuropathy may appear in SLE as a vasculitic mononeuropathy or mononeuritis multiplex, or as an ischemic symmetric distal sensorimotor deficit. Myositis occurs in 25% of patients with SLE, but is a serious complication only when the myocardium is involved.

Adelman DC, et al: The neuropsychiatric manifestations of systemic lupus erythematosus: An overview. Semin Arthritis Rheum 15:185–199, 1986.

90. Do the neurologic sequelae of SLE adversely affect patient survival?

Neurologic symptoms and signs appear as manifestations of SLE in 50% of afflicted patients. The mean 5-year survival for such patients is 30% less than that found for SLE patients without neurologic problems. Vasculitis with CNS hemorrhage accounts for a large portion of this difference.

Rosner S, et al: A multicenter study of the outcome in systemic lupus erythematosus. II. Cause of death. Arthritis Rheum 25:612–617, 1982.

91. What are the neurologic effects of rheumatoid arthritis (RA) on the peripheral nervous system?

The major sequelae of RA are limited to the peripheral nervous system. Neuropathy may be the result of nerve entrapment near inflamed joints, direct inflammation of the perineurium resulting in distal demyelinating sensory neuropathies, and vasculitic destruction of larger nerves, resulting in asymmetric sensorimotor neuropathies. Diffuse nodular polymyositis may occur in 30% of patients with RA, although classic polymyositis is rare (5%). Disuse muscle atrophy is a common finding in severely affected individuals who are bedridden. Focal ischemic myositis occurs as a result of vasculitic attack on the muscle vasculature.

Chamberlain MA, et al: Clinical and electrophysiological features of rheumatoid arthritis. Ann Rheum Dis 29:609–616, 1970.

Sokolf L, et al: Diagnostic value of histologic lesions in striated muscle in rheumatoid arthritis. Am J Med Sci 219:174–182, 1950.

92. What are the neurologic effects of RA on the CNS?

Effects include a rare polyarteritis-nodosa-like vasculitis that may affect cerebral vasculature, an even rarer hyperviscosity syndrome that produces focal ischemic and hemorrhagic lesions throughout the CNS, and rheumatoid cervical disease with myelopathy.

Brick JE: Neurologic manifestations of rheumatologic disease. Neurol Clin 7:629–639, 1989.

93. What causes myelopathy in patients with RA?

Myelopathy may result from atlantoaxial subluxation, vertical subluxation of the odontoid into the foramen magnum, backward subluxation of the atlas on the axis, or subaxial subluxation, most commonly occurring at C4–C5. Compression or laceration of the spinal cord may be the direct result of odontoid impaction or subluxation of one or more vertebral bodies or rings against the cord. Vascular compression syndromes may also be found in RA patients with cervical disease, especially involving the anterior spinal artery. These syndromes lead to ischemic central gray destruction and to necrosis of the dorsal columns and corticospinal tracts.

Bland JH: Rheumatoid arthritis of the cervical spine. J Rheumatol 1:319–342, 1974.

94. Which neuromuscular diseases may be associated with Sjögren's syndrome?

Sjögren's syndrome is an autoimmune disease that combines connective tissue disease (often rheumatoid arthritis), xerostomia, and keratoconjunctivitis sicca. It is the second most common rheumatic disease (after rheumatoid arthritis). Most of its neurologic complications are the result of vasculitis, but it is also associated with several (probably autoimmune) neurologic diseases. Thus, increased incidence for myasthenia gravis, polymyositis, inclusion body myositis, and ALS have been noted in patients with Sjögren's disease.

Fox RI, Kang H-I: Sjögren's syndrome. In Kelley WN, Harris ED, Ruddy S, et al (eds): Textbook of Rheumatology, 4th ed. Philadelphia, W.B. Saunders, 1993, pp 931–942.

95. Trigeminal neuropathy is found in which rheumatic diseases?

Isolated trigeminal neuropathy may be the presenting sign in 10% of patients with neurologic manifestations of scleroderma and occurs in 4–5% of all patients with scleroderma. Fibrosis with nerve entrapment is the likely cause for this and other cranial neuropathies in progressive systemic sclerosis. Vasculitic damage to the trigeminal nerve is found in SLE and less commonly in mixed connective tissue disorder (MCTD).

Ashworth B, et al: Trigeminal neuropathy in connective tissue disease. Neurology 21:609–614, 1971.

Farrell DA, et al: Trigeminal neuropathy in progressive systemic sclerosis. Am J Med 73:57–62, 1982.

96. What is the most common neurologic manifestation of Behçet's disease?

CNS disease is found in 10–30% of patients afflicted with this disease. An initially relapsing and remitting focal meningoencephalitis that predominantly affects the brainstem is the most common finding in Behçet's disease. Cranial nerve and long tract signs may eventually lead to spastic quadriplegia and pseudobulbar palsy. Subcortical dementia, pseudotumor cerebri, vasculitis with cerebral infarction, and peripheral neuropathy have also been reported in this disease.

Chajek T, et al: Behçet's disease: Report of 41 cases and a review of the literature. Medicine 54:179–196, 1975.

VASCULITIDES

97. Which vessels are affected by primary vasculitic disease?

Although all vessels may be damaged in vasculitis, different vasculitides affect different vessel types. The aorta is selectively damaged in Takayasu's arteritis, whereas giant cell arteritis more commonly affects the temporal, vertebral, and carotid arteries. Medium-sized muscular intracerebral arteries are affected in polyarteritis nodosa (PAN), allergic granulomatosis, and granulomatous angiitis, whereas small muscular arteries are thrombosed in Wegener's granulomatosis. Hypersensitivity angiitis selectively involves capillaries and venules, sparing the arterial system.

98. What are the peripheral nervous system effects of PAN?

Half of patients diagnosed with polyarteritis nodosa have evidence of peripheral neuropathy. Five different peripheral neuropathy syndromes have been identified: (1) mononeuritis multiplex, involving both sensory and motor nerves; (2) extensive mononeuritis multiplex, with severe, primarily distal weakness and sensory deficits; (3) isolated small cutaneous sensory nerve involvement; (4) distal symmetric sensorimotor neuropathy; and (5) radiculopathy. Myalgias have also been reported in 25% of patients with PAN, usually associated with weakness. Histologic assessment of muscle biopsies acquired from these patients reveals evidence of inflammatory myopathy in roughly half of the affected individuals.

Moore PM, et al: Neurologic manifestations of systemic vasculitis: A retrospective and prospective study of the clinicopathologic features and responses to therapy in 25 patients. Am J Med 71:517–524, 1981.

99. What are the CNS effects of PAN?

CNS manifestations of vasculitic disease can be found in 40–45% of patients with PAN. Central neurologic complications may be grouped into those producing a diffuse encephalopathy, usually with seizures (50%), and those leading to focal deficits that are suggestive of infarction of the cerebrum, cerebellum, or brainstem (50%). Additionally, 15% of patients present to their physicians with isolated cranial neuropathies, most commonly involving cranial nerves II, III, and VIII. Hypertensive CNS changes with papilledema and focal hemorrhages are observed in 10% of patients with an acute confusional state, and often signify a poorer prognosis. Peripheral neuropathy is a common and early finding of

PAN, whereas CNS sequelae are often late manifestations of this disease, occurring 2–3 years after the initial diagnosis.

Ford RG, et al: Central nervous system manifestations of polyarteritis nodosa. Neurology 15:114–122, 1965.

Travers RL, et al: Polyarteritis nodosa: A clinical and angiographic analysis of 17 cases. Semin Arthritis Rheum 8:184–199, 1979.

100. Which diseases may be clinically confused with necrotizing vasculitis (PAN or necrotizing angiitis)?

The clinical diagnosis of necrotizing angiitis is based on the presence of constitutional symptoms with multisystem involvement. PAN may be difficult to separate clinically from multiple cholesterol emboli syndrome, which usually appears days after an arteriographic procedure and includes hematologic changes such as visceral infarctions, eosinophilia with leukocytosis and thrombocytopenia. Multiple embolizations from an atrial myxoma may also give the appearance of PAN-like CNS disease, although the time course of onset and progression of symptoms is wrong for PAN. Lyme disease and tertiary syphilis may also be considered in the differential diagnosis of PAN, although the concomitant presence of rheumatic disease, hepatitis, or intravenous drug abuse should strongly suggest PAN.

Rosansky RJ: Multiple cholesterol emboli syndrome. South Med J 75:677–680, 1982.

101. What is the prognosis for necrotizing vasculitis?

Untreated, only one-sixth of patients survive 5 years from the time of diagnosis, with half of the deaths occurring within the first year. Treatment with steroids reduces the overall 5-year mortality to 50%; a combination of high-dose steroids with other immunosuppressive agents further decreases mortality to 20%. Immediate benefits of plasmapheresis are often noted, and this initial treatment modality may be considered in patients with severe acute exacerbation or deterioration while awaiting onset of action of the above mentioned therapies. The majority of patients in the latter group achieve stable remissions within 24 months of treatment. With treatment, encephalopathy and seizures are usually reversible. The presence of residual sequelae of CNS disease does not significantly affect mortality.

Frohnert PP, et al: Long-term follow-up study of polyarteritis nodosa. Am J Med 43:8–21, 1967.

Leib ES, et al: Immunosuppressive and corticosteroid therapy of polyarteritis nodosa. Am J Med 67:941–948, 1979.

102. Does Churg-Strauss syndrome cause neurologic damage?

Two-thirds of patients with allergic granulomatosis (Churg-Strauss syndrome) have CNS manifestations similar to those seen in PAN, commonly including encephalopathy, seizures, and coma, and almost all patients have mononeuritis multiplex. Hemorrhage is more common in this disorder than in PAN, but the clinical distinction between these two diseases rests on the almost invariable presence of pulmonary involvement with asthma in patients with Churg-Strauss syndrome, and the tremendous eosinophilia and elevated IgE levels found in this latter disease.

Chumbley LC, et al: Allergic granulomatosis and angiitis: Report and analysis of 30 cases. Mayo Clin Proc 52:177–184, 1977.

103. Are the neurologic sequelae of hypersensitivity angiitis usually central or peripheral?

Hypersensitivity vasculitides include cutaneous vasculitis, drug-induced allergic vasculitis, postinfectious vasculitis, serum sickness, Henoch-Schonlein purpura, hypocomplementemic vasculitis, cryoglobulinemia, neoplastic angiitis, connective tissue disease-associated vasculitis, and Zeek angiitis. Neurologic complications are rare in hypocomplementemic vasculitis and in Henoch-Schonlein purpura, although both stroke and intracranial hemorrhage have been reported in the latter disease. With the exception of the hypersensitivity angiitis of Zeek and serum sickness, only peripheral nerve involvement is typically observed with the other forms of hypersensitivity angiitis.

Zeek angiitis, also called leukocytoblastic vasculitis, resembles PAN clinically, but is less likely to involve the nervous system, and has prominent skin disease. In both this disease and serum sickness, neurologic sequelae can include encephalopathy, coma, and seizures, as well as peripheral neuropathy and brachial plexopathy.

In all forms of hypersensitivity angiitis, biopsy of the skin lesions will provide the diagnosis, and treatment of the underlying disorder with identification and removal of any sensitizing agent, combined with immunosuppression (when there is evidence of progression), usually cures the disease.

Moore PM, et al: Neurologic complications of vasculitis. Ann Neurol 14:155–167, 1983.

104. What are the neurologic effects of Wegener's granulomatosis?
Wegener's granulomatosis presents as a triad of focal segmental glomerulonephritis, granulomas of the respiratory tract, and necrotizing vasculitis. Neurologic complications occur in 25–50% of affected individuals, with peripheral vasculitic mononeuritis multiplex being the most common sign. CNS manifestations of the disease are more often the result of granulomatous invasion from the sinuses or nasal passages, and may appear as exophthalmos, pituitary disease, or basilar meningitis with cranial neuropathies. Up to 5% of patients will have intracranial hemorrhages secondary to either focal vasculitis or intragranulomatous hemorrhage.

Drachman DA: Neurologic complications of Wegener's granulomatosis. Arch Neurol 8:155–165, 1963.

Fauci AS, et al: Wegener's granulomatosis: Prospective clinical and therapeutic experience with 85 patients for 25 years. Ann Intern Med 98:76–85, 1983.

105. Describe the triad of clinical findings often found in temporal arteritis.
Headache, jaw claudication, and constitutional symptoms compose the triad of clinical symptoms often found in temporal arteritis. The headache is typically boring, throbbing, or lancinating, radiating from one or both temples to the neck, jaw, tongue, or back of the head. Fever, malaise, nightsweats, and anorexia with weight loss usually present early in the disease. Patients with temporal arteritis are almost invariably over 50 years of age, and half will have evidence of concomitant polyarthralgia rheumatica. Mononeuritis multiplex may occur in 10% of afflicted patients, but should always suggest the possibility of PAN or an overlap syndrome.

Goodman BW Jr: Temporal arteritis. Am J Med 77:839–852, 1979.

106. What are the neurologic complications of temporal arteritis?
Untreated, one-third of patients will develop amaurosis fugax, monocular or binocular blindness, diplopia, or ophthalmoplegia. Cerebral infarctions or transient ischemic attacks that often involve the vertebral distribution are likewise common late complications of the disease.

Wilkinson IMS, et al: Arteries of the head and neck in giant cell arteritis: A pathological study to show the pattern of arterial involvement. Arch Neurol 27:378–383, 1972.

Caselli RJ, et al: Neurologic disease in biopsy-proven giant cell (temporal) arteritis. Neurology 38:352–358, 1988.

107. How is temporal arteritis diagnosed and treated?
Evidence of an elevated sedimentation rate (>60 mm/hr by the Westergren method) and characteristic findings of arteritis on biopsy of the temporal artery are helpful in making the diagnosis, but biopsy is frequently negative (70% diagnostic after bilateral biopsy). Treatment of temporal arteritis is with steroids and should not await biopsy (biopsy should be performed within the first few days of therapy). Treatment should

continue at least 2 years, with regulation of steroid therapy usually on the basis of sedimentation rates.

Hunder GG, et al: Daily and alternate-day corticosteroid regimens in treatment of giant cell arteritis: Comparison in a prospective study. Ann Intern Med 82:613–618, 1975.

108. What are four vasculitides whose effects are localized to the CNS?
Cogan's syndrome produces vestibular and/or auditory dysfunction with episodic acute interstitial keratitis, scleritis or episcleritis. **Eale's syndrome** is an isolated peripheral retinal vasculitis. Both of these rare syndromes tend to afflict young adults. **Spinal cord arteritis** is a diagnosis of exclusion, since many diseases may present with myelopathy. Among those diseases is **granulomatous angiitis of the nervous system (GANS),** the most severe isolated CNS vasculitic syndrome.

Sigal LH: The neurologic presentation of vasculitic and rheumatologic syndromes: A review. Medicine 66:157–180, 1987.

109. What are the nervous system manifestations of granulomatous angiitis?
GANS is also called isolated angiitis of the CNS, because the disease is almost always restricted to the CNS. This syndrome is likely a collection of vasculitides. An associated hematologic malignancy, especially Hodgkin's lymphoma, occurs in almost 50% of affected patients. Hodgkin's GANS typically begins as a subacute illness with progressive confusion, disorientation, and headache, leading to focal cerebral involvement, seizures, coma, and death. A spinal tap reveals an elevated opening pressure in 30% of patients, CSF pleocytosis in 65% of patients, and increased protein in 80% of patients. Cerebral angiography and brain biopsy may each be diagnostic in 50% of cases. The differential diagnosis includes other vasculitides, tuberculosis, MS, strokes due to emboli, sarcoidosis, syphilis, Lyme disease, drug abuse associated CNS vasculopathy, neoplasm, and lymphomatoid granulomatosis.

Cupps TR, et al: Isolated angiitis of the nervous system: Prospective diagnostic and therapeutic experience. Am J Med 74:97–105, 1983.

NEOPLASTIC DISEASE

110. How does cancer usually affect the brain?
Cancer produces most of its neurologic symptoms as a result of direct invasion of the nervous system. Between 20 and 30% of patients with primary neoplasms in other tissues have brain metastases. In these patients, the most commonly identified neoplasms are adenocarcinomas from lung, colon, and breast. Symptoms usually correspond to the focal loss of function in the region of the metastasis, although irritation of surrounding cortical regions may produce seizures.

Delattre JY, et al: Distribution of brain metastases. Arch Neurol 45:741–744, 1988.

111. How do cancers cause stroke?
Up to 8% of patients with systemic cancer have symptomatic cerebrovascular complications, whereas an additional 8% have evidence of cerebrovascular disease at autopsy. Stroke may result from tumor embolus, metastatic venous occlusion, coagulopathy-induced thromboembolism, diffuse or disseminated intravascular coagulation, septic infarction, or therapy-related complications (especially cisplatin treatment and irradiation). Hemorrhage into a metastatic parenchymal solid tumor is the most common cause for intracranial bleeding from cancer, although leukemic coagulopathy, subdural hemorrhage from metastases to the meninges, leukemic leukostasis, and L-asparaginase-induced bleeding are other causes for neoplastic hemorrhage.

Graus F, et al: Cerebrovascular complications in patients with cancer. Medicine 64:16–25, 1985.

112. Which tumors are most commonly responsible for neoplastic meningitis?

Symptomatic leptomeningeal disease develops in 5–10% of patients with solid tumors, 15–25% of patients with non-Hodgkin's lymphoma, and up to 50% of patients with leukemia. Adenocarcinomas—especially breast and lung adenocarcinoma, and melanoma—are the most common solid tumors to metastasize to the meninges. Some primitive neuroectodermal tumors may also metastasize, producing meningeal involvement. Of lymphomas, those with diffuse, Burkitt's, and lymphoblastic histologies are most likely to produce neoplastic meningitis. Acute lymphoblastic and acute myelogenous leukemias have a high propensity for meningeal spread. Half of patients with chronic lymphocytic leukemia have asymptomatic meningeal involvement diagnosed at autopsy.

Grossman SA, et al: Neoplastic meningitis. Neurol Clin 9:843–856, 1991.

113. How does cancer usually affect the spinal cord?

Cancer may either arise locally or metastasize to the spinal cord, resulting in spinal cord compression. Classic symptoms of cord compression include paraparesis, a sensory level, and bowel and bladder dysfunction.

114. Which tumors most commonly cause epidural spinal cord compression?

Tumors metastasizing to vertebrae and producing compression of the spinal cord can be remembered by the mnemonic SMUG Pb (lead) KETTLE. Thus, sarcoma (accounting for 5% of epidural metastases), myeloma (5%), unknown sites (10–15%), cancer of the genitourinary or gastrointestinal tracts (each 5%), prostate (10%), breast (25%), kidney (5%), medullary thyroid (<2%), lung (20%) or lymphoma (10%) can all produce epidural cord compression. Seventy percent of metastases effect the thoracic spine, and one third of patients have multiple levels of involvement at the time of presentation.

Grant R, et al: Metastatic epidural spinal cord compression. Neurol Clin 9:825–841, 1991.

115. How does cancer usually affect cranial and peripheral nerves?

Peripheral nerve involvement in cancer usually results from direct tumor extension. This can be seen as direct invasion by schwannomas of the auditory or optic nerves, Horner's syndrome or brachial plexopathy resulting from extension of a pancoast tumor, or facial palsy occurring in a person with a parotid tumor. Sometimes carcinomatous meningitis results in cranial neuropathies by direct extension of tumor along the roots as they emerge from the CNS.

116. What is the most common cause of neuropathy in patients with cancer?

Cancer treatment (irradiation and chemotherapy) causes more peripheral nerve injury than do direct or remote effects of cancer. Cisplatin, misonidazole, and rarely cytosine arabinoside primarily produce sensory neuropathies, while hexamethylmelamine, vincristine, and taxol can each cause sensorimotor and/or autonomic neuropathies. Radiation-induced peripheral nerve injury is most commonly manifest as a plexopathy, secondary to local radiation-induced scarring.

Macdonald DR: Neurologic complications of chemotherapy. Neurol Clin 9:955–967, 1991.

117. What central nervous system disorders can result from the remote effects of cancer?

Paraneoplastic syndromes constitute only a tiny percentage of the CNS effects of cancer. Known paraneoplastic disorders with CNS symptoms include:

1. Subacute cerebellar degeneration
2. Limbic encephalitis
3. Brainstem encephalitis
4. Opsoclonus-myoclonus
5. Retinal degenerations
6. Optic neuritis
7. Necrotizing myelopathy
8. Subacute motor neuropathy
9. Motor neuron disease
10. Myelitis

Posner JB, et al: Paraneoplastic syndromes. In Waksman BH (ed): Immunologic Mechanisms in Neurologic and Psychiatric Disease. New York, Raven Press, 1990, pp 187–219.

118. Which peripheral nervous system disorders can result from the remote effects of cancer?

Individually, each syndrome is rare, but collectively they account for a significant proportion of the peripheral nervous system effects of cancer:

1. Subacute sensory neuropathy
2. Sensorimotor neuropathy
3. Subacute motor neuronopathy
4. Mononeuritis multiplex
5. Autonomic neuronopathy
6. Guillain-Barré syndrome
7. Neuromyotonia
8. Myasthenia gravis
9. Lambert-Eaton myasthenic syndrome
10. Dermatomyositis/polymyositis
11. Acute necrotizing myopathy
12. Carcinomatous neuromyopathy
13. Stiff man syndrome

Posner JB: Paraneoplastic syndromes. Neurol Clin 9:919–936, 1991.

PREGNANCY AND SEXUAL DYSFUNCTION

119. What is the most common neurologic symptom found during pregnancy?

Headache is the most common neurologic symptom. Although pregnancy is generally thought to have a somewhat protective effect against headache in patients with an established diagnosis, it is still the most common neurologic complaint of the pregnant patient.

Headaches beginning during pregnancy are a cause for concern about serious underlying illnesses that occur with higher frequency in pregnant women. These include subarachnoid hemorrhage, rapid expansion of a tumor, cortical venous thrombosis, pseudotumor cerebri, *Listeria monocytogenes* meningitis, or preeclampsia and eclampsia. History and physical examination can usually exclude serious problems. Other headaches that may begin during pregnancy include migraines, even though the majority of female migraneurs improve during pregnancy. Onset of benign bifrontal nonmigranous headaches is also seen in pregnancy, and is most common during the first trimester. Postpartum headache is the most common self-limited headache of the puerperium, and occurs in up to 40% of all women.

Reik L Jr: Headaches in pregnancy. Semin Neurol 8:187–192, 1988.

120. What is eclampsia?

Eclampsia, which means "to shine forth," is a state characterized by the neurologic complications of seizures and/or coma, presenting in a pregnant patient with preeclampsia (i.e., with signs of hypertension and proteinuria with or without edema). It occurs in 0.05–0.2% of all pregnancies extending beyond the 20th week of gestation. Seizures or coma develop in 50% of eclamptic patients prior to the onset of labor, with an additional 25% becoming symptomatic during labor. The remaining 25% of eclamptic patients have onset of symptoms after delivery, usually within the first 24 hours postpartum. The differential diagnosis for eclampsia includes cerebrovascular accidents, hypertensive encephalopathy, epilepsy, brain neoplasms and abscesses, meningitis/encephalitis, and metabolic diseases such as hypoglycemia or hypocalcemia.

Fox MW, et al: Selected neurologic complications of pregnancy. Mayo Clin Proc 65:1595–1618, 1990.

121. What is the cause of associated mortality in eclampsia?

If present, eclampsia results in a maternal mortality of up to 14%, with associated fetal mortality of up to 28%. Maternal death from eclampsia is caused by complications of sustained intracranial and systemic hypertension. Death can be due to intracerebral hemorrhage, vasospasm, pulmonary edema, disseminated intravascular coagulation, abruptio placentae, the HELLP syndrome (hemolysis, elevated liver enzymes, and low platelet count), or renal or hepatic failure from decreased organ perfusion. Fetal mortality results from decreased uteroplacental perfusion.

Sibai BM, et al: Eclampsia. In Goldstein PJ (ed): Neurological Disorders of Pregnancy. New York, Futura Publishing Company, 1986, pp 1–18.

122. How is eclampsia treated?

Because the maternal morbidity and mortality of eclampsia appear to derive from complications of loss of cerebral autoregulation due to sustained relative hypertension, the primary objective of treatment is to reduce blood pressure without compromising uteroplacental or maternal renal perfusion. Intracranial hypertension is usually present in patients with encephalopathy or coma, and thus ICP should be monitored in such persons, with treatment by intubation and hyperventilation. These patients should also be imaged by CT to check for intracranial hemorrhage or the degree of cerebral edema.

Because eclamptic seizures result in high fetal mortality and potentially further increases in intracranial pressure, they must be aggressively controlled. Diazepam may be used without alterations in fetal pH, PCO_2 or PO_2 after administration of 5 or 10 mg to the mother. Phenytoin or phenobarbital are usually given concomitantly to provide longer term prophylaxis. Although intravenous administration of magnesium sulfate is often given by obstetricians to treat seizures, its use complicates anesthesia, suppresses uterine contractions, produces weakness in the fetus, is lethal in accidental infusions of too-high doses, and usually is used to the exclusion of effective anticonvulsants.

However, the definitive treatment for eclampsia occurring before birth is termination of the pregnancy by delivery of the fetus. Therefore, preparations for immediate cesarean section should begin while attempting to control hypertension and seizures. The risk of recurrent seizures decreases within 24 hours following delivery, and long-term prophylaxis of eclampsia-induced seizures is unnecessary. Although hypertension resolves more slowly, normalization of blood pressure occurs in the first postpartum week.

Donaldson JO: Eclamptic hypertensive encephalopathy. Semin Neurol 8:230–233, 1988.

123. What is the recurrence risk for preeclampsia and eclampsia?

The recurrence rate of preeclampsia in a young primigravid woman who was normotensive before and after pregnancy is approximately 25%. For older multiparous women with pregestational hypertension, this risk increases to 70%. Risk for preeclampsia increases with severity of the previous preeclamptic episode, presence of antiphospholipid antibodies and/or platelet dysfunction, new paternity, and parity of the patient. While approximately 2% of preeclamptic patients develop eclampsia, the risk of recurrence of eclampsia may be ten-fold higher in a previously eclamptic patient.

Anderson GD: Eclampsia. In Rivlin ME, et al (eds): Manual of Clinical Problems in Obstetrics and Gynecology. Boston, Little, Brown and Co., 1982, pp 36–39.

Branch DW, et al: The association of antiphospholipid antibodies with severe preeclampsia. Obstet Gynecol 73:541–545, 1989.

124. Is the risk for stroke altered in pregnancy?

Cerebrovascular ischemic events occur 13 times more frequently in pregnant patients than in age-matched nonpregnant women, with an overall stroke risk of 1 in 3000 pregnancies. Stroke accounts for 10% of all maternal deaths during pregnancy, and 35% of all strokes in female patients aged 15 to 45 years occur during pregnancy or in the puerperium. Atherosclerotic disease is less commonly a cause for stroke in this population than is arterial embolus or cerebral venous thrombosis.

Wiebers DO: Ischemic cerebrovascular complications of pregnancy. Arch Neurol 42:1106–1113, 1985.

Stern BJ: Cerebrovascular disease and pregnancy. In Goldstein PJ (ed): Neurological Disorders of Pregnancy. New York, Futura, 1986, pp 19–40.

125. How does the physician clinically distinguish puerperal cerebral venous thrombosis from arterial thrombosis?

Central venous thrombosis usually occurs in the first three postpartum weeks and commonly presents with headache, focal or generalized seizures, stupor or coma, transient focal deficits, and/or signs of increased intracranial pressure. Rare but often discussed named vein thromboses include superior sagittal sinus thrombosis, which may present with paraplegia and sensory deficits of the leg with associated bladder dysfunction, and rolandic vein thrombosis, which causes sensory and motor deficits of the leg, hip, and shoulder, sparing the face and arm. Mortality in sagittal sinus thrombosis approaches 40% when diagnosis is delayed, but may be reduced to 20% with intensive care and, in some cases, anticoagulants. Recovery of survivors is usually complete.

Arterial thrombosis is more rare than arterial embolus or venous thrombosis, is more likely to occur in the second or third trimester than in the puerperium, and commonly presents with persistent focal deficit, such as hemiparesis, without alteration of consciousness, seizures, or signs of increased intracranial pressure.

Recently an immune mechanism has been hypothesized for a significant percentage of pregnancy-related venous and arterial thromboses. The presence of antiphospholipid antibodies should be sought, especially when a history of previous miscarriages or preeclampsia is obtained.

Srinivasan K: Puerperal cerebral venous and arterial thrombosis. Semin Neurol 8:222–225, 1988.

Branch DW: Antiphospholipid antibodies and pregnancy: Maternal implications. Semin Perinatol 14:139–146, 1990.

Coull BM, et al: The role of antiphospholipid antibodies in stroke. Neurol Clin 10:125–143, 1991.

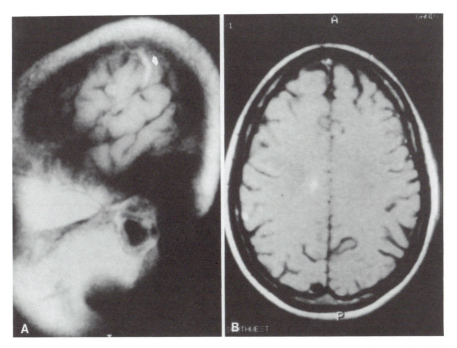

T1-weighted sagittal view of the superficial cerebral cortex of the parietal lobe, showing a cerebral vein thrombosis (*A*, arrow). The axial T1 view (*B*) shows the small hemorrhagic infarction caused by the venous thrombosis.

126. What is the differential diagnosis for seizures during childbirth?

As cause for seizures, **eclampsia, HELLP syndrome,** and thrombotic thrombocytopenic **purpura** are most commonly observed during the third trimester. **Amniotic fluid embolism, water intoxication, autonomic stress in patients with upper spinal cord injury,** and **toxicity from local anesthetics** are all intrapartum causes for seizures. **Cerebral vein thrombosis** usually occurs postpartum and may present with seizures.

Subarachnoid hemorrhage may occur at any time during pregnancy to produce seizures, although aneurysms most commonly rupture during the third trimester, with greatest risk for rebleeding in the postpartum period. Arteriovenous malformations are more likely to rupture in the second trimester and rebleed during delivery or with subsequent pregnancies. **Epilepsy** may manifest at any time before, during, or after pregnancy, and may require lifelong therapy. However, such patients must be distinguished from those with **gestational epilepsy,** which requires therapy only during pregnancy.

127. How should therapy of epilepsy change during pregnancy?

First, all anticonvulsants have some potential to be teratogenic or in some other way harmful to the fetus, and complications to the fetus increase as the number of therapeutic agents used to control seizures increases. Thus, in patients who require pharmacologic anticonvulsant therapy, monotherapy at the lowest functionally effective dose is best.

Second, a number of physiologic changes occur in pregnant patients which alter the pharmacokinetics of anticonvulsants. Effective pre-pregnancy anticonvulsant levels should be used as the target levels during pregnancy. Drug levels should be measured as soon as pregnancy is diagnosed, since blood concentrations of anticonvulsants may drop precipitously during the first trimester, as a result of alterations in drug absorption, metabolism, or protein binding. This is especially true for phenytoin, with its nonlinear kinetics, in which doses may need to be increased by 50–100% during pregnancy to maintain pre-pregnancy levels. Routine drug levels should be measured each trimester, and more frequently if seizure control worsens, of if patients have a history of previous alterations in drug levels during pregnancy. Since drug clearance returns to pre-pregnancy norms within three to six weeks postpartum, pre-pregnancy anticonvulsant doses should be gradually introduced during this period.

Leppik IE, Rask CA: Pharmacokinetics of antiepileptic drugs during pregnancy. Semin Neurol 8:240–246, 1988.

128. What neuropathies are commonly associated with pregnancy and childbirth?

Whether due to peripheral edema, birth trauma, or other causes, certain neuropathies occur more commonly in pregnancy. Prior to birth, carpal tunnel syndrome is most common. This neuropathy is usually treated conservatively with wrist splinting, since it commonly resolves within 3 months postpartum. Meralgia paresthetica (numbness or dysesthesia of the anterolateral thigh due to obturator compression along the pelvic wall or obturator canal) occurs as the fetus enlarges, and is also a self-limited process, typically resolving within 3 months of delivery. Bell's palsy is seen with increased frequency (45.1/100,000) in pregnant women, relative to nonpregnant women of childbearing age (17.4/100,000). The use of corticosteroids during pregnancy for treatment of Bell's palsy is still controversial.

Traumatic mononeuropathy usually occurs during childbirth. Trauma involving the obturator nerve may result from compression by the fetal head, from misplaced forceps, or from hyperflexion in the lithotomy position. Compression injuries during delivery have also been reported involving the femoral, saphenous, common peroneal, or sciatic nerves. Postpartum foot drop is an interesting example of traumatic mononeuropathy with generally excellent prognosis, most typically observed in short primigravid women with large infants.

Aguayo AJ: Neuropathy due to compression or entrapment. In Dyck PJ, et al (eds): Peripheral Neuropathy. Philadelphia, W.B. Saunders, 1975.

129. What is postpartum depression?

Postpartum depression is a common transient state in which affected individuals develop fatigue, myalgias, and symptoms and signs suggesting depression. Correlations between the presence of antimicrosomal antibodies in pregnancy and subsequent manifestation of postpartum depression led some researchers to believe that this entity is actually the result of transient hypothyroidism. Recently, a transient form of lymphocytic thyroiditis, termed postpartum thyroiditis, has been found to affect between 5 and 10% of all pregnant women, and may be responsible for a substantial proportion of cases of postpartum depression.

Dussault JH, et al: Immunologically mediated hypothyroidism. Endocrinol Metab Clin 16:417–427, 1987.

130. Is male impotence caused by neurologic disease?

Organic disease is responsible for about half of all cases of impotence assessed by physicians. Of patients with organic disease, primary or secondary neurologic causes can be identified in an additional half. Although neuropathy (especially diabetic neuropathy) is the most common neurologic explanation for impotence, other causes may include spinal stenosis, myelopathy, cerebrovascular accident, multiple sclerosis, or neoplasm of the brain, pituitary gland, or spinal cord. In 85% of these cases, the underlying neurologic cause was unsuspected until the evaluation for impotence.

Grotta J, et al: Screening for neurologic disease in impotent patients. Texas Med 81:44–47, 1985.
Morley JE: Impotence. Am J Med 80:897–905, 1986.

131. Is female sexual dysfunction caused by neurologic disease?

This question has unfortunately not been addressed by a significant number of clinician researchers. However, because both male and female sexual response and behaviors have been shown to involve activation of specific portions of the neuroendocrine axis, it must be assumed that a woman who reports dyspareunia or loss of ability to achieve orgasm should have a similar risk for organic cause of her complaints as is found in the male population. A search for similar neurologic etiologies as identified for male impotence would thus seem appropriate in the assessment of these complaints.

BIBLIOGRAPHY

1. Goldstein PJ (ed): Neurological Disorders of Pregnancy. New York, Futura, 1986.
2. Kakulas BA, Adams RD (eds): Diseases of Muscle, 4th ed. Philadelphia, Harper Row, 1985.
3. Kelley WN, Harris ED, Ruddy S, et al (eds): Textbook of Rheumatology, 4th ed. Philadelphia, W.B. Saunders, 1993.
4. Maxwell MH (ed): Clinical Disorders of Fluid and Electrolyte Metabolism, 5th ed. New York, McGraw-Hill, 1987.
5. Waksman BN (ed): Immunologic Mechanisms in Neurologic and Psychiatric Disease. New York, Raven Press, 1990.

23. INFECTIOUS DISEASES, INCLUDING AIDS

E. Patricia Gill, M.D., and Richard L. Harris, M.D.

BACTERIAL INFECTIONS

1. What clinical findings differentiate meningitis from encephalitis?
Patients with meningitis have nuchal rigidity, headache, photophobia, and fever. Patients with encephalitis have disruption of cognitive function that may include altered consciousness, disorientation, behavioral or speech difficulties, and focal neurologic signs such as seizures or hemiparesis. In reality, the majority of infections cause meningoencephalitis; bacterial meningitis leads to predominant meningeal symptomatology (MENINGOencephalitis) and processes such as herpes encephalitis produce predominant cerebral symptomatology (meningoENCEPHALITIS).

Whitley RJ: Viral encephalitis. N Engl J Med 323:242–250, 1990.

2. When may a bacterial infection produce CSF results identical to aseptic meningitis?
Aseptic meningitis is often a viral infection and typically produces a lymphocytic pleocytosis, normal glucose, mildly elevated protein, negative Gram stain, and sterile bacterial cultures. Similar cerebrospinal fluid (CSF) findings can occur in partially treated bacterial meningitis or parameningeal foci such as epidural, subdural, or brain abscesses.

3. Bacterial meningitis is the most common cause of hypoglycorrhachia. What are the other most common causes?
1. Cryptococcal meningitis
2. Tuberculous meningitis
3. Syphilitic meningitis
4. Neurosarcoidosis
5. Meningeal carcinomatosis

4. A patient presents with probable acute bacterial meningitis but you are unable to obtain an informed consent for a lumbar puncture until after a CT scan. You wisely decide to start antibiotics immediately and not wait for the lumbar puncture. What tests can you still perform that may identify the etiologic agent?

1. Blood cultures can almost always be obtained before stat antibiotics are given. Approximately 50% of patients with bacterial meningitis will have a positive blood culture.

2. Serologic studies, such as latex agglutination or counter immunoelectrophoresis (CIE), for *Streptococcus pneumoniae*, *Neisseria meningitidis*, *Hemophilus influenzae*, and *Listeria monocytogenes* may be positive on the blood, urine, and CSF (even after antibiotics).

3. Culture of CSF, even after antibiotics are given, will likely still be positive for hours.

5. Who should receive prophylaxis after coming into contact with a patient with meningitis?
Prophylaxis depends on the organism and the age of the person exposed to the patient:
1. *H. influenzae,* **type B**—all children who have close contact with the patient.
2. **Neisseria meningitis**—all close contacts regardless of age.
Rifampin is usually considered the drug of choice for prophylaxis.

6. What are the most common gram-negative bacilli causing meningitis after the neonatal period?
Klebsiella, *E. coli*, and Pseudomonas account for 75–90% of gram-negative bacillary meningitis after the neonatal period. Eighty percent of these cases of gram-negative meningitis occur in conjunction with head trauma or neurosurgical procedures.

7. Which organisms are most likely causes of meningitis after neurosurgical procedures?
Gram-negative bacilli and staphylococci are the most common organisms, but virtually any kind of bacteria and even fungi such as Candida can gain access to the subarachnoid space.

8. In a patient with a ventriculoatrial or ventriculoperitoneal shunt, what is the msot common cause of bacterial meningitis?
Coagulase-negative staphylococci account for >50% of cases of meningitis in patients with ventricular shunts, followed by *S. aureus*, *Propionibacterium acnes*, gram-negative bacilli, and enterococci.

9. What bacteria is the most common cause of meningitis in patients with a CSF leak?
Streptococcus pneumoniae.
> Hand WL, Sanford JP: Posttraumatic bacterial meningitis. Ann Intern Med 72:869–874, 1970.

10. What is the most common cause of meningitis following blunt head trauma?
Streptococcus pneumoniae.

11. What are the commonest four clinical settings in which brain abscesses develop?
1. Contiguous suppurative foci such as otitis media or sinusitis
2. Hematogenous spread from a distant focus
3. Penetrating cranial injuries or neurosurgical procedures
4. Cryptogenic (20% of cases)

12. What is the most common bacterial agent involved in spinal epidural abscess?
Staphylococcus aureus accounts for approximately 62% of cases, followed by aerobic gram-negative rods (18%) and aerobic streptococci (8%). *Staphylococcus epidermidis* and anaerobes each cause about 2% of cases, and unknown (6%) or other organisms (1%) cause the remainder. Empirical antibiotic coverage (pending results of operative cultures) must include a first-line antistaphylococcal agent. Gram-negative coverage may be warranted when there is a history of a spinal procedure, intravenous drug abuse, or recent gastro-intestinal or genitourinary infection. Antibiotic therapy will be required for 4–8 weeks.
> Danner RL, Hartman BJ: Update of spinal epidural abscess: 35 cases and review of the literature. Rev Infect Dis 9:265–274, 1987.

13. What is the clinical course of an untreated spinal epidural abscess?
The first symptom noted is usually focal vertebral pain, followed by root pain, then deficits of motor, sensory, or sphincter function, and finally paralysis.

14. What conditions predispose to recurrent bacterial meningitis?
1. Anatomic communications with paranasal sinuses, nasopharynx, the middle ear, skin (such as congenital midline dermal sinus tracts), or prosthetic devices such as ventriculoperitoneal shunts.
2. Parameningeal foci may either drain into the meninges or lead to repeated inflammatory reactions and meningeal signs or symptoms.
3. Immunologic defects such as hypogammaglobulinemia, splenectomy, leukemia and lymphoma, sickle cell anemia and other hemoglobinopathies, or complement deficiencies.

15. Name conditions that predispose to polymicrobial meningitis.
    1. Infections at contiguous foci
    2. Tumors in close proximity to the central nervous system
    3. Fistulous communications
    4. Rarely, disseminated strongyloidiasis (enteric organisms carried "piggy-back" from the gut through the bloodstream to the subarachnoid space)

16. A 72-year-old man was hospitalized one week ago for a stroke. He has a dense right hemiplegia and is incontinent of bowel and bladder. Today, he developed a fever of 101° F, along with shaking chills. What sources are most likely responsible?
The cause of fever is probably a nosocomial infection. A urinary tract infection is most likely—whether he has a Foley catheter, a condom catheter, or a neurogenic bladder that does not fully empty, the lower urinary tract is the best bet. Other good possibilities include pneumonia (especially aspiration pneumonia) or venous catheter–related infection.

17. A 14-year-old boy whose only medical problem is acne presents with diplopia, photophobia, and right periorbital edema. His neurologic examination reveals a midposition, fixed right pupil, decreased sensation over the upper face, right ophthalmoplegia, and papilledema on the right. What's wrong?
His symptoms and signs are consistent with an infectious cavernous sinus thrombosis on the right, most likely from squeezing a pimple. Untreated, he may develop progressive exophthalmos, loss of corneal reflex, retinal hemorrhage, and visual loss. As the infection spreads to the contralateral cavernous sinus, similar findings appear in the opposite eye. Cranial nerves III, IV, V and VI are affected as they pass through the cavernous sinuses.

18. A 57-year-old diabetic man presents with a right facial nerve palsy, otalgia, and otorrhea. What is the most likely organism?
The condition is most often due to *Pseudomonas aeruginosa*, producing the syndrome of necrotizing or "malignant" external otitis.

19. A 42-year-old hypertensive woman who has been poorly compliant with her medications is found unconscious at home by her husband. In the ER, she is noted to have decorticate posturing and papilledema. While undergoing a head CT scan, she begins to vomit. Does she need antibiotics? What organisms would you cover for?
Opinions vary on whether or not this patient needs antibiotics. Acidic gastric contents are sterile but can cause a chemical pneumonitis. Aspirated oral contents in a nonhospitalized, healthy person contain primarily anaerobic and aerobic gram-positive organisms. Some experts would not treat acute aspiration unless the patient develops fever or purulent sputum. If the patient had been hospitalized (especially if intubated and in an ICU) when she aspirated, her oral flora would also likely contain gram-negative bacilli, possibly multiply-resistant to antibiotics.

20. In what clinical situations would a CNS infection merit the use of systemic steroids?
    1. An infant with *H. influenzae* meningitis
    2. A severely ill adult with tuberculous meningitis
    3. A patient with neurocysticercosis and increased intracranial pressure

21. What is the clinical presentation of a patient receiving excessive doses of beta-lactam antibiotics?
Toxicity can cause confusion, jitteriness, myoclonic jerks, and seizures.

22. In addition to aminoglycosides, what other drugs cause ototoxicity?
1. Ethacrynic acid—probably the highest risk
2. Furosemide
3. Erythromycin—usually reversible hearing loss with high-dose therapy
4. Vancomycin—listed as ototoxic, but if so, very, very rarely

23. Which conditions predispose to peripheral neuropathy in patients who take isoniazid?
Peripheral neuropathy is especially likely to occur in patients who are slow acetylators, are poorly nourished, or have an underlying neuropathy secondary to diabetes, uremia, or alcoholism. Concomitant administration of pyridoxine (vitamin B6) may prevent the neuropathy.

TOXINS

24. What three bacteria produce exotoxins that affect peripheral nerves either directly or indirectly?
1. The B subunit of diphtheria toxin binds to cell membranes and allows the A subunit to enter nerves, where it inhibits protein synthesis and causes a noninflammatory demyelination. Cranial nerves are affected more frequently than peripheral nerves.
2. Tetanus toxin is transported up the axon and binds to the presynaptic endings on motor neurons in the anterior horns of the spinal cord. Inhibitory input is blocked, resulting in muscle spasms.
3. Botulinum toxin binds to the presynaptic axon terminal of the neuromuscular junction, preventing acetylcholine release and producing a flaccid paralysis.

25. What is the clinical presentation of botulism?
Botulinum toxin prevents presynaptic acetylcholine release. The patient is usually alert, oriented, and afebrile, but with nausea, vomiting, dizziness, dry mouth, orthostatic hypotension, and urinary retention. Ptosis, dilated pupils, and diplopia are common. Over the first day the patient may develop progressive weakness, including respiratory muscle paralysis. The sensory examination remains normal.

26. What are the manifestations of ciguatera? How does one acquire this illness?
Patients ingest ciguatoxin, produced by the dinoflagellate *Gambierdiscus toxicus*, when they eat large, carnivorous reef fish such as grouper or snapper. Within about 6 hours, GI symptoms of nausea, vomiting, diarrhea, and cramps begin. Bizarre neurologic symptoms may appear early or after the GI complaints and resolve in 24–48 hours. Neurologic manifestations include numbness and tingling of lips and extremities, a reversal of hot-cold sensation, and tooth pain. Paresthesias may not follow dermatomal patterns. Vertigo, hypersalivation, blurred vision, tremor, ataxia, and coma may occur.
Eastaugh J, Shepherd S: Infectious and toxic syndromes from fish and shellfish consumption: A review. Arch Intern Med 144:1735–1740, 1989.

27. What illness is caused by eating puffer fish?
Tetrodotoxication occurs within 3 hours of eating a tetrodotoxic fish such as puffer fish, porcupine fish, ocean sunfish, blue-ringed octopus, and some species of newts and salamanders. Symptoms include lethargy, paresthesias, hyperemesis, salivation, weakness, ataxia, and dysphagia. Ascending paralysis, respiratory failure, hypotension, and bradycardia may occur. Diagnosis is clinical, and treatment is supportive. Gastric lavage, activated charcoal, and anticholinesterase inhibitors may be helpful.
Eastaugh J, Shepherd S: Infectious and toxic syndromes from fish and shellfish consumption: A review. Arch Intern Med 144:1735–1740, 1989.

28. What are the symptoms of scombroid poisoning?
Scombroid poisoning symptoms begin within minutes to hours of ingestion of toxic fish. The fish are usually of the family *Scombridae*, which includes tuna, mackerel, and jacks, but cases are also reported from nonscombroid fish. Victims experience flushing and a hot sensation of the skin, headache, dizziness, burning sensation in the mouth and throat, and palpitations. Nausea, diarrhea, and occasionally vomiting occur. A sunburn-like skin rash appears. In severe cases, bronchospasm, palpitations, supraventricular arrhythmias, and occasionally mild hypotension may occur. The diagnosis is clinical; treatment is supportive. Deaths have not been reported.

29. What is the "scombrotoxin"?
The "scombrotoxin" is formed when surface bacteria (Proteus and Klebsiella) proliferate on the flesh of the fish because of improper refrigeration. Free histidine, present in increased quantities in dark meat fish, is degraded to histamine by the bacteria. The exact role of histamine is unclear because orally ingested histamine is degraded in the gastrointestinal tract, but a histamine-like substance such as saurine produces the clinical effects.

Eastaugh J, Shepherd S: Infectious and toxic syndromes from fish and shellfish consumption: A review. Arch Intern Med 144:1735–1740, 1989.

SPIROCHETAL INFECTIONS

30. How frequent are abnormalities in the CSF of patients with primary or secondary syphilis?
Abnormalities in the CSF are found in 15–40% of patients who have primary or secondary syphilis and are usually asymptomatic.

Musher DM, Hamill RJ, Baughn RE: Effect of human immunodeficiency virus (HIV) infection on the course of syphilis and on the response to treatment. Ann Intern Med 113:872–881, 1990.

31. At what stage of syphilis (primary, secondary, or tertiary) does neurosyphilis occur?
Neurosyphilis may occur in any stage of syphilis. CNS invasion by *T. pallidum* occurs in nearly one-third of patients with primary and secondary syphilis.

Hook EW: Treatment of syphilis: Current recommendations, alternatives, and continuing problems. Rev Inf Dis 11(Suppl 6):S1511–S1517, 1989.

32. What circumstances predispose to early neurosyphilis?
Inadequate treatment of early syphilis and HIV infection both predispose to early neurosyphilis.

Musher DM, Hamill RJ, Baughn RE: Effect of human immunodeficiency virus (HIV) infection on the course of syphilis and on the response to treatment. Ann Intern Med 113:872–881, 1990.

33. Which cranial nerves are most often involved in syphilitic meningitis?
Syphilis affects the seventh and eighth cranial nerves most often (40%), and the second, third, and fourth cranial nerves less frequently (25%).

34. What are the neurologic complications of Lyme disease?
Early in the course, meningitis, cranial neuritis, Bell's palsy, motor or sensory radiculoneuritis, subtle encephalitis, mononeuritis multiplex, myelitis, chorea, or cerebellar ataxia may occur. Chronically, patients may develop encephalitis, spastic paraparesis, ataxic gait, subtle mental disorders, chronic axonal polyradiculopathy, or dementia.

Steere AC: Lyme disease. N Engl J Med 321:586–596, 1989.

35. What is the most likely clinical presentation of *Borrelia burgdorferi* (Lyme disease)?
A patient with a 10-cm erythematous lesion with central clearing on his back. The presence of the typical tick-bite wound is a more reliable guide to infection than serologic titers or (often vague) clinical symptoms.

36. What is the clinical presentation of infection with leptospirosis?
Leptospirosis often develops after a camping trip and may present as aseptic meningitis (with normal CSF glucose), bulbar conjunctivitis, erythematous rash, adenopathy, hepatosplenomegaly, and renal insufficiency.

FUNGAL, PARASITIC, AND OTHER PROCESSES

37. What is the clinical presentation of infection with *Acanthamoeba* or *Naegleria*?
These infections usually present as severe persistent frontal headache after swimming in a fresh-water lake.

38. Which species of plasmodium may cause cerebral malaria?
Plasmodium falciparum infection may be complicated by cerebral malaria.

39. What neurologic abnormalities occur with cerebral malaria? What does the spinal fluid show?
Neurologic abnormalities include disturbances of consciousness, acute organic brain syndromes, seizures, meningismus, and rarely, focal neurologic signs. A lumbar puncture usually reveals an elevated opening pressure with normal CSF. Occasionally CSF protein is elevated and low-level pleocytosis occurs, but hypoglycorrhachia does not occur.

40. Are corticosteroids beneficial in cerebral malaria?
No. In a double-blind trial comparing placebo to high-dose dexamethasone, mortality was not different, but duration of coma was longer and complications such as gastrointestinal bleeding were more frequent in the dexamethasone-treated group.

Warrell DA, et al: Dexamethasone proves deleterious in cerebral malaria: A double-blind trial in 100 comatose patients. N Engl J Med 306:313–319, 1982.

41. What is the epidemiology of neurocysticercosis?
Infection with eggs of the pork tapeworm, *Taenia solium*, can lead to neurocysticercosis. In the intermediate stage, it is referred to as *Cysticercus cellulosae*, but *T. solium* and *C. cellulosae* are the same parasite. Ingestion of measled (infected) pork → intestinal tapeworm (often asymptomatic) → fecal excretion → human fecal-oral contamination → egg ingestion and penetration of intestinal wall → oncospheres → larvae that encyst → neurocysticercosis.

42. A 21-year-old archeology student complains of headache, fever, lethargy, and difficulty concentrating in class. He had been well until 2 months previously, when he had a brief illness with fever, arthralgias, cough, and sputum production just after he returned from a dig in Arizona. He was again well until his current symptoms began 2 weeks ago. What is his probable diagnosis? How should he be treated?
The most likely diagnosis is coccidioidomycosis meningitis. He will need intrathecal amphotericin B, as well as small doses of systemic amphotericin. Treatment will be long-term and relapses are common. Newer drugs that may have a role are fluconazole and itraconazole.

43. Which antifungal agents are most useful in CNS infections because of their good spinal fluid penetration?
Amphotericin B and fluconazole enter the CSF adequately. Ketaconozole has poor penetration.

44. An 82-year-old white woman presents with fever, sweats, generalized body aches, weakness, severe headache, and weight loss. She describes intermittent cough and painful jaw muscles while chewing food. Her laboratory studies show anemia, elevated alkaline phosphatase, and a sedimentation rate of 92 mm/hr. What is the diagnosis?
Temporal arteritis. This granulomatous arteritis often mimics an infectious disease.

45. A patient you diagnosed 1 year previously with temporal arteritis has done well on her therapy. Today, she returns for an office visit and complains of dysphagia and weight loss. What do you suspect?
Suspect infectious esophagitis. Candida, or perhaps herpes simplex virus, is the most likely pathogen in a patient who has been on long-term steroids.

46. What is Vogt-Koyanagi-Harada syndrome?
This syndrome consists of subacute meningoencephalitis with severe, protracted granulomatous uveitis and depigmentary skin changes. The cause is unknown, but it is noninfectious.

PRIONS

47. What is a prion? Why is it important in neurologic disease?
A prion is a small proteinaceous infectious particle that resists inactivation by procedures that modify nucleic acids. The concept of an infectious agent that does not require DNA or RNA is novel. This type of agent is thought to be responsible for scrapie and possibly Creutzfeldt-Jakob disease and kuru.
  Prusiner SB: Prions and neurogenerative disease. N Engl J Med 317:1571–1581, 1987.

48. A 45-year-old patient presents with myoclonus and dementia that have progressed rapidly over the past 6 months. His CSF is normal. What is his likely diagnosis? What would his EEG show?
The patient has findings characteristic of Creutzfeldt-Jakob disease. Dementia progresses rapidly over months and death usually occurs in less than a year. The EEG characteristically (though not always) has periodic-appearing, biphasic or triphasic, high-amplitude sharp waves. CSF is usually normal, although a mild elevation in protein is occasionally found.

49. What is the pathologic lesion in Creutzfeldt-Jakob disease?
The pathologic lesion is a spongiform encephalopathy. There is a loss of neurons, with astrocytic proliferation and gliosis, swelling, and intracytoplasmic vacuolization of neuronal and astroglial processes.

50. What infection control measures should be observed for a patient with Creutzfeldt-Jakob disease?
Blood, brain, cornea, visceral organs, and CSF are infectious. Autoclaving for 1 hour at 250° F and 15 psi, exposure to 1 N or 0.1 N sodium hydroxide for 1 hour at room temperature, or exposure to 0.5% sodium hypochlorite will kill the causative agent. Of note, neither boiling, ultraviolet radiation, ionizing radiation, 70% ethyl alcohol, formaldehyde, glutaraldehyde, nor 10% formalin will destroy the agent. The patient need not be isolated, but blood and body fluid precautions should be observed.

51. How is kuru transmitted?
Kuru, another disease caused by prions, is transmitted by cannibalism. New Guinea natives practicing ritualistic consumption of dead kinsmen (including their brains) as a rite of mourning developed this illness. Clinically, kuru presents as a progressive fatal dementia with severe ataxia.

VIRAL INFECTIONS

52. When may aseptic meningitis be confused with bacterial meningitis? How do you resolve the confusion?
Early in viral meningitis, the spinal fluid may have a predominance of polymorphonuclear (PMN) leukocytes. The Gram stain will be negative and CSF glucose will be normal. The PMN predominance will quickly change to a mononuclear cell predominance, so a repeat lumbar puncture 6–12 hours later will clarify the issue.

Feigin RD, Shackelford PG: Value of repeat lumbar puncture in the differential diagnosis of meningitis. N Engl J Med 289:571–574, 1973.

53. Other than culture results, which of the routine studies performed on CSF is the most useful for distinguishing between meningitis due to tuberculosis and that due to a virus, such as ECHO 9? What does ECHO stand for?
The glucose is most useful. The glucose is usually low in tuberculous infections, but normal in viral infections. ECHO = enteric cytopathic human orphan [virus].

54. Worldwide, what is the most common cause of epidemic encephalitis?
Japanese B encephalitis is the most common epidemic infection outside North America. It is a major medical problem in China, Southwest Asia, and India.

Whitley RJ: Viral encephalitis. N Engl J Med 323:242–250, 1990.

55. What is the most common sporadic encephalitis in the U.S.?
Herpes simplex causes encephalitis most frequently.

Whitley RJ: Viral encephalitis. N Engl J Med 323:242–250, 1990.

56. What is La Crosse encephalitis?
La Crosse, a type of California encephalitis, is the most common arthropod-borne encephalitis in the United States. It occurs in the central and eastern U.S., and primarily affects children. It has a mortality of <1% and sequelae are rare.

57. What are the other common arthropod-borne viral encephalitides in the United States?
   1. **St. Louis encephalitis** occurs in the central, western, and southern U.S. and affects older adults.
   2. **Venezuelan encephalitis** occurs in the South, affects adults, and has very low mortality and sequelae rates.
   3. **Western equine encephalitis** occurs in the West and Midwest, affecting people at extremes of age. Mortality is 5–15% and sequelae are more common in infants than in older survivors.
   4. **Eastern equine encephalitis** affects children in the East, South, and Gulf Coast. Mortality is 50–75% and 80% of survivors have sequelae.

Whitley RJ: Viral encephalitis. N Engl J Med 323:242–250, 1990.

58. What are some differences between Western, Eastern, and Venezuelan equine encephalitis?
   1. **Eastern:** A summertime disease, it causes less than 15 human cases per year, but has a 50–75% mortality rate. It strikes mainly in the Gulf/Atlantic states.
   2. **Venezuelan:** It occurs in epidemics that have caused tens of thousands of cases, but with a fatality rate of only 0.6%. It occurs mainly in Central and South America.
   3. **Western:** It occurs in the summer months also, usually in states west of the Mississippi. It causes 0–200 cases/year and infants are most susceptible. The risk is greatest in rural areas. The case fatality rate is 3–5%.

59. A patient presents with aphasia, right-sided weakness, fever, and confusion. A lumbar puncture reveals CSF with 400 RBC/mm³, 30 WBC/mm³ (predominantly mononuclear cells), glucose of 70 mg/dl, and protein of 60 mg/dl. His EEG shows periodic high-voltage spike wave activity from the left temporal region. What is the most likely causative agent?

This clinical picture suggests herpes simplex encephalitis. The main clue to herpes versus other causes of viral encephalitis is focality, especially to the temporal lobe.

Whitley RJ: Viral encephalitis. N Engl J Med 323:242–250, 1990.

60. What are typical CSF findings in herpes encephalitis?

Normal CSF cell counts and chemistries can occasionally be seen in herpes simplex virus (HSV) encephalitis. Typical CSF findings are lymphocytic predominance, elevated protein, and the presence of RBCs. In the majority of cases, HSV cannot be cultured from the CSF.

61. What histopathologic finding is pathognomonic for herpes encephalitis?

The Cowdry type A inclusion body is an eosinophilic, intranuclear particle and is pathognomonic for herpes.

Whitely RJ: Viral encephalitis. N Engl J Med 323:242–250, 1990.

62. What is the recommended therapy for HSV encephalitis?

Treatment requires acyclovir 30 mg/kg/day in three divided doses, for at least 14 days. Acyclovir is cleared by the kidney so the dose will require adjustment for renal insufficiency, and patients with normal renal function should be encouraged to take in generous amounts of free water each day.

63. An animal handler at a scientific laboratory is bitten on the left thumb by a macaque monkey. Five days later, he develops numbness in his left arm, fever, and myalgias, and eventually becomes comatose. His physical examination shows grouped vesicles at the bite site. What is the diagnosis?

His infection is caused by *Herpes virus simiae*. This strain has a high fatality, even with acyclovir therapy. Person to person spread is rare.

64. A 32-year-old woman presents with painful genital vesicular lesions, urinary retention, and severe headache. Her CSF shows lymphocytic pleocytosis. The neurologic examination is otherwise unremarkable. What is the probable diagnosis?

Herpes simplex virus II meningitis. Genital lesions usually recur but the meningitis usually does not. It has an excellent prognosis neurologically. This benign form of "aseptic" meningitis should not be confused with the potentially fatal, necrotizing form of HSV I encephalitis.

65. What is the Ramsey-Hunt syndrome?

It is herpes zoster involving the VII and VIII cranial nerve. A patient presents with vertigo, ipsilateral hearing deficit, and facial palsy, plus vesicles in the external auditory canal.

66. What are the most important neurologic complications of primary varicella infections?

1. Reye syndrome. This acute, noninflammatory encephalopathy is characterized by fatty destruction of the liver, hypoglycemia, and increased intracranial pressure. It has a 20% fatality rate. Aspirin use with varicella and influenzae has been associated with Reye syndrome in children.
2. Aseptic meningitis
3. Transverse myelitis
4. Guillain-Barré syndrome

   5. Cerebellar encephalitis. In children, this results in ataxia, nausea, and rigidity, but most make a full recovery. In adults, this results in altered sensorium, seizures, focal signs, and a mortality up to 35%.

   Straus SE, et al: Varicella-zoster virus infection: Biology, natural history, treatment, and prevention. Ann Intern Med 108:221–237, 1988.

67. Which two viruses enter the CNS by peripheral intraneural routes to cause encephalitis?

Herpes simplex and rabies viruses enter the nervous system by peripheral intraneuronal routes. One route for HSV may be the olfactory tract.

   Whitley RJ: Viral encephalitis. N Engl J Med 323:242–250, 1990.

68. Who should receive postexposure rabies prophylaxis?

Postexposure prophylaxis for rabies is recommended for all persons bitten or scratched by wild or domestic animals that may be carrying the disease, or who have an open wound or mucous membrane contaminated with saliva or other potentially infectious material from a rabid animal. It is also recommended for persons who report a possibly infectious exposure to a human with rabies. Potentially rabid animals include (but are not limited to) dogs, cats, skunks, raccoons, foxes, and bats.

   Human rabies—Texas, Arkansas, Georgia, 1991. JAMA 266:2956–2958, 1991.

69. Which infections may lead to a postinfectious encephalomyelitis?

Varicella, influenza, and measles may all cause an irreversible demyelinating syndrome.

   Whitley RJ: Viral encephalitis. N Engl J Med 323:242–250, 1990.

70. What clinical features characterize the postpolio syndrome?

The main symptoms of the postpolio syndrome are the new onset of weakness, pain, and fatigue occurring years after acute poliomyelitis. About 25% of survivors of polio are affected. EMG and muscle biopsy show evidence of both chronic and recent denervation, although these changes are nonspecific; asymptomatic survivors of polio also exhibit these changes.

   Cashman NR, et al: Late denervation in patients with antecedent paralytic poliomyelitis. N Engl J Med 317:7–12, 1987.

71. What infections are associated with facial palsy?

The cause of lower motor neuron lesions affecting the facial nerve is seldom identified. Evidence exists, however, for infectious causes, including the following:

Herpes simplex virus	Epstein-Barr virus	Lyme disease
Varicella zoster virus	Rubella	Syphilis
Cytomegalovirus	Mumps	HIV

   Morgan M, Nathwani D: Facial palsy and infection: The unfolding story. Clin Infect Dis 14:263–271, 1992.

AIDS

72. Both HIV infection and zidovudine (AZT) therapy appear capable of causing myopathy clinically expressed as proximal muscle weakness, atrophy, weight loss, and elevated levels of creatine kinase (CK). How can the clinician distinguish between these two entities?

   1. Give the patient a drug-free holiday for 2 weeks to see if the symptoms improve off of the medication.

   2. A muscle biopsy shows abnormal mitochondria in AZT-induced myopathy, but not in primary HIV myopathy.

73. A new nucleotide analog dideoxyinosine (DDI, or Videx) is now available for the therapy of the patient with HIV infection who is intolerant of AZT or is clinically declining. The most frequent adverse effects of DDI have been abdominal cramps and diarrhea. What is the most frequent neurologic toxicity that limits treatment?
Acute painful neuropathy can occur with DDI therapy.

74. What is the most common type of peripheral neuropathy in patients with HIV infection?
A chronic, distal, symmetric polyneuropathy is most common. It is predominantly sensory, with painful dysesthesias, numbness, and paresthesias. Weakness or autonomic dysfunction occur, but less frequently. Occasionally, a chronic or acute inflammatory demyelinating polyneuropathy is seen.

75. How is the acute, inflammatory demyelinating neuropathy of HIV infection distinguished from Guillain-Barré syndrome?
In the HIV-related disorder, there is a CSF pleocytosis ranging from 10–50 cells/mm³ along with CSF protein elevation. In Guillain-Barré, pleocytosis generally does not occur.

76. What CSF findings do you expect to see in a patient with HIV-associated aseptic meningitis?
Similar to other causes of viral meningitis, HIV infection can produce a mononuclear pleocytosis with 20–300 cells/mm³ and a protein elevation in the range of 50–100 mg/dl. Meningeal signs, headache, fever, and cranial nerve palsies, especially of fifth, seventh, and eighth cranial nerves, also occur.

Gabuzda DH, Hirsch MS: Neurologic manifestations of infection with human immunodeficiency virus: Clinical features and pathogenesis. Ann Intern Med 107:383–391, 1987.

77. What are the most common causes of new-onset seizures in patients with HIV infection?
Toxoplasmosis, HIV encephalopathy, cryptococcus, and lymphoma.

Holtzman DM, Kaku DA, So YT: New-onset seizures associated with human immunodeficiency virus infection: Causation and clinical features in 100 cases. Am J Med 87:173–177, 1989.

78. What clinical feature distinguishes the AIDS-dementia complex from Creutzfeldt-Jakob disease?
In AIDS dementia, a normal level of consciousness is usually maintained, even late in the disease, unless some other systemic disease intervenes. This is not true of Creutzfeldt-Jakob disease, which is otherwise clinically similar to AIDS dementia.

Hodd et al: The acquired immunodeficiency syndrome (AIDS) dementia complex. Ann Intern Med 111:400–410, 1989.

79. A patient with known AIDS complains of decreased visual acuity. What infectious agents are most likely responsible?
Cytomegalovirus (CMV) retinitis is most common, occurring in about 30% of patients with AIDS. Toxoplasmosis is probably the second most common retinal infection, accounting for only 4% of retinitis cases. Ocular syphilis may manifest as iridocyclitis, neuroretinitis, optic perineuritis, and retrobulbar neuritis. HIV infection itself may cause cotton-wool spots that are usually not visually significant. A rare cause of retinitis is tuberculosis.

de Smet MD, Nussenbatt RB: Ocular manifestations of AIDS. JAMA 266:3019–3022, 1991.

80. What are the diagnostic features of toxoplasma encephalitis in patients with AIDS?.
Most patients have elevated IgG antibodies to toxoplasma. The absence of toxoplasma IgG in a patient with suspected toxoplasma encephalitis militates strongly against the diagnosis. Routine analyses of the CSF may be normal. Contrast-enhanced CT scans demonstrate

nodular or ring-enhancing lesions in greater than 90% of patients. The treatment of choice is high-dose pyrimethamine and sulfadiazine.

81. Numerous patients with AIDS are sulfa allergic. In a patient with sulfa allergy, what would be the treatment of choice for toxoplasma encephalitis?
Clindamycin, 1200 mg intravenously every 6 hours, plus pyrimethamine 200 mg then 75–100 mg/day PO, plus folinic acid, at least 10 mg/day PO.

Dannemann B, McCutchan JA, Israelski D, et al: Treatment of toxoplasmic encephalitis in patients with AIDS. Ann Intern Med 116:33–43, 1992.

82. What are the most common presentations of neurosyphilis in patients with HIV infection?
  1. Acute meningitis
  2. Cranial neuropathy
     a. Optic neuritis
     b. VIII nerve palsy
  3. Meningovascular, causing strokes

83. How does syphilis differ in HIV-infected patients compared to normal hosts?
  1. Slower response to therapy
  2. Higher rate of treatment failure
  3. Higher rate of false-negative serologic tests
  4. Early neurosyphilis is rare in normal hosts.

84. How does HIV infection affect the diagnosis of syphilis?
Patients with HIV infection, especially with a very low T_4 lymphocyte count, may lose reactivity to treponemal tests for syphilis. Both FTA-ABS and MHA-TP tests may be negative in patients with prior syphilis infection and HIV infection.

Haas JS, et al: Sensitivity of treponemal tests for detecting prior treated syphilis during human immunodeficiency virus infection. J Infect Dis 162:862–866, 1990.

85. How does HIV affect the course of syphilis?
HIV infection may cause a failure of syphilis to respond to treatment within the expected time, a relapse of infection after treatment, and the frequent appearance of early neurosyphilis. Conventional doses of penicillin may not be adequate. Three doses of benzathine penicillin, 2.4 million units at weekly intervals, has been suggested for treatment of primary or secondary infection. Alternative regimens have been suggested—amoxicillin (up to 6 gm/day), or supplementing three doses of benzathine penicillin with oral penicillin or amoxicillin for a 2- to 3-week period, or ceftriaxone 500 mg or 1 gm, given daily or every other day for 5 to 10 days.

Musher DM, Hamill RJ, Baughn RE: Effect of human immunodeficiency virus (HIV) infection on the course of syphilis and on the response to treatment. Ann Intern Med 113:872–881, 1990.

BIBLIOGRAPHY

1. Mandell Gl, Douglas RG, Bennett JE: Principles and Practice of Infectious Disease. 3rd ed. New York, John Wiley, 1991.

24. PEDIATRIC NEUROLOGY

Angus A. Wilfong, M.D., FRCPC

NORMAL NEUROLOGIC GROWTH AND DEVELOPMENT

1. In addition to the routine questions asked during a neurologic interview, what additional questions are important for a complete pediatric neurology history?

Pediatric Neurology History

I. Antenatal
  A. Maternal parity
  B. Previous miscarriages or abortions
  C. Illnesses during the pregnancy
  D. Maternal nutrition and supplementation
    1. Weight gain
    2. Uterine size
  E. Medications taken during the pregnancy
    1. Prescription
    2. Over-the-counter
  F. Illicit drug abuse
  G. Alcohol use
  H. Cigarette use
  I. Toxic exposures
    1. Occupational
    2. Industrial
    3. Agricultural
    4. Irradition
  J. Accidents and trauma
  K. Travel abroad
  L. Fetal movements
  M. Premature labor contractions
  N. Vaginal spotting or bleeding
  O. Premature rupture of the membranes

II. Perinatal
  A. Spontaneous or induced labor
  B. Duration of labor
  C. Fetal monitoring during labor
  D. Type of delivery
    1. Vaginal
      a. Vertex
      b. Breech
      c. Forceps or vacuum assisted
        (1) failure to progress
        (2) fetal distress
    2. Cesarean section
      a. Repeat
      b. Failure to progress
      c. Fetal distress

II. Perinatal *(Cont.)*
  E. Type of anesthesia, if any
    1. Local
    2. Spinal
    3. Epidural
    4. General
  F. Estimated gestational age at time of delivery
  G. Intant's appearance at birth and need for resuscitation—Apgar score if recalled.
  H. Birth weight, length, fronto-occipital circumference (FOC)

III. Neonatal Complications
  A. Jaundice
  B. Temperature
  C. Breathing
  D. Feeding: breast, bottle, tube
  E. How long in hospital until released home

IV. Neurodevelopment
  A. Progressing or regressing
  B. Development of handedness
  C. Attainment of major milestones
  D. Academic performance in school

V. Immunizations
  A. DPT
  B. MMR
  C. BCG
  D. HIB

VI. Behavior
  A. Peer relations
  B. Interpersonal skills
  C. Conduct

VII. Family History—Consanguinity

VIII. Social History
  A. Intrafamilial psychosocial stressors
  B. Pets

2. What are some of the important features of the physical examination of infants and young children that may not be included in the examination of adults?

Pediatric Neurology Physical Examination

1. Measurement of the FOC and comparison with previous values	6. Limb asymmetries and malformations (including dermatoglyphics)
2. Palpation of cranial sutures and fontanelles if open	7. Abnormal cutaneous lesions
3. Cranial and ocular auscultation	8. Assessment of developmental reflexes
4. Documentation of any craniofacial dysmorphology	9. Evaluation of developmental progress
5. Funduscopic examination with careful attention to the retina, not just to the optic disc	10. Motor tone—appendicular and axial
	11. Gowers' maneuver

3. What are some of the common developmental reflexes? When do you expect them to be present?

Developmental Reflexes

REFLEX	APPEARS	DISAPPEARS
Lateral incurvation of trunk	Birth	1–2 months
Rooting	Birth	3 months
Moro	Birth	5–6 months
Tonic neck reflex	Birth	5–6 months
Palmar grasp	Birth	6 months
Crossed adduction with knee jerk	Birth	7–8 months
Plantar grasp	Birth	9–10 months
Extensor plantar responses	Birth	6–12 months
Parachute response	8–9 months	Persists
Landau reflex	10 months	24 months

4. What is the average FOC for a term newborn? What is the rate of growth over the first year?

Average FOC for a term newborn is 35 cm.

Average FOC growth: 2 cm/month for first 3 months
1 cm/month for next 3 months
0.5 cm/month for the last 6 months

5. What are the important developmental milestones for the first 5 years of life?

Developmental Milestones

AGE	REFLEX	AGE	REFLEX
0–4 weeks	Flexed posture Brief visual fixation and following Preference for human face Active Moro, stepping, placing, grasping, rooting	8 weeks	Head level with ventral suspension Tonic neck posture Follows through 180° Social smile, coos, listens
4 weeks	Legs extended Tonic neck posture when supine Follows moving objects	12 weeks	Lifts head and chest off bed Head above horizontal with ventral suspension Listens to music

Table continued on next page.

Developmental Milestones (Continued)

AGE	REFLEX	AGE	REFLEX
16 weeks	Symmetric posture Reaches and grasps for objects Hands in midline	2 years *(Cont.)*	Imitates horizontal strokes on paper 3 word sentences Holds spoon well
28 weeks	Rolls over, sits briefly Transfers objects hand to hand Babbles, enjoys mirror	3 years	Walks up stairs alternating feet Rides tricycle Stands momentarily on one foot
40 weeks	Pulls to stand Crawls, pincer grasp "Mama," "dada" Peek-a-boo, pat-a-cake		Tower of 9 cubes and bridge of cubes Knows name and sex Counts 3 objects
12 months	Cruises or walks with one hand held 2 or 3 single words		Parallel play and washes hands
15 months	Walks independently Tower of 2 cubes Makes line with crayon 2 word sentences	4 years	Hops on one foot Throws ball overhand Uses scissors Copies cross and square on paper
18 months	Runs, walks up stairs with one hand held Explores drawers, wastebaskets Tower of 3 cubes 10 single words, names pictures Identifies 1 or 2 body parts Feeds self with fingers		Draws man with 2–4 parts Counts 4 pennies accurately Role playing Goes to toilet alone
2 years	Runs well, walks up and down stairs alone Tower of 6 cubes	5 years	Skips Copies triangle, names 4 colors Counts 10 pennies Dresses and undresses self

PRENATAL DISEASES AND DEVELOPMENTAL DEFECTS

6. What is the Apgar score?

The Apgar score is a clinical vitality rating scale applied to newborn infants in an attempt to identify those at risk for certain neonatal complications. Apgar is an eponym (Virginia Apgar, U.S. anesthesiologist), although it is often used as an acronym.

Apgar Score

	SCORE		
SIGN	0	1	2
A Appearance (color)	Blue, pale	Acrocyanosis	Pink
P Pulse (heart rate)	Absent	<100	>100
G Grimace (reflex irritability in response to nasal suctioning)	No response	Grimace	Cry
A Activity (muscle tone)	Limp	Some flexion of limbs	Active motion
R Respiration (respiratory effort)	Absent	Slow and irregular	Strong crying

Infants are routinely scored at 1 and 5 minutes following birth. Further scores may be made at 10 and 20 minutes if the infant appears to have been compromised.

7. Is the Apgar score useful in determining neurologic prognosis?

The 1-minute Apgar score reflects whether the newborn requires cardiopulmonary resuscitation and correlates little with long-term neurologic outcome. Five-minute Apgar scores of less than 5, particularly in infants with hypotonia, apnea, or feeding difficulties, raise the possibility of neurologic disability. One-third of infants with Apgar scores of 3 or less beyond 10 minutes will have severe neurologic sequelae, one-fifth will not survive the neonatal period, and the remainder will have milder disabilities or be normal.

8. How would you classify neonatal intraventricular hemorrhage (IVH)?

Classification of IVH

Grade I	Localized subependymal hemorrhage into the germinal matrix
Grade II	Subependymal hemorrhage with extension into the ventricles (less than 50% of the ventricular volume filled with blood)
Grade III	Subependymal hemorrhage with extension into the ventricles and acute ventricular dilatation (greater than 50 % of the ventricular volume filled with blood)
Grade IV	Subependymal, intraventricular, and extension into the surrounding cerebral parenchyma

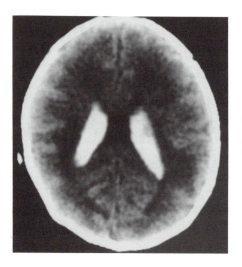

Unenhanced axial CT: grade III, IVH in a premature newborn (32 weeks' gestation). Note acute ventricular distention with blood filling more than 50% of the ventricular volume. There is no parenchymal extension of the hemorrhage.

9. What risk factors are thought to play a role in the genesis of these lesions?

The most important risk factor for the development of an IVH is prematurity. Up to 40–50% of neonates weighing less than 1500 gm will experience an IVH. Other risk factors include mechanical ventilation, pneumothoraces, rapid expansion of intravascular volume (large or rapid IV infusions), rapid or wide fluctuations in blood pressure, hypoxic-ischemic injury, hypernatremia and hyperosmolality, and administration of certain medications such as indomethacin.

10. What complications may arise secondary to an IVH?

The most common complications of IVH include posthemorrhagic hydrocephalus, seizures, and the parenchymal cerebral injury associated with grade IV bleeds.

11. Does the neurologic prognosis correlate with the different IVHs?

Long-term follow-up studies of neonates grouped with all grades of IVH who reached kindergarten age revealed that 40% survived and 60% were neurologically abnormal. Approximately 30% now have a static encephalopathy (cerebral palsy), 30% have hydrocephalus, most of which required a shunting procedure, and 30% are multi-handicapped with combinations of blindness, paresis, spasticity, delayed fine motor and language skill, hydrocephalus, hearing loss and seizures. Generally, grades I and II IVH are relatively benign, grade III has more significant hydrocephalus and seizures, and grade IV has by far the greatest likelihood of severe neurologic sequelae such as spastic quadriparesis, blindness, and mental retardation.

12. What is the clinicopathologic classification for perinatal hypoxic-ischemic brain injury?

Neuropathologic findings associated with perinatal asphyxia are of four principal types. Each type has a rather characteristic clinical presentation:

　　1. **Neuronal necrosis**—may be restricted to certain regions of the brain or may be more widespread and multifocal. This is typically the most severe form of insult, and children who survive are left with quadriplegia or hemiplegia, mental retardation, and seizures.

　　2. **Status marmoratus**—occurs only in term infants and is characterized by gliosis and hypermyelination of the basal ganglia. Clinically this is associated with choreoathetoid cerebral palsy.

　　3. **Watershed infarction**—in term infants results in neuronal injury in the border zones between anterior, middle and posterior cerebral arteries and often involves the motor cortex, resulting in hemiparesis.

　　4. **Periventricular leukomalacia**—a form of watershed infarction that occurs in premature infants and involves the white matter adjacent to the lateral ventricles. Clinically this is associated with a spastic paresis of the lower extremities termed spastic diplegia.

13. What are the common antenatal risk factors for developing a static encephalopathy?

Antenatal Risk Factors for Encephalopathy

1. Hypoxic-ischemic encephalopathy	6. Multiple gestations
2. Intrauterine infections	7. Maternal factors
3. Exposure to teratogens, including	a. Diabetes
illicit drugs, alcohol, and smoking	b. Malnutrition
4. Congenital malformations	c. Toxemia
5. Genetic anomalies	

14. What are the most common perinatal/neonatal risk factors for developing a static encephalopathy?

Perinatal Risk Factors for Encephalopathy

1. Prematurity	4. Trauma
2. Hypoxic-ischemic encephalopathy	5. Sepsis, including
3. Kernicterus	meningitis

15. What is TORCH?

This acronym refers to the agents most commonly responsible for intrauterine infection:

　　　　　　TO = toxoplasmosis,
　　　　　　R　= rubella,
　　　　　　C　= cytomegalovirus (CMV), and
　　　　　　H　= herpes simplex virus.

16. What are the neuroanatomical structures which, if damaged, could result in infantile hypotonia (floppy baby)?

Differential Diagnosis of a Floppy Baby

STRUCTURES	EXAMPLES
Muscle	Congenital myopathies, congenital myotonic dystrophy, type II glycogenosis (Pompe's)
Neuromuscular junction	Congenital myasthenic syndromes, transient neonatal myasthenia gravis, botulism, hypermagnesemia
Peripheral nerve	Giant neuroaxonal dystrophy, familial dysautonomia (Riley-Day), hypomyelinative neuropathy
Anterio horn cell	Type I spinal muscular atrophy (Werdnig-Hoffmann)
Spinal cord	Myelodysplasias (meningomyeloceles, diplomyelia, diastematomyelia), traumatic transection
Cerebellum, brainstem, basal ganglia, cerebral hemispheres	Malformations, infections, toxic encephalopathies, metabolic encephalopathies, hypoxic-ischemic encephalopathies, genetic and chromosomal anomalies, neurodegenerative disorders

17. What are the commonest causes of a floppy baby? What are the least common?
By far the overall commonest are the "central" causes involving the cerebellum, brainstem, basal ganglia, and cerebral hemispheres. The least common causes of infantile hypotonia are those that afflict the peripheral nerves.

18. Which syndromes are associated with agenesis of the corpus callosum?
Formation of the corpus callosum takes place over days 60–120 of gestation, but myelination continues after birth. Agenesis of the corpus callosum may be partial or complete. Many cases of this malformation appear to be sporadic; however, autosomal dominant and X-linked recessive inheritance has been described. In addition, agenesis of the corpus callosum is a feature of Aicardi's syndrome, which only affects females (X-linked dominant inheritance) and also includes infantile spasms with a hypsarrhythmic EEG pattern, severe psychomotor retardation, and characteristic chorioretinal lacunae.

19. What is the difference between macrocephaly and megaloencephaly?
Macrocephaly refers to a large head, whereas megaloencephaly refers specifically to a large brain.

20. What is the differential diagnosis of macrocephaly in an infant?

Differential Diagnosis of Macrocephaly

I. Hydrocephalus
  A. Obstructive
  B. Communicating
	III. Thickened skull
	  A. Anemia with increased marrow space
	  B. Osteopetrosis
	  C. Rickets
	  D. Osteogenesis imperfecta

II. Extra-axial fluid collections
  A. Subdural effusions
  B. Subdural hematomas
	IV. Megaloencephaly

21. What is the differential diagnosis of megaloencephaly?

Differential Diagnosis of Megaloencephaly

I. Toxic/metabolic	II. Structural
A. Cerebral edema	A. Cerebral gigantism
1. lead	(Sotos syndrome)
2. pseudotumor cerebri	B. Familial megaloencephaly
B. Canavan's disease	C. Neurofibromatosis
C. Alexander's disease	D. Tuberous sclerosis
D. Tay-Sachs disease	E. Fragile X syndrome
E. Metachromatic leukodystrophy	
F. Mucopolysaccharidoses	

22. In evaluating a child with microcephaly, what are some important questions to ask in the history?

Is the microcephaly congenital or acquired? Serial measurements of fronto-occipital circumference (FOC) are very helpful. Is the FOC getting progressively worse (Rett syndrome in girls) or is it returning to normal (catchup growth after a serious illness or prematurity) or is it remaining on the same percentile line (static process)? Review the antenatal history carefully for evidence of intrauterine infection. Did the infant appear healthy at birth? Any postnatal CNS infections or trauma? Family history of microcephaly?

23. What are some of the more important features of the physical examination to review in children with microcephaly?

Palpate the fontanelles and sutures for the presence of craniofacial dysmorphology suggestive of the craniosynostosis syndromes (premature closure of the cranial sutures), chromosomal anomalies (trisomy 13, 18, 21), or other nonchromosomal hereditary syndromes (Rubinstein-Taybi, Cornelia de Lange). The retinal exam may show chorioretinitis associated with the TORCH agents. Focal or lateralizing neurologic deficits suggest CNS damage or malformation.

24. Which laboratory tests, if any, would you order in a child with microcephaly?

Plain skull x-rays evaluate premature closure of the cranial sutures. A heat CT scan will survey for evidence of CNS malformations, abnormal calcification (which may indicate infection with a TORCH agent or earlier hypoxic-ischemic injury), or massive destruction of the cerebrum as in hydranencephaly. The EEG is sometimes helpful in evaluating developmental characteristics and may also suggest the presence of certain malformations, encephaloclastic events, and chromosomal anomalies. In addition, TORCH titers may be measured if such an infection is suspected, or a chromosomal analysis may be used to evaluate genetic causes.

25. How would you evaluate and manage a newborn with spina bifida?

Perform a careful neurologic examination to estimate the level of spinal cord and nerve root involvement, including assessment of bowel and bladder function. Cranial neuroimaging (ultrasound, CT, MRI) is essential to determine the presence of other CNS conditions that are frequently present. Plain spine x-rays evaluate the bony extent of the lesion.

Immediately following birth, sterile saline soaked gauze pads must be gently applied to the myelomeningocele membrane and all attempts should be made to keep the membrane intact during transfer to a tertiary center. Bladder catheterization may be necessary to ensure adequate drainage. Neurosurgical closure of the dysraphic defect should be performed within the first day or two of life.

26. What are some of the common complications that may confront a child with myelomeningocele?

Virtually all children with lumbosacral myelomeningoceles have an associated type II Arnold-Chiari malformation that results in hydrocephalus. The hydrocephalus may be congenital or may occur following closure of the dysraphic defect. Many children will require a shunting procedure. CNS infectious complications are common and devastating. Infants at highest risk are those with large defects, the covering membrane of which has been ruptured. Out of infancy, one of the commonest causes of mortality in these individuals is renal failure due to chronic and repeated urinary tract infections and obstructive uropathy. Many children with myelomeningoceles will experience progressive seizures at some point, some of which may be related to the placement of ventriculoperitoneal shunts. Some children, after years of static neurologic deficits, experience progressive spasticity and weakness in their legs, worsening bladder and bowel function, progressive scoliosis, and/or increasing low back pain and stiffness. With CT myelography or MRI, these children are found to have a low-lying conus medullaris and are said to have a "tethered cord." Some of these children have improved neurologic function with surgical release of the filum terminale and freeing of the cord.

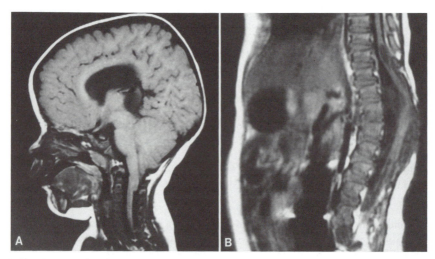

A, Unenhanced midsagittal T1-weighted MRI in a 6-month-old boy with type II Arnold-Chiari malformation. Note "herniation" or downward displacement of the cerebellar tonsils through the foramen magnum to the level of C2 and the associated obstructive hydrocephalus. *B,* Unenhanced midsagittal T1-weighted MRI lumbosacral spine: extensive thoracolumbar myelomeningocele associated with the Arnold-Chiari malformation in *A.* Note the dorsal kyphosis, absence of posterior elements of the vertebrae and the malformed spinal cord at the level of the defect. A small syrinx in the cord is present above the defect.

27. Classify the Arnold-Chiari malformations.

Type I—characterized by downward displacement of the cerebellum with elongation of the medulla such that the cerebellar tonsils egress through the foramen magnum into the cervical spinal canal. It is not associated with other nervous system malformations and clinically may be asymptomatic or may present with recurrent headaches, neck pain, and unsteady gait. The function of certain lower cranial nerves may be compromised, producing dysphagia and dysarthria. Cerebellar function may be affected, producing progressive ataxia and disordered ocular movements. The pyramidal tracts may be compressed, producing spasticity and extensor plantar responses. The posterior columns are often affected, resulting in impaired proprioception and vibratory sensation.

Type II—by definition, this type is associated with a lumbosacral myelomeningocele and with numerous other nervous system malformations. The posterior fossa is small and, as in Type I, there is downward displacement of the cerebellar tonsils through the foramen magnum. The medulla is elongated and thinned and often kinked so that it may lie beside the upper segments of the cervical cord. A characteristic beaking appearance of the quadrigeminal plate is present. Hydrocephalus frequently occurs, but its exact mechanism is unclear. Syringomyelia and occasionally syringobulbia also occur, along with a number of other malformations. These include a curious interdigitation of gyri along the interhemispheric fissure, polymicrogyria, gray matter heterotopias, craniocervical junction anomalies, and craniolacunia.

Type III—an occipital encephalocele with protrusion of cerebellar remnants into the overlying sac.

Type IV—isolated hypoplasia of the cerebellum not associated with other nervous system malformations.

28. What is Down's syndrome?
A chromosomal anomaly characterized by trisomy 21. The majority of cases result from chromosomal nondisjunction, a phenomenon increasingly more likely to occur as maternal age advances. Clinically, it is characterized by marked infantile hypotonia with hyperflexibility of joints, mental deficiency, brachycephaly with flat occiput, upslanting palpebral fissures, late closure of fontanelles, flattened nasal bridge, epicanthal folds, speckling of iris (Brushfield's spots), fine lens opacities, small ears, hypoplastic teeth, short neck, brachydactyly with clinodactyly of fifth fingers, simian creases with distal axis triradius, wide space between first and second toes, congenital heart disease (in 40%), and hypogonadism.

NEURODEGENERATIVE DISORDERS

29. In general terms, how would you expect a neurodegenerative disease affecting white matter to present?
These diseases are classically described as presenting with loss of motor skills, spasticity, and ataxia.

30. In general terms, how would you expect a neurodegenerative disease affecting gray matter to present?
These diseases are classically described as presenting with loss of intellectual skills, seizures, and blindness.

31. What are the seven clinical variants of metachromatic leukodystrophy (MLD)?
Metachromatic leukodystrophy is an autosomal recessively inherited metabolic disorder of myelin due to a deficiency of arylsulfatase A. The disorder has been linked to chromosome 22. The seven clinical variants are:

1. Congenital MLD—onset at birth with apnea, seizures and weakness. Very rare.

2. Late-infantile MLD—commonest and the classic form. Onset between 1 and 2 years of age.

3. Juvenile MLD—onset from 3–16 years of age, often presents with school or behavioral problems.

4. Adult MLD—onset in fourth decade with dementia and psychiatric disturbances.

5. Multiple sulfatase deficiency—clinically a combination of late-infantile MLD and Hurler's syndrome.

6. Pseudo-arylsulfatase deficiency—clinically asymptomatic but enzyme assays are positive for MLD. These patients have a mutated but functional variant of arylsulfatase A.

7. Activator protein deficiency—clinically, patients have late-infantile MLD but a normal enzyme assay. They have normal arylsulfatase A but lack a critical protein necessary for the enzyme to perform its function.

Polten A, Fluharty AL, Fluharty CB, et al: Molecular basis of different forms of metachromatic leukodystrophy. N Engl J Med 324:18–22, 1991.

32. Which leukodystrophy is virtually always associated with a particular endocrinologic deficiency?

Adrenoleukodystrophy, an X-linked recessive disorder, is one of the peroxisomal disorders. It is characterized by impaired beta-oxidation of the very long-chain (C26) fatty acids, leading to their accumulation. In addition to neurodegeneration typical of the leukodystrophies, patients also have adrenocortical insufficiency. Onset is usually between 4 and 6 years of age. An adult form of the disease called adrenomyeloneuropathy is characterized by progressive spastic paraparesis and peripheral neuropathy.

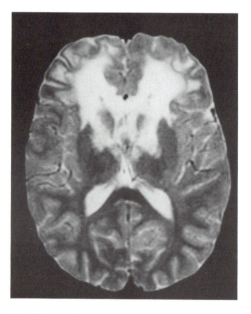

Unenhanced axial T2-weighted MRI in a 9-year-old boy with adrenoleukodystrophy. Note extensive dysmyelination involving the anterior centrum semiovale, subcortical white matter, genu of the corpus callosum, and internal capsule. The cerebral cortex, basal ganglia, and thalami are unaffected.

33. Which of the leukodystrophies is characterized in early infancy by hyperirritability with an exaggerated startle response, marked spasticity with *decreased* tendon reflexes, and a normal FOC?

Globoid cell leukodystrophy, or Krabbe's disease, is an autosomal recessive disorder due to a deficiency of galactocerebroside beta-galactosidase. Onset is between 3 and 8 months and clinical presentation is as outlined above.

34. Which leukodystrophies have prominent megaloencephaly?

1. **Canavan's disease** (spongy degeneration)—autosomal recessive disorder recently shown to be secondary to a deficiency of aspartoacylase. The classic infantile form has its onset within the first few weeks of life and is characterized by initial hypotonia, followed at 6 months by hypertonia, megaloencephaly, visual loss with optic atrophy, nystagmus, mixed seizures, choreoathetosis, vomiting, transient increases in intracranial pressure, and hyperpyrexia. Death occurs by 3–4 years of age. Rare neonatal-onset and juvenile-onset forms are described.

2. **Alexander's disease**—sporadic occurrence; etiopathogenetic origin unknown. Infantile or juvenile onset with spasticity, psychomotor retardation, seizures, ataxia, and prominent megaloencephaly with or without hydrocephalus. The pathologic hallmark is prominent Rosenthal fibers throughout the brain.

35. Pathologically, most of the leukodystrophies are characterized by a process referred to as dysmyelination. Due to metabolic derangements, myelinogenesis is disturbed and the resulting myelin is defective in structure and function. In contrast to having demyelination, which leukodystrophy has virtual amyelination (absence of any myelin)?

Pelizaeus-Merzbacher disease is an X-linked recessive disorder that is caused by a lack of proteolipid protein in myelin. Proteolipid protein is one of two principal structural components of myelin, the other being myelin basic protein. In addition to psychomotor retardation, spasticity, and ataxia, children with this disease also have marked choreoathetosis and pendular nystagmus.

36. How often does multiple sclerosis occur in children?

In only approximately 2% of all patients with multiple sclerosis (MS) is the onset of symptoms in childhood. The majority of affected children (approximately 80%) are greater than 10 years of age, but MS cases have been described in patients less than 3 years old. The clinical spectrum of disease is just as broad in children as it is in adults.

37. What is a cherry-red spot?

It is the bright red appearance of the fovea centralis of the eye as seen by funduscopy in children with certain gray-matter storage diseases, classically Tay-Sachs disease. As the storage material accumulates in the nerve fiber layer, the retina takes on a grayish-white appearance. Because there are very few fibers traversing the fovea, it retains its normal color and continues to reflect the bright red vascular choroid underneath.

38. Tay-Sachs is often thought of as the prototypical gray-matter neurodegenerative disease. What are its principal clinical features?

Tay-Sachs is an autosomal recessive disorder due to a deficiency of hexosaminidase A. Until recently, the highest prevalence was in the Ashkenazi Jewish community. However, due to an aggressive and very successful screening program, most cases diagnosed today are in non-Jewish individuals. Onset is within 3-5 months of age with extreme irritability, hyperacusis, global developmental delay, and hypotonia. Often a hypsarrhythmia pattern develops on the EEG and seizures are prominent within the first 6 months of life (usually myoclonic). Decreasing vision develops by 12 months of age and a cherry-red spot appears. Spasticity occurs late in the course and death is by 2-4 years of age. There are also juvenile-onset and adult-onset forms of the disease. The adult form may have an amyotrophic lateral sclerosis (ALS) type of presentation.

39. In which neurodegenerative diseases would you expect to find an enlarged liver and/or spleen?

Neurodegenerative Diseases with Hepatosplenomegaly

DISEASE	INHERITANCE	FEATURES
Niemann-Pick disease	Autosomal recessive	Deficiency of sphingomyelinase
Gaucher's disease	Autosomal recessive	Deficiency of glucocerebrosidase
Mucopolysaccharidoses Hurler's disease (severe expression)	Autosomal recessive	Deficiency of alpha-L-iduronidase

Table continued on next page.

Neurodegenerative Diseases with Hepatosplenomegaly

DISEASE	INHERITANCE	FEATURES
Mucopolysaccharidoses Hunter's disease (mild expression)	X-linked recessive	Deficiency of iduronate-2-sulfatase
Zellweger's syndrome	Autosomal recessive	Peroxisomal disorder
Wilson's disease	Autosomal recessive	Deficiency of ceruloplasmin which leads to accumulation of copper in brain (predominantly basal ganglia) and liver causing cirrhosis
Galactosemia	Autosomal recessive	Deficiency of galactose-1-phosphate uridyltransferase

40. What are the neuronal ceroid lipofuscinoses (NCL)?

NCL is a group of autosomal recessively inherited disorders characterized by excessive neuronal accumulations of the lipid pigments, ceroid, and lipofuscin. These compounds are normally present in small amounts as cells become senescent. However, excessive and premature accumulation, as occurs in these diseases, leads to cell dysfunction and death.

Types of Neuronal Ceroid Lipofuscinoses

I. Infantile NCL (Santavuori-Haltia)
   A. Onset 8–18 months, death 5–10 years
   B. Dementia, seizures, myoclonus, blindness
	III. Juvenile NCL (Spielmeyer-Vogt-Sjogren)
	   A. Onset 5–10 years, death 15–25 years
	   B. Dementia, seizures, blindness

II. Late-infantile NCL (Jansky-Bielschowsky)
   A. Onset 3–4 years, death 8–12 years
   B. Dementia, seizures, myoclonus, blindness, ataxia
	IV. Adult NCL (Kuff's)
	   A. Variable onset, slow course, variable age at death
	   B. Extrapyramidal signs, ataxia, myoclonus, dysarthria, no dementia

41. What are ragged red fibers?

In some of the mitochondrial cytopathies, mitochondria become clumped beneath the skeletal muscle sarcolemmal membrane. When the muscle biopsy specimen is prepared with modified Gomori's trichrome stain and viewed by light microscopy, the clumps of mitochondria stain red and give the muscle fibers a ragged appearance—hence the term ragged red fibers.

42. What is the mode of inheritance and biochemical defect in each of the three principal mitochondrial encephalomyopathies?

1. **Kearns-Sayre syndrome** occurs sporadically and has dysfunction of complex I of the respiratory chain. The predominant clinical features include progressive encephalopathy, external ophthalmoplegia, pigmentary retinopathy, ptosis, weakness, sensorineural deafness, ataxia, spasticity, cardiac conduction abnormalities, and respiratory insufficiency. Laboratory study reveals elevated blood lactate and pyruvate, increased CSF protein, and ragged red fibers on muscle biopsy.

2. Myoclonus, epilepsy, encephalomyopathy, and ragged red fibers are characteristics of the **MERRF syndrome**. This disorder has a maternal pattern of inheritance (mitochondrial genetic defect) and affects complex IV of the respiratory chain.

3. Mitochondrial encephalomyopathy with lactic acidosis and stroke-like episodes occur in the **MELAS syndrome**. This syndrome has maternal inheritance and affects complex I.

Tulinius MH, Holme E, Kristiansson B, et al: Mitochrondrial encephalomyopathies of childhood. II. Clinical manifestations and syndromes. J Pediatr 119(2):251–259, 1991.

43. A fair-skinned, blue-eyed, and blonde-haired infant was normal at birth. He now presents at 6–8 months of age with progressive psychomotor retardation, infantile spasms, microcephaly, dystonia, vomiting, and has a "musty" odor. What would be first on your list of differential diagnoses?
This is a classic description of phenylketonuria (PKU); however, other aminoacidurias and some of the organic acidurias may present similarly. The three main types of PKU are (1) deficiency of phenylalanine hydroxylase; (2) deficiency of dihydropteridine reductase (DHPR); and (3) deficient synthesis of dihydrobiopterin (DH_2).

44. Which endocrinologic disorder may present as a gray-matter neurodegenerative disease if it is missed on neonatal screening?
Congenital hypothyroidism (cretinism) is extremely difficult to detect clinically at birth and the diagnosis may not be suspected until it is too late for replacement therapy to be maximally efficacious. Left untreated, these children develop prolonged jaundice, abdominal distention with umbilical hernia, large fontanelles, hypotonia, impaired bony development, large tongue, psychomotor retardation, seizures, spasticity, ataxia, and deafness.

45. Which neurodegenerative disorder results in excessive accumulation of iron in the basal ganglia?
Hallervorden-Spatz disease is an autosomal recessive disorder due to a deficiency of cysteine dioxygenase. This deficiency leads to increased concentrations of cysteine, whose thiol group chelates iron. This promotes the formation of free radicals, which cause cell damage and death. Affected individuals present before 10 years of age with psychomotor regression, extrapyramidal signs followed by pyramidal signs, optic atrophy, and pitmentary retinopathy. Neuroimaging reveals dense deposits of iron in the basal ganglia.

NEUROCUTANEOUS SYNDROMES

46. What is the commonest neurocutaneous syndrome? What are its clinical characteristics?
Neurofibromatosis (NF) type I (von Recklinghausen's disease of the nerves) has an incidence of 1/3,000–4,000 population. Inheritance is autosomal dominant and the spontaneous mutation rate is very high (30–50%). The mutation has been linked to chromosome 17. Clinical characteristics include café-au-lait spots, neurofibromas, axillary/ inguinal freckling, optic gliomas, iridic Lisch nodules, megaloencephaly, mental retardation, seizures, and characteristic bony lesions.

Neurofibromatosis type II is much less common (1/50,000) than NF-I. Inheritance is autosomal dominant and it has been linked to chromosome 22. The principal clinical manifestation is bilateral acoustic neurinomas.

Berg BO: Current concepts of neurocutaneous disorders. Brain Dev 13:9–20, 1991.

47. When evaluating an infant with hypsarrhythmia and infantile spasms, which neuro-cutaneous syndrome must be specifically sought?
Tuberous sclerosis (TS) is highly correlated with the occurrence of infantile spasms (more than 25% of infants with infantile spasms will later express other signs of TS). TS is an autosomal dominant disorder linked to chromosome 9. Its incidence is 1/30,000 with a high spontaneous mutation rate.

Clinical manifestations include mental retardation, seizures, adenoma sebaceum, ash-leaf spots, shagreen patches, café-au-lait spots, subungual/periungual fibromas (Koenen's tumors), gingival fibromas, dental enamel pits, retinal tumors (mulberry tumor of the optic disc), cardiac rhabdomyomata, renal angiomyolipomata, and CNS cortical tubers and subependymal hamartomas that calcify and occasionally become malignant (subependymal giant-cell astrocytomas).

48. Of the more common neurocutaneous syndromes, which one has no clear pattern of inheritance?

Sturge-Weber syndrome (encephalofacialangiomatosis) has no clear pattern of inheritance. Prevalence and incidence is unknown, but it is less common than NF or TS. Patients have a characteristic congenital facial port-wine stain (nevus) that is usually unilateral and involves the V_1 segment of the trigeminal nerve (may be much larger and involve the entire side of the face and body). The nevus may involve the nasopharyngeal mucosa and ocular choroidal membrane, causing glaucoma. Other findings include iridic heterochromia, optic atrophy, progressive dementia, and steadily worsening partial motor seizures, with longer duration of postictal paralysis eventually leading to permanent hemiplegia and hemianopsia. Arteriography reveals extensive arteriovenous malformation involving the ipsilateral cerebral hemispheric dura. Vascular "steal" phenomenon leads to chronic ischemia of the underlying cerebral cortex. The characteristic "tram" or "railroad track" sign seen on skull films is due to mineralization of adjacent gyri.

49. In addition to brain and skin involvement, which neurocutaneous syndrome also has immunologic abnormalities, impaired DNA repair mechanisms, and a high propensity for various neoplasms?

Ataxia telangiectasia is an autosomal recessive disorder with an incidence of 1/100,000. Affected individuals develop telangiectasias by 2–4 years of age on exposed areas of skin and conjunctiva. Other skin lesions include premature aging, frequent infections with poor healing, vitiligo, café-au-lait spots, and occasionally scleroderma-like lesions. Progressive cerebellar ataxia begins within the first few years of life. Muscle bulk becomes diffusely diminished and tendon reflexes are reduced. Choreoathetosis is common but sensory changes are rare. Patients have decreased or absent IgA and IgE and decreased IgG_2 and IgG_4. Tonsils, lymphoid tissues, and thymus gland are abnormal or absent. Defective cellular DNA repair leads to increased spontaneous and radiation-induced chromosomal aberrations, inducing various neoplasia. Patients also have elevated alpha-fetoprotein levels, which can be used as a screening technique, including antenatal detection.

50. Which neurocutaneous syndrome has no skin lesions?

Von Hippel-Lindau disease has autosomal dominant inheritance and no skin lesions. Clinical manifestations include retinal and cerebellar hemangioblastomas, polycythemia, elevated CSF protein, pheochromocytomas, and cystic changes in the pancreas, liver, and epididymis.

INFECTIONS AND INFESTATIONS

51. Infectious etiologies account for what percentage of prenatally and postnatally acquired cerebral palsy?

Infectious disease accounts for approximately 50–60% of postnatally acquired cerebral palsy (CP), as opposed to only 10–20% of prenatally acquired CP.

52. What are the most common bacterial pathogens responsible for meningitis at different ages?

Commonest Bacterial Pathogens

NEONATAL	CHILDHOOD
Group B beta-hemolytic streptococci	*Hemophilus influenzae* type B
Escherichia coli	*Streptococcus pneumoniae*
Listeria monocytogenes	*Neisseria meningitidis*
Klebsiella pneumoniae	

53. What are the usual signs and symptoms of neonatal meningitis?

Clinical Features of Neonatal Meningitis

1. Lethargy	6. Poor feeding
2. Irritability	7. Hypothermia or hyperthermia
3. Apnea	8. Seizures
4. Hypotonia or hypertonia	9. Bulging fontanelle
5. Opisthotonos	10. Cranial nerve palsies

54. What factors predict a poor outcome at the time of admission for neonatal bacterial meningitis?

Poor Prognostic Features for Neonatal Meningitis

1. Coma	5. High CSF protein
2. Shock	6. High concentration of type III
3. Peripheral neutrophil count	capsular antigen in CSF
$<2 \times 10^9/L$	7. Birth weight <2500 gm
4. Thrombocytopenia	8. Age at diagnosis <1 day

55. What are the usual signs and symptoms in the older infant and child with bacterial meningitis?

Clinical Features of Childhood Meningitis

1. Fever	7. Full or bulging fontanelle
2. Altered mental status	8. Seizures
3. Meningismus	9. Focal neurological signs
4. Headache	10. Papilledema
5. Nausea and vomiting	11. Syndrome of inappropriate secretion
6. Irritability	of antidiuretic hormone (SIADH)

56. How does herpes encephalitis in neonates differ from that in the older child or adult?
Two strains of herpes simplex virus (HSV) may infect the neonatal CNS, types I and II. In older children and adults, non-CNS disease caused by HSV-I usually manifests as a mucocutaneous infection (herpes labialis or ocular herpes), whereas non-CNS disease caused by HSV-II usually manifests as a genital infection. As a result, the vast majority of neonatal HSV encephalitis is due to type II infection. Neonatal HSV infection produces a panencephalitis with high mortality and morbidity. Neonates with HSV-II tend to present with a higher frequency of seizures, greater pleocytosis and protein concentrations in the CSF, and more frequent evidence of structural damage on neuroimaging studies than those with HSV-I infection. Recent widespread availability of the antiviral agent acyclovir has improved the outcome considerably. Children who survive neonatal HSV encephalitis will develop significantly disabling static encephalopathies in up to 64% of cases. HSV-I encephalitis tends to respond more favorably to acyclovir than does HSV-II encephalitis.

Cameron PD, Wallace SJ, Munro J: Herpes simplex virus encephalitis: Problems in diagnosis. Dev Med Child Neurol 34:134–140, 1992.

57. A child from Central America presents with a prolonged partial motor seizure. Neurologic examination the following day demonstrates no focal or lateralizing findings; however, funduscopic examination reveals early papilledema. CT scanning of the brain discloses a number of small, densely calcified lesions scattered along the gray-white junction

of the cerebral hemispheres. **Contrast administration reveals two additional lesions that were not calcified and have bright ring enhancement and surrounding edema. What is the most likely diagnosis and how might you confirm your suspicions?**

The pork tapeworm, *Taenia solium*, is endemic in Central America. When man inadvertently becomes the intermediate host (rather than the pig), he may develop neurocysticercosis. This occurs when the ingested *T. solium* ova become partially digested, releasing oncospheres that gain access to the circulation and are carried throughout the body. They then become larvae (cysticerci) in subcutaneous tissue, muscle, and brain. The majority of the CNS cysticerci die spontaneously and become densely calcified. The commonest clinical manifestation is seizures, although focal neurologic deficits, hydrocephalus, and meningitis are also encountered. Rarely, in disseminated cases, progressive massive cerebral edema with increasing intracranial pressure may occur, leading to coma and death.

The diagnosis can be confirmed by serum or CSF antibody and antigen detection methods and in certain cases by tissue biopsy.

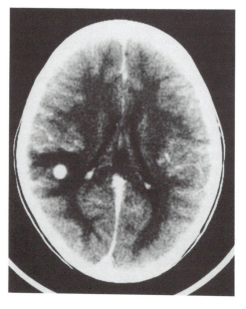

Enhanced axial CT: neurocysticercosis in a 7-year-old girl. Note the solitary, densely enhancing lesion with surrounding edema.

Takayanagui OM, Jardim E. Therapy for neurocysticercosis. Arch Neurol 49(3):290–294, 1992.

58. Which parainfectious neurologic diseases are known to result in cerebral palsy?

Parainfectious Cerebral Palsies

1. Acute disseminated encephalomyelitis
2. Acute hemorrhagic leukoencephalitis
3. Acute cerebellar ataxia
4. Reye syndrome

VASCULAR DISORDERS

59. Which laboratory investigations may be important in the evaluation of acute infantile hemiplegia (childhood stroke)?

Laboratory Evaluation of Childhood Stroke

I. CBC with Differential and Platelets	VIII. Viral Titers for Postexanthem
A. Polycythemia, thrombocytosis,	Vasculitis and Varicella
thrombocytopenia	IX. CSF Analysis
B. Leukemia	A. Infection
II. PT and PTT for Coagulopathies	B. Vasculitis
III. ESR, RF, ANA, RPR, SPEP	X. EKG/Echocardiography
for Vasculitides	A. Septal defects
IV. Hemoglobin Electrophoresis for	B. Endocarditis
Hemoglobinopathies	C. Valvular disease
V. Serum Cholesterol, Triglycerides,	D. Thrombus
Lipoprotein, Electrophoresis for	XI. CT Scan/MRI: Infarct vs. Hemorrhage
Familial Hyperlipoproteinemias	XII. Angiography
VI. Serum Amino Acids, Especially	A. AVM
Homocystinuria	B. Vasculitis
VII. Alpha-galactosidase A for	C. Fibromuscular dysplasia
Fabry's Disease	D. Thrombosis/embolism

Lanska MJ, Lanska DJ, Horwitz SJ, Aram DM: Presentation, clinical course, and outcome of childhood stroke. Pediatr Neurol 7:333–341, 1991.

60. What is the commonest hemoglobinopathy associated with cerebrovascular disease?

Approximately one-fourth of all individuals with sickle cell disease will experience cerebrovascular complications, the vast majority of these patients being children. When strokes do occur in adults, they are more likely to be intracerebral hemorrhages as opposed to the infarctions that affect children. In addition to small vessel occlusion by sickled red cells, endothelial proliferation is also thought to be an important mechanism in the genesis of these strokes.

61. How does the prognosis for neurologic recovery following a stroke relate to age?

As a broad generalization, the younger a particular CNS insult occurs, the better is the prognosis for meaningful neurologic recovery. The developing brain can assume the function of areas that have been damaged. This has been quite convincingly demonstrated in children who develop a slow-growing neoplasm in a temporal lobe. For example, a patient may start out being right-handed, but as a tumor damages the left temporal lobe, he or she gradually becomes left-handed. Neuropsychological tests reveal either a transference of language and memory to the opposite side as well, or "crowding" within the left temporal lobe.

62. How do vein of Galen malformations commonly present?

This type of arteriovenous malformation may present in one of three ways.

    1. Newborns may present in florid high-output congestive cardiac failure due to direct shunting of blood from the carotid circulation into the vein of Galen, which becomes massively dilated. The majority of these infants have severe cerebral ischemic damage due to the "steal" phenomenon of blood being diverted into the AVM. Prognosis is extremely grave.

    2. Another group of patients have less marked malformation and present in later infancy. They develop hydrocephalus due to the aneurysmal compression of the cerebral aqueduct. Prognosis in these patients is also poor because of progressive enlargement of the aneurysm and its propensity for rupture.

    3. A third group of patients presents in later childhood with subarachnoid hemorrhages, hydrocephalus, or signs of brainstem compression.

Pavlakis SG, Gould RJ, Zito JL: Stroke in children. Adv Pediatr 38:151–179, 1991.

NEOPLASMS

63. Are infratentorial or supratentorial tumors more common in infants? Children? Adults?
In infants less than 1 year of age, supratentorial brain tumors predominate. In children older than 1 year, infratentorial tumors are more common. Then again in adults, supratentorial tumors are more frequently encountered.

64. What is meant by the term PNET?
PNET is an acronym for primitive neuroectodermal tumor. These are highly malignant small, blue-cell tumors. They are part of a newer classification of CNS tumors and replace the term "blastoma." If a PNET is completely undifferentiated and is in the midline posterior fossa, it would previously have been referred to as a medulloblastoma. PNETs may show varying degrees of differentiation along different cell lines, including glial, ependymal, pineal, and neuronal.

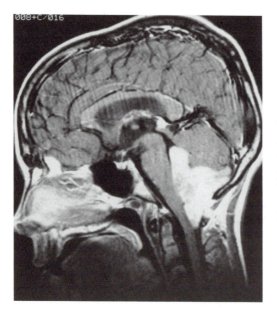

Enhanced midsagittal T1-weighted MRI reveals a posterior fossa primitive neuro-ectodermal tumor (PNET) in a 5-year-old boy. Note the brightly enhancing tumor mass extending upward through the fourth ventricle into the cerebral aqueduct and downward through the foramen magnum. There is compression of the medulla and marked displacement of the cerebellum. Early obstructive hydrocephalus is developing.

Pigott TJ, Punt JA, Lowe JS, et al: The clinical, radiological and histopathological features of cerebral primitive neuroectodermal tumors. Br J Neurosurg 4:287–297, 1990.

65. What are some of the common complications associated with PNETs?
PNETs have an extremely high propensity to metastasize along CSF pathways, which may lead to complete filling of the subarachnoid space over the surface of the cerebrum or cerebellum (so-called sugar coating), obstructive hydrocephalus, drop metastases along the spinal cord, and intra-abdominal spread via ventriculoperitoneal shunts.

66. A school-aged child complains of recurrent headaches and recent onset of marked polyuria/polydipsia. Examination reveals bitemporal homonymous hemianopsia and papilledema. Laboratory tests are consistent with diabetes insipidus. Where is the lesion? What is the differential diagnosis?
The anatomic location of this lesion must be in the parasellar region. The visual field defect is produced by compression of the optic chiasm. The diabetes insipidus is produced by compression of the pituitary stalk.

Differential Diagnosis of Parasellar Lesions

I. Neoplasm
   A. Craniopharyngioma
   B. Germ-cell tumor, including teratoma
   C. Pituitary tumor
   D. Optic glioma (astrocytoma) with
      or without neurofibromatosis
   E. Hypothalamic glioma
   F. Meningioma
   G. Chordoma of the clivus
   H. Metastatic tumor

II. Inflammatory: Chronic Basilar Meningitis
   A. Tuberculosis with or without
      tuberculoma
   B. Fungal
   C. Neurosarcoidosis

III. Structural
   A. Rathke's pouch cyst
   B. Enlarging arachnoid cyst
   C. Aneurysm

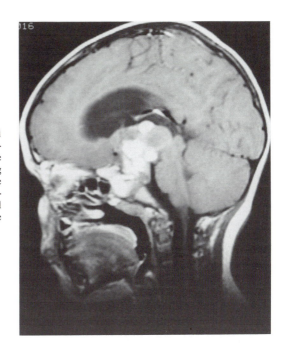

Enhanced midsagittal T1-weighted MRI demonstrates a craniopharyngioma in a 3-year-old girl. Note the large, multilobulated tumor extending from the parasellar region through the midbrain. The tumor has brightly enhancing solid areas and fluid-filled cysts. There is associated obstructive hydrocephalus.

67. What are the implications if a patient with a parasellar lesion also developed wasting of subcutaneous tissue despite apparently normal, or even increased, food intake, an usually euphoric disposition, and Collier's sign (upper eyelid retraction)?
This constellation of features is typical of the diencephalic syndrome (Russell's syndrome) and implies dysfunction of the hypothalamus. Thus the lesion may have originated in the hypothalamus or may be invading or compressing it.

68. How do posterior fossa tumors commonly present in the younger child?

Clinical Features of Posterior Fossa Tumors

1. Irritability/altered mental status	4. Head tilt
2. Unsteadiness/ataxia	5. Cranial nerve palsies
3. Headache/vomiting/progressive obtundation/ bulging fontanelle due to hydrocephalus	

69. Most posterior fossa tumors in children portend a grave prognosis. However, one particular posterior fossa tumor has an excellent prognosis. What is it?

Juvenile cerebellar pilocystic astrocytoma has virtually a 100% 5-year survival rate. This tumor develops in the cerebellar hemispheres of school-aged children. Histologically, the tumor cells are hair-like (pilocystic) and there is a microcyst formation and often Rosenthal fibers. The tumor is well circumscribed without local invasiveness. Neurosurgical resection is usually complete and recurrence is very uncommon.

70. An older child with medically intractable complex partial seizures has an MRI scan performed. The scan reveals a partially calcified mass in the right mesial temporal lobe without associated edema. What is the most likely diagnosis?

Gangliogliomas are slow-growing benign neoplasms that are increasingly being recognized as a cause for intractable seizures.

INJURY BY PHYSICAL AGENTS AND TRAUMA

71. Does age have any effect on whether or not cranial irradiation would be considered as treatment for cancer?

Children who received cranial x-ray therapy (XRT) prior to 3 years of age have significantly reduced intelligence quotients.

72. What are some of the other adverse effects that may be encountered in children who receive cranial XRT?

Many children experience transient somnolence, headaches, and anorexia 6–8 weeks after initiation of XRT. However, a severe and potentially life-threatening side effect may occur 1–3 years after the XRT has stopped, and is termed radiation necrosis (radionecrosis). This phenomenon may mimic a mass effect, and it may be difficult to distinguish tumor recurrence from radionecrosis. Pathologically the lesion involves hyalinization of blood vessels with massive infarction and encrosis of brain tissues.

Children may also experience hypothalamic-pituitary dysfunction following XRT. This usually involves decreased production of growth hormone and thyroid-stimulating hormone. The formation of cataracts is also common if the ocular globes were exposed to irradiation. Finally, XRT may induce a second malignancy that appears years later. These are usually meningiomas, sarcomas, thyroid tumors, and parotid gland tumors.

Duffner PK, Cohen ME: The long-term effects of central nervous system therapy on children with brain tumors. Neurol Clin 9:479–495, 1991.

73. Children with acute lymphoblastic leukemia receive CNS prophylaxis in the form of cranial XRT and/or intrathecal methotrexate and occasionally cytosine-arabinoside. What is the severe neurologic complication that some of the children experience?

Some of these children develop a leukoencephalopathy with progressive dementia, seizures, and focal neurologic deficits. Neuroimaging reveals cerebral atrophy, extensive white matter lesions, and scattered calcifications.

74. A 6-month-old infant presents to the emergency room with obtundation and a history of recent onset of seizures. Examination reveals no fever, anterior fontanelle slightly bulging, depressed level of consciousness, and hypotonia. A partial motor seizure is witnessed. On funduscopic examination, extensive, bilateral retinal hemorrhages and mild papilledema are observed. What is your leading diagnosis?

Child abuse, specifically the shaken-baby syndrome, needs to be first on the list of diagnostic possibilities. Due to the violent shaking of the body and head, these infants sustain massive subarachnoid hemorrhages and associated retinal hemorrhages. This commonly leads to seizures and may cause cortical infarctions as the cerebral vessels spasm.

75. What is a growing skull fracture?
This is a rather rare complication of linear skull fractures, usually occurring in children less than 3 years of age. Because of brain and CSF pulsations, the opposing edges of bone along the fracture do not fuse. Resorption of bone along the edges occurs, so that the fracture opening progressively enlarges, producing a "growing skull fracture."

SEIZURES AND OTHER PAROXYSMAL DISORDERS

76. What is a simple febrile seizure?
A simple febrile seizure is a convulsion that occurs in a child between 6 months and 5 years of age in association with a fever greater than 38°C, but not in the presence of a CNS infection. The seizure must last less than 15 minutes, not have any focal features, and not occur in a series that has a total duration of greater than 30 minutes.

77. What is a complex febrile seizure?
The convulsion has focal features, lasts greater than 15 minutes or a series of convulsions lasts greater than 30 minutes, or occurs in a child younger than 6 months or older than 5 years of age.

78. Does having had a simple febrile convulsion increase the risk for later development of epilepsy (recurrent nonfebrile seizures)?
Yes, the risk of developing epilepsy increases to about 1%, double the risk for the general population.
 Verity CM, Golding J. Risk of epilepsy after febrile convulsions: A national cohort study. Br Med J 303(6814):1373–1376, 1991.
 Odievre M, Huguet P, Congard B. Febrile convulsions in children: Management. Ann Pediatr 37:570–573, 1990.

79. What is the incidence of neonatal seizures? How do they usually present?
The incidence of neonatal seizures is approximately 0.5%. Because of maturational factors such as lack of myelination of commissural fiber tracts, neonates do not experience the bilaterally synchronous generalized tonic-clonic seizures common in older children and adults. Clinically, neonatal seizures can be classified into one of five main types:
 1. Subtle seizures with eye deviation, eye fluttering, sucking, drooling, tonic posturing, or apnea
 2. Multifocal clonic seizures that exhibit clonic activity of one or more extremities that often randomly and irregularly migrate to another part of the body
 3. Focal clonic seizures
 4. Tonic seizures with decerebrate posturing
 5. Myoclonic seizures with rapid synchronous single or multiple flexion jerks of the extremities

80. An 18-month-old child is referred for evaluation of possible epilepsy. The mother relates a history of several paroxysmal spells that have occurred over the past month or so. Each spell has been similar in nature and consists of the child turning red, then blue in the face, and then passing out with a few clonic jerks of the extremities. Detailed questioning reveals that immediately preceding each spell, the child had been startled, frightened, or frustrated and began crying. This was soon followed by the sequence of events outlined above. What is the probable diagnosis?
This is a typical history of blue breathholding spells, a form of infantile syncope. Breath-holding spells occur in 4–5% of children; there is a positive family history in 25% of cases. Two-thirds have cyanotic or blue breathholding spells, 20% have pallid breathholding

spells, and the remainder have a mixture of the two. The peak incidence is between 1 and 2 years of age and resolution occurs by 6 years of age. The spells follow minor injuries, fright, or frustration. Twenty percent of these children will have syncope as older children or adults, but there is no increased risk for epilepsy.

DiMauro FJ Jr: Breath-holding spells in childhood. Am J Dis Child 146(1):125–131, 1992.

81. Other than syncope, what are some other spells which may be confused with seizures?

Differential Diagnosis of Childhood Seizures

1. Classic and complicated migraines	6. Benign nocturnal myoclonus
2. Pavor nocturnus (night terrors)	7. Motor tics/Tourette's syndrome
3. Paroxysmal dyskinesias/dystonias	8. Gastroesophageal reflux in infants
4. Benign paroxysmal vertigo of childhood	9. Attention deficit disorder/daydreaming
5. Narcolepsy/cataplexy	10. Pseudoseizures
	11. Munchausen's syndrome by proxy

HEAD PAIN

82. What are the features of a headache that would raise concern about the presence of an intracranial mass lesion?

Headaches from Intracranial Masses

1. Recent onset of headaches or change in character of chronic headaches
2. Headaches that awaken the patient from sleep or are present upon awakening in the morning
3. Association with altered mental status, vomiting, constriction of visual fields (papilledema), or focal neurologic deficits

83. What are the clinical features of childhood migraine headaches?

Migraine headaches in children are not uncommon. Approximately 50% of all individuals who develop migraine had the onset of their attacks before 20 years of age. Boys are more frequently affected until puberty, after which time the incidence is considerably higher in females. Younger children usually complain of a generalized or bifrontal/bitemporal headache, rather than the hemicranial pain characteristically present in the older child or adult. The pain may or may not be described as throbbing or pulsatile. Abdominal distress with nausea and sometimes vomiting is prominent. While experiencing a migraine, the child often appears pale and will frequently stop all activities and lie down. Photophobia and acousticophobia are usually present. If the child is able to fall asleep, the headache is virtually always gone upon awakening. The family history for migraine is positive in 70–90% of cases.

Elser JM, Woody RC: Migraine headache in the infant and young child. Headache 30:366–368, 1990.

84. What are the different types of migraine headaches?

1. **Common migraine**—account for up to three-quarters of all migraine attacks. Clinical manifestations are those listed in the preceding answer.

2. **Classic migraine**—same as above except these individuals experience an aura just prior to the onset of the headache. The aura is usually visual but rarely can be somatosensory in nature.

3. **Complicated migraine**—migraine headache associated with various transient neurological phenomena. These include hemiplegic migraine, ophthalmoplegic migraine, vertebrobasilar migraine, and acute confusional migraine.

4. **Migraine variants or equivalents**—benign paroxysmal vertigo of childhood and cyclical vomiting of childhood are two syndromes thought to be related to migraine. Both are paroxysmal in nature and patients with these syndromes often develop typical migraine headaches in later life.

85. What is the syndrome of alternating hemiplegia?

A special subtype of hemiplegic migraine is the syndrome of alternating hemiplegia. Affected individuals present with recurrent episodes of hemiplegia which occur on each side of the body at different times. Each hemiplegic episode may last hours to days, and one may merge into the next. The headache component is usually not prominent. One clue to the diagnosis is that during a particular episode of weakness, the hemiplegia usually resolves during sleep, only to return moments after awakening.

86. What are some of the therapeutic strategies used in treating migraines?

Biofeedback and relaxation techniques seem to work well for some individuals. In addition, avoidance of particular foods that appear to precipitate migraines in a small percentage of patients is helpful. Foods that have been implicated include chocolate, caffeine, nitrites, monosodium glutamate, and sharp cheeses.

87. What are the most important pharmacologic agents used in treating migraine?

1. **Symptomatic treatments.** These medications are basically painkillers that have no action on the underlying cause of the migraine headache. Medications included here are acetaminophen, codeine, meperidine, etc. It is usually best to avoid narcotic preparations in the treatment of chronic illnesses if at all possible.

2. **Abortive therapies.** These medications are vasoactive agents and modify the vasculature so the migraine headache is aborted before becoming fully developed. Medications in this group include the ergotamine preparations and isometheptene mucate.

3. **Prophylactic medications.** These are drugs that the patient takes every day in an attempt to prevent the migraine headaches from occurring at all. Medications in this group include nonsteroidal anti-inflammatory agents (aspirin), beta blockers, calcium channel blockers, antiepileptic medications (phenobarbital and phenytoin), tricyclic antidepressants (amitriptyline), and the serotonin antagonists (cyproheptadine and methysergide).

88. What is occipital neuralgia?

Occipital neuralgia is a childhood syndrome of recurrent occipital headaches. Clinical manifestations include pain and numbness in the C2 distribution, loss of the cervical lordotic curve, tenderness of the C2 spinous process, and limitation of cervical range of motion. The syndrome is thought to be due to C2 root irritation caused by excessive mobility of the C1 vertebra on the C2 vertebra.

NEUROMUSCULAR DISORDERS

89. What is the gene product of the Xp21 portion of the X chromosome?

The gene product is a protein called **dystrophin**. Dystrophin is a structural protein that is important in several tissues, including skeletal muscle, cardiac muscle, and brain. Certain mutations of the dystrophin gene lead to essentially no dystrophin production and result in Duchenne muscular dystrophy. Other mutations allow for the production of some dystrophin and cause the less severe and later-onset Becker muscular dystrophy.

Dickson G, Love DR, Davies KE, et al: Human dystrophin gene transfer: Production and expression of a functional recombinant DNA-based gene. Hum Genet 88:53–58, 1991.

90. What are the clinical manifestations of Duchenne muscular dystrophy (DMD)?
Estimates of the incidence of DMD range from 10–30 cases per 100,000 live male births. Affected children are normal through the first year of life. The first clue is that the child may walk later than expected, but detectable weakness is not present until 3–4 years of age. The pelvic girdle weakens first and gives rise to the characteristic Gowers' sign. Soon widespread weakness is apparent and relentless progression ensues. Most children become unable to walk by the end of their first decade. Once the patient is wheelchair bound, the disease seems to progress rapidly, with development of flexion contractures and progressive scoliosis. Cardiac involvement, as evidenced by EKG abnormalities, is invariable. Mild intellectual impairment is also common in these patients. Death from pulmonary infection, respiratory failure, and/or cardiac failure usually occurs by age 30 years.

91. How is the clinical diagnosis of DMD confirmed?
Electromyography and routine muscle biopsy can reveal the characteristic but nonspecific changes of a dystrophy. True confirmation can be obtained, however, with immunocytochemical studies of muscle biopsy specimens, in which the dystrophin levels are directly quantitated. In addition, molecular genetic analysis is possible, which can assay for the specific gene mutations.

92. What are some of therapeutic strategies currently being investigated for DMD that hold promise for the future?
There are currently two active areas of research. The first is the myoblast transfer project. Here healthy myoblasts are injected into individual muscles of a DMD patient. Because skeletal muscle is a syncytium, the dystrophin produced by the donor cells should mix with the deficit cells and reverse disease progression in that particular muscle. The disadvantages are the impracticality of injecting all the muscles in the body, and the inability to affect the cardiac and CNS involvement. The second area of research is to introduce a normal copy of the dystrophin gene throughout the affected patient, theoretically by using a retrovirus vector.

Grompe M, Mitani K, Lee CC, et al: Gene therapy in man and mice: Adenosine deaminase deficiency, ornithine transcarbamylase deficiency, and Duchenne muscular dystrophy. Adv Exp Med Biol 309B:51–56, 1991.

93. What are the most common congenital myopathies?
(1) Central core disease, (2) centronuclear myopathy, (3) nemaline myopathy, (4) minimal change myopathy, and (5) congenital fiber type disproportion.

94. What are the clinical manifestations of myotonic muscular dystrophy?
Myotonic dystrophy is an autosomal dominant disease that has been linked to chromosome 19. Clinical manifestations usually begin in adolescence or early adult life; however, there is variable expressivity. Clinical features include distal muscle weakness and myotonia. Muscle wasting about the face and sternocleidomastoids, in combination with facial weakness, leads to the distinctive "hatchet-face" appearance. Patients have partial ptosis, swan-like posture of the neck, enlarged paranasal sinuses, early prominent male-pattern balding in both sexes, cataracts, cardiac conduction abnormalities, hypogonadism with testicular atrophy, and abnormal glucose tolerance.

Aslanidis C, Jansen G, Amemiya C, et al: Cloning the essential myotonic dystrophy region and mapping of the putative defect. Nature 355(6360):548–551, 1992.

95. What is a common and potentially life-threatening complication that may befall neonates born to mothers with myotonic muscular dystrophy?
Some newborns who have inherited the myotonic dystrophy gene from their mothers experience profound weakness, with respiratory failure and bulbar insufficiency requiring

endotracheal intubation and mechanical ventilation. Mortality may be as high as 30–40%. Should the neonate survive, the weakness resolves spontaneously. The occurrence of the neonatal syndrome has no effect on the severity of the adult expression of the disease.

96. What are the two types of myasthenia that may affect the newborn or young infant?
    1. **Transient neonatal myasthenia gravis.** Affected neonates are born to mothers with autoimmune myasthenia gravis. The newborns experience transient weakness and hypotonia, which may be severe and life-threatening, due to the transplacental transfer of maternal antiacetylcholine receptor antibodies.
    2. **Nonautoimmune congenital myasthenia syndromes.**

97. Which types of myasthenia are not due to autoimmune production of antibodies against the acetylcholine receptor?
    1. Defects in acetylcholine (Ach) synthesis or mobilization
    2. End-plate acetylcholinesterase deficiency
    3. Slow-channel syndrome
    4. End-plate Ach receptor deficiency

Engel AG, Walls TJ, Nagel A, Uchitel O: Newly recognized congenital myasthenic syndromes. I. Congenital paucity of synaptic vesicles and reduced quantal release. II. High-conductance fast-channel syndrome. III. Abnormal acetylcholine receptor (AChR) interaction with acetylcholine. IV. AChR deficiency and short channel-open time. Prog Brain Res 84:125–137, 1990.

LEARNING DISABILITIES

98. What is meant by the term "learning disability"?
A learning disability is present when a child with overall normal intellect has a deficit in acquiring the skills needed to perform a specific cognitive task. For example, the commonest learning disability is dyslexia, a disorder manifested by difficulty in learning to read despite conventional instruction, adequate intelligence, and sociocultural opportunity.

99. A school-aged child is referred for evalution of possible absence epilepsy because of constant "day-dreaming" and worsening grades. The mother and teachers relate a history of short attention span for school work, but not for television or video games, easy distractibility, impulsiveness, constant supervision needed to complete homework and chores, adventurous and risk-taking behavior, and constant physical activity (as if driven by a motor). What is the most likely diagnosis?
This is the usual presentation of a child with attention-deficit hyperactivity disorder (ADHD). Some children have the attention deficit without the hyperactivity. This is a troublesome disorder and not infrequently leads to conduct problems. Affected children have unusually short attention spans and are simply unable to concentrate for more than a few minutes for all but the most stimulating and enjoyable activities. Their constant distractibility and day-dreaming may be confused with the seizures of absence epilepsy.

If resources are available, many of these children do very well with individualized instruction. However, for most of the more severely affected children, pharmacotherapy is necessary and generally works very well. CNS stimulants, which greatly enhance the ability to concentrate and pay attention, such as methylphenidate (Ritalin), dextroamphetamine (Dexedrine), and pemoline (Cylert) are used.

100. What are the clinical manifestations of infantile autism?
The onset of autism usually occurs by the end of the first year of life and is manifested by social and language developmental regression and a relative lack of communication. Motor development is generally not affected. These children reject or ignore virtually all

interpersonal interactions. They are often disturbed by even the slightest change in their environment, such as rearranging the furniture or books on a shelf. Repetitive self-stimulation behaviors are common and consist of rocking, head banging, whirling, and flapping of hands in front of face. Many of these children appear to have normal intelligence. The etiopathogenetic basis remains unknown and the prognosis for meaningful recovery is very poor.

BIBLIOGRAPHY

1. Behrman RE, Vaughan VC III (eds): Nelson Textbook of Pediatrics, 14th ed. Philadelphia, W.B. Saunders Co., 1992.
2. Brooke MH: A Clinician's View of Neuromuscular Diseases, 2nd ed. Baltimore, Williams & Wilkins, 1986.
3. Fishman MA (ed): Pediatric Neurology. Orlando, Grune & Stratton Inc., 1986.
4. Jones KL: Smith's Recognizable Patterns of Human Malformation, 4th ed. Philadelphia, W.B. Saunders Co., 1988.
5. Menkes JH (ed): Textbook of Child Neurology, 4th ed. Philadelphia, Lea & Febiger, 1990.
6. Miller G, Ramer JC (eds): Static Encephalopathies of Infancy and Childhood. New York, Raven Press, 1992.
7. Oski FA, DeAngelis CD, Feigin RD, Warshaw JB (eds): Principles and Practice of Pediatrics. Philadelphia, J.B. Lippincott Co., 1990.
8. Swaiman KF (ed): Pediatric Neurology: Principles and Practice. St. Louis, CV Mosby Co., 1989.
9. Volpe JJ: Neurology of the Newborn, 2nd ed. Philadelphia, W.B. Saunders Co., 1987.

25. ELECTROENCEPHALOGRAPHY

Richard A. Hrachovy, M.D.

1. What is believed to be the source of the electrical activity recorded by scalp electrodes in the electroencephalogram (EEG)?
The best available evidence indicates that surface- and scalp-recorded electrical activity results from extracellular current flow associated with summation of excitatory postsynaptic potentials and inhibitory postsynaptic potentials.

2. What are the different frequencies recorded on an EEG?
Four frequency bands are recorded: delta = <4 Hz, theta = 4–7 Hz, alpha = 8–13 Hz, and beta = >13 Hz.

3. What are the features of an EEG in an awake, normal adult?
The EEG reveals a dominant rhythm in the occipital leads bilaterally. The frequency of this rhythm in most adult individuals is between 9 and 11 Hz. This rhythm is variously referred to as the occipital dominant rhythm, the occipital dominant alpha rhythm, or simply the alpha rhythm. The occipital dominant rhythm is best seen with the eyes closed and the individual relaxed. This rhythm usually attenuates when the eyes are opened. In the anterior regions, alpha frequency activity is also present but is lower in voltage and generally less continuous than that in the posterior regions. There is also low-voltage 18–22 Hz activity present in the anterior leads.

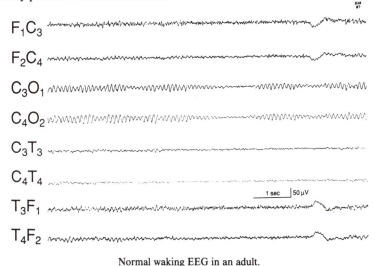

F_1C_3

F_2C_4

C_3O_1

C_4O_2

C_3T_3

C_4T_4

T_3F_1

T_4F_2

Normal waking EEG in an adult.

4. What are the EEG features of the various sleep stages in the adult?

NREM SLEEP
   Stage 1: The first change in the EEG as an individual becomes drowsy is the disappearance of the occipital dominant alpha rhythm, followed by increasing amounts of theta frequency activity in all regions. During stage 1, diphasic sharp waves also appear in the EEG, occurring maximally at the vertex. These sharp waves are referred to as vertex transients.

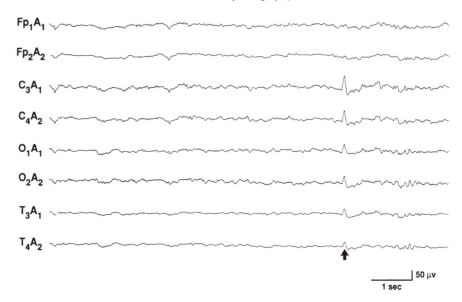

Stage 1 NREM sleep. Arrow denotes vertex transient.

Stage 2: The onset of stage 2 NREM sleep is characterized by the appearance of sleep spindles. Sleep spindles consist of bursts of 12–14 Hz activity, maximally expressed over the central regions of the head. These bursts generally last less than 2 seconds in the adult. The background activity during stage 2 sleep consists of relatively low-voltage, mixed frequency EEG background activity, with delta activity comprising less than 20% of the sleep period.

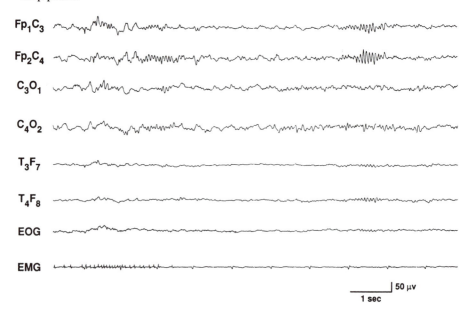

Stage 2 NREM sleep.

Stage 3: As the patient enters deeper NREM sleep, the amount of delta activity increases in voltage and quantity. During stage 3 NREM sleep, the amount of delta activity comprising the record varies between 20 and 50%. Sleep spindles persist into stage 3 sleep.

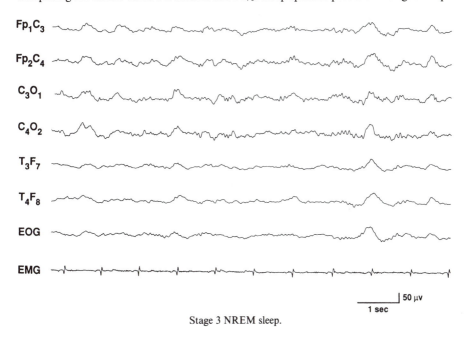

Stage 3 NREM sleep.

Stage 4: During stage 4 NREM sleep, the amount of delta activity comprises more than 50% of the record. Spindles persist into stage 4 NREM sleep.

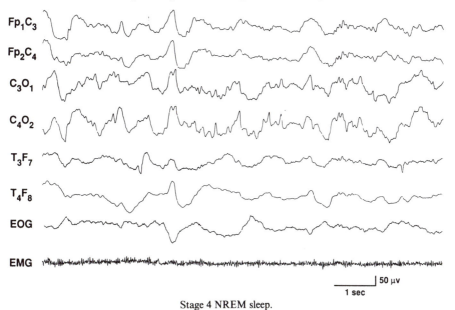

Stage 4 NREM sleep.

REM SLEEP

This state is also referred to as paradoxical sleep. The EEG during REM sleep reveals a generally lower voltage record similar in appearance to stage 1. However, in some individuals, runs of alpha frequency activity may appear in the occipital leads identical to the alpha rhythm in the awake tracing. During this stage of sleep, the individual has spontaneous rapid eye movements and tonic motor activity is suppressed.

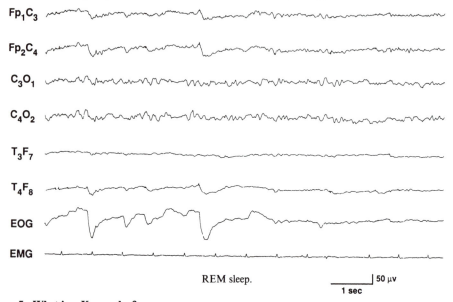

REM sleep.   50 μv

1 sec

5. What is a K complex?

A K complex is a high-voltage diphasic slow wave that may be preceded or followed by a spindle burst, maximally expressed in the frontocentral regions bilaterally. K complexes occur spontaneously during sleep, but may be elicited by sudden sensory stimuli, such as loud noises.

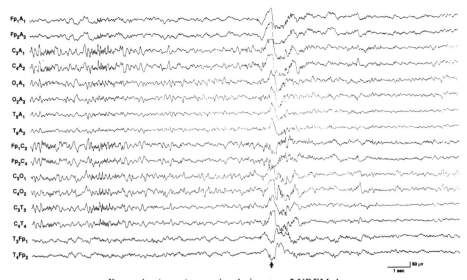

K complex (arrow) occurring during stage 2 NREM sleep.

6. What is the *tracé discontinu* pattern?

Tracé discontinu refers to the EEG pattern seen in premature infants. When the brain's electrical activity first appears, it is discontinuous, with long periods of quiescence or flattening. Initially, it is present in all states of waking and sleep. In early prematurity (26–28 weeks), the periods of flattening may last up to 20–30 seconds. As age increases, the periods of inactivity shorten, and, at 30 weeks' conceptional age, the EEG activity becomes continuous during REM sleep. At about 34 weeks, the EEG activity becomes continuous in the awake state. Continuity appears last in NREM, or quiet sleep, at about 37–38 weeks.

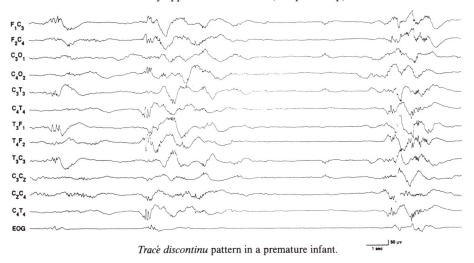

Tracé discontinu pattern in a premature infant.

7. What does the EEG show in an awake term infant?

The typical awake pattern in a term infant is characterized by a mixture of alpha, beta, theta, and delta frequencies, and is often referred to as a poly frequency record.

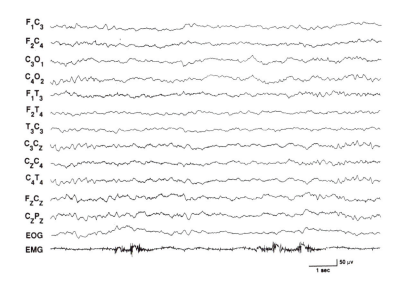

Normal awake pattern in a term infant.

8. What is the *tracé alternant* pattern? At what age is it seen?

The *tracé alternant* pattern is seen from about 37–38 weeks' conceptional age to about 5–6 weeks postterm. This pattern occurs during NREM sleep and is characterized by bursts of slow waves mixed with low-voltage sharp activity, separated by episodes of generalized voltage attenuation lasting from 3–15 seconds, but not absolute quiescence.

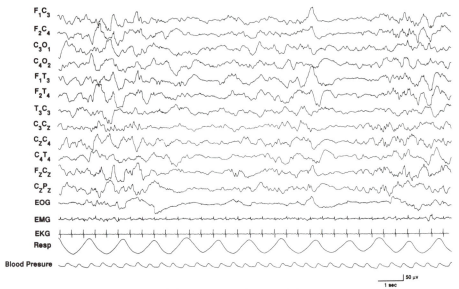

Tracé alternant pattern in a term infant.

9. At what age do vertex transients appear in the EEG? At what age are these transients synchronous? At what age are they symmetrical?

Vertex transients first appear in the EEG at 6–8 weeks postterm. They are synchronous and symmetrical from the time they first appear.

10. At what age do sleep spindles first appear in the EEG? At what age are they synchronous? At what age are they symmetrical?

Like vertex transients, sleep spindles first appear in the EEG at 6–8 weeks postterm. From the time they first appear, they are symmetrical on the two sides; however, spindle synchrony does not occur until approximately 12 months of age.

11. At what age does the occipital dominant rhythm first appear? At what age does the occipital dominant rhythm attain a frequency of 8 Hz?

At approximately 3 months of age, a rhythm that blocks with eye opening and disappears with drowsiness appears in the occipital leads bilaterally. The frequency of this rhythm when it first appears is 3–4 Hz. At 1 year of age, the occipital dominant rhythm is approximately 6 Hz. It does not reach 8 Hz until the age of 3 years.

12. What are the differences in the EEG of an awake child or young adolescent compared with an adult?

- The background activity in the child's EEG is usually higher in voltage.
- The occipital dominant rhythm in children is mixed, with slower fused waveforms referred to as slow waves of youth.
- There is more theta frequency activity in the anterior leads of a child's EEG.

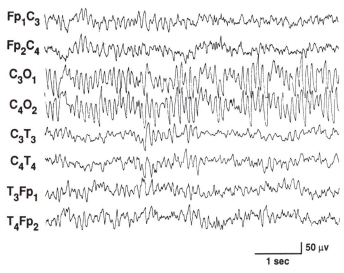

Normal waking EEG in a 9-year-old child.

13. What is the mu rhythm?

The mu rhythm is a normal central rhythm of alpha-activity frequency, usually in the range of 8–10 Hz, which occurs during wakefulness. This rhythm is detectable in approximately 20% of young adults, but is less common in older individuals and children. The mu rhythm is blocked or attenuated by movement, or thought of movement, of the contralateral extremity.

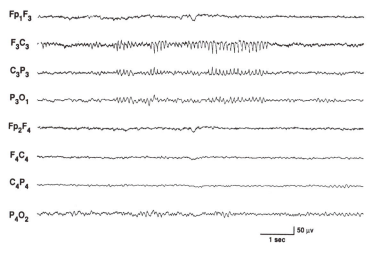

Mu rhythm.

14. What is a breach rhythm?

A breach rhythm typically refers to a high-voltage, sharply contoured rhythm appearing over an area of a skull defect. It is important to realize that this is an accentuated normal rhythm and should not be reported as a focal abnormality.

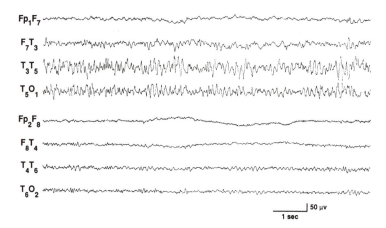

Breach rhythm in the left posterior temporal (T_5) region.

15. What is the most common finding in pseudotumor cerebri?

Although there may be a variety of nonspecific findings in patients with pseudotumor cerebri, the EEG is usually normal.

16. If you were recording the EEG at the time a patient experienced a middle cerebral artery infarction, what would be the sequence of EEG changes you would expect to see?

The initial change following an ischemic episode is depression of the background rhythms over the ipsilateral hemisphere, followed by the appearance of continuous polymorphic slow activity over this hemisphere, maximally expressed in the temporofrontal region.

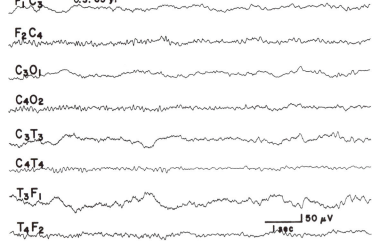

EEG of a patient with a left middle cerebral artery infarction. Note depression of activity over the left hemispheric leads and left temporal slowing.

17. An EEG is obtained 3 years after a person has experienced a hemispheric infarction. What EEG findings may be seen in this patient?

As in the acute state, the EEG recorded years after a hemispheric infarction may continue to show depression of background activity over the ipsilateral hemisphere. Focal slow-wave activity may also continue ipsilaterally. However, the focal slow-wave activity is not as continuous as it is in the acute state. The patient may continue to show depression of the occipital dominant rhythm on the side of the infarct. However, in many patients, the amplitude of the occipital dominant rhythm returns to normal ipsilaterally, and in some patients the occipital dominant rhythm becomes enhanced on the side of the infarction (so-called paradoxical enhancement of the alpha rhythm). A small number of patients may reveal a spike focus ipsilaterally. Finally, a large percentage of patients will show a normal EEG years after a hemispheric infarction.

18. What are the typical EEG changes seen with a small lacunar infarct?
Small lacunar infarcts usually produce no change in the background EEG activity; the EEG in such infarcts is usually normal.

19. What types of EEG findings may be seen with a subdural hematoma?
Depression of background activity over the ipsilateral hemisphere and/or focal slow-wave activity over the ipsilateral hemisphere are the findings most frequently seen with a subdural hematoma. Episodic bifrontal slow activity may also occur. However, it is important to remember that the EEG may be normal.

20. A 6-year-old child presents with headache and ataxia. A posterior fossa tumor is suspected. What EEG findings suggest this diagnosis?
The most common EEG finding associated with posterior fossa tumors in children is paroxysmal bioccipital delta activity.

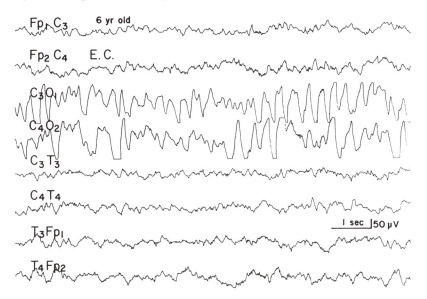

Rhythmic occipital slow activity in a child with a posterior fossa tumor.

21. What is the significance of triphasic waves in the EEG?
Triphasic waves usually appear in the EEG when there has been diffuse slowing of background rhythms. Although triphasic waves may be seen with a variety of encephalopathies (infectious, toxic, postanoxic, etc.), they most often are associated with metabolic encephalopathies, most commonly hepatic or renal.

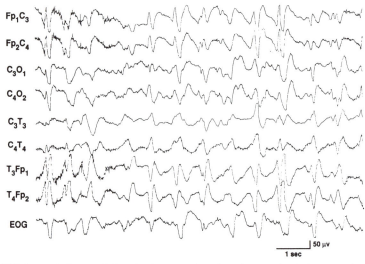

EEG in metabolic encephalopathy demonstrating triphasic waves in the frontal regions.

22. What is the relationship between clinical improvement and EEG improvement in children with various encephalopathies?

Although in older individuals with various types of encephalopathies, clinical and EEG improvement usually occur simultaneously, in children the clinical status of the patient may improve more rapidly than the EEG.

23. What is the usual progression of EEG changes in Alzheimer's disease (AD)?

During the early stages of AD, the EEG may be normal. As the disease progresses, the EEG initially shows slowing of the occipital dominant rhythm, which, in turn, is followed by increasing amounts of theta-frequency activity and then by the appearance of bifrontal and, in some patients, bioccipital delta activity. Occasional sharp waves may appear in the frontal and posterior head regions in severely demented patients; however, these sharp waves never develop the periodic character of the sharp waves seen with Creutzfeldt-Jakob disease. Marked asymmetries of the background activity and focal slow wave activity are not features of AD.

24. What are the major differences between the periodic pattern seen with Creutzfeldt-Jakob disease and that seen with subacute sclerosing panencephalitis (SSPE)?

Creutzfeldt-Jakob Disease vs. SSPE

	C-J	SSPE
Complex morphology	Di- or triphasic sharp waves	Slow waves or groups of slow waves; may have sharp component
Period	Classically, 1 sec	4–14 sec
Distribution	Generalized but may begin focally or lateralized to one hemisphere	Usually generalized but maximal in frontcentral leads
Background activity	Diffusely slow when complexes first appear	May be normal when complexes first appear

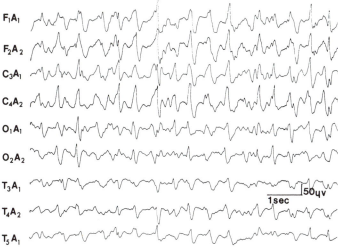

Periodic pattern in Creutzfeldt-Jacob disease.

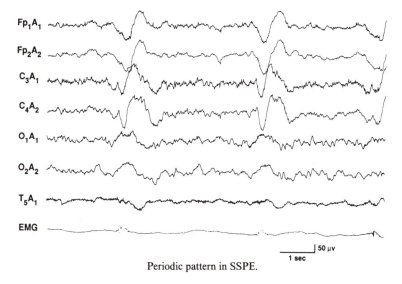

Periodic pattern in SSPE.

25. What other disease processes may produce a periodic pattern similar to that seen with Creutzfeldt-Jakob disease?

The periodic pattern consisting of generalized, high-voltage diphasic and triphasic sharp waves recurring with a period of 1 second is highly suggestive of Creutzfeldt-Jakob disease. However, a pattern indistinguishable from that seen in Creutzfeldt-Jakob disease may occur in the postanoxic state. Also, a similar type of pattern may be seen with lithium intoxication.

26. What is the significance of periodic lateralizing epileptiform discharges (PLEDs)? What is the most common etiology?

PLEDs signify the presence of a large destructive lesion involving one hemisphere. They may be seen with a variety of lesions, including tumors, abscesses, hematomas, and herpes encephalitis. However, the most common cause of PLEDs is acute cerebral infarction.

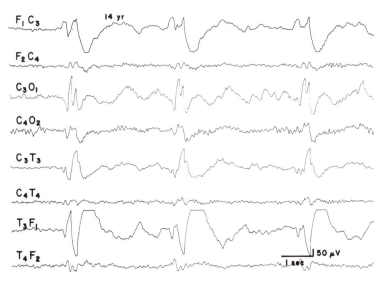

Periodic lateralizing epileptiform discharges (PLEDs).

27. What classes of drugs produce increased amounts of voltages of beta activity in the EEG at therapeutic doses?

The most common classes of drugs that produce increased fast activity in the EEG are the sedatives, anxiolytic agents, CNS stimulants, and antihistamines. Antidepressants may increase the amount of beta activity in the EEG at therapeutic doses but also result in an increase in the amount of theta-frequency activity.

Excessive beta activity in a patient receiving a benzodiazepine.

28. What is hypsarrhythmia?

Hypsarrhythmia is the interictal EEG pattern usually seen in infants who experience infantile spasms. The pattern consists of random, high-voltage slow waves mixed with high-voltage, multifocal spike and sharp waves arising from all cortical regions. The triad of infantile spasms, hypsarrhythmia, and mental retardation is often referred to as West's syndrome.

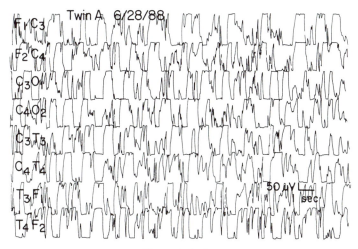

Hypsarrhythmia.

29. What are the characteristics of the 3 per second spike and slow-wave pattern?

This pattern is bilateral, symmetrical, and usually maximally expressed in the frontocentral regions. However, in some patients the bursts of 3 per second spike and wave activity may be restricted to or maximally expressed in the occipital regions. The discharges appear and disappear suddenly. The frequency of the spike and wave complexes may vary slightly during the burst. The first few complexes of the bursts may occur at a frequency of 3.5–4.0 Hz, whereas the last few may slow to 2.5 Hz. As soon as the 3-Hz spike and wave bursts stop, the EEG returns to its interictal state immediately with no postictal depression or slowing.

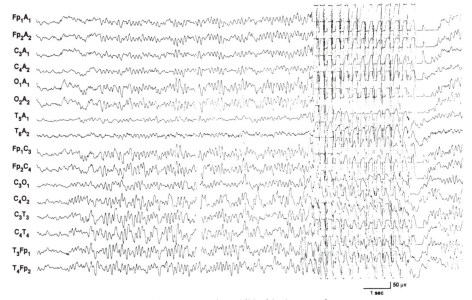

3-Hz spike and wave in a child with absence seizures.

30. A 10-year-old girl with staring spells is referred for an EEG. What routine activating procedures should be performed on this patient?
The common activating procedures usually performed on patients with suspected seizures are hyperventilation, photic stimulation, and sleep. Generalized spike and wave activity may be activated by any of these three activating procedures, whereas focal spikes are usually activated only by sleep.

31. Which two normal patterns are frequently confused with generalized spike and wave activity in children?
The first is **hypnagogic hypersynchrony**. This pattern appears at 3–4 months of age and persists until 10–12 years of age. It consists of paroxysmal rhythmic 3–5 Hz activity, maximally expressed in the central and centrofrontal regions. This activity may occur in long runs; however, it may also appear in brief paroxysms. Faster components may be mixed with the paroxysmal slower activity. The second pattern often confused with generalized spike and slow-wave activity is the **normal hyperventilation response**. Children, particularly between the ages of 5 and 15 years, often show a buildup of high-voltage, frontal dominant, generalized 3–4 Hz activity. This high-voltage, rhythmic slow activity may be continuous or occur in a paroxysmal fashion while the child is deep-breathing. This pattern may be easily confused by the novice electroencephalographer with the 3-Hz spike and slow-wave pattern, which may also occur during hyperventilation in children.

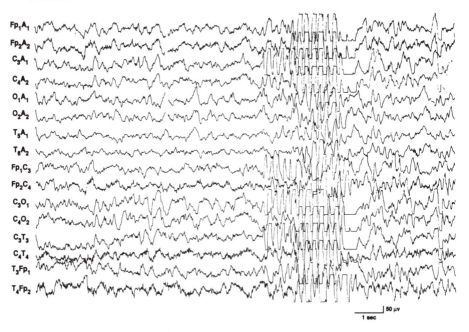

Hypnagogic hypersynchrony.

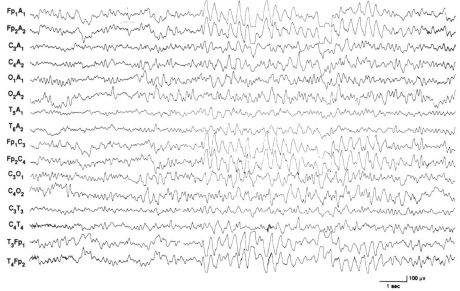

Hyperventilation response in a child.

32. What are the characteristics of focal epileptiform spikes?

A spike is an EEG transient with a duration of less than 70 ms. The transient may occur alone, but frequently a slow wave follows, forming a spike and slow-wave complex. The duration of the slow wave may last from 150–350 milliseconds. The spike transient may be monophasic or polyphasic. The polarity of most focal epileptiform spikes recorded at the scalp is surface negative. Surface positive spikes rarely occur in patients with epilepsy.

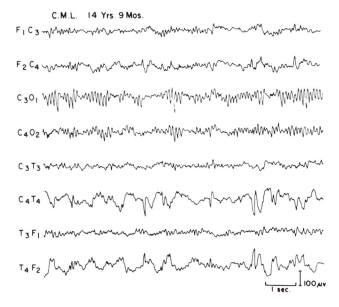

Right temporal spikes mixed with slow waves in a child with complex partial seizures.

33. Which three normal EEG patterns may be confused with focal epileptiform spikes in the EEG?

    1. Vertex transients = synchronous diphasic sharp waves that appear at the vertex.

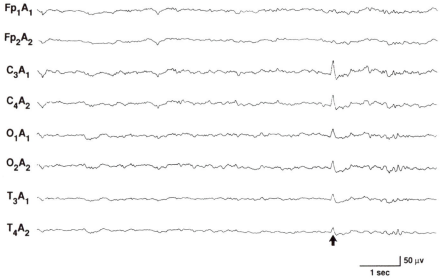

Stage 1 NREM sleep. Arrow denotes vertex transient.

    2. Lambda waves = multiphasic spikes that appear in the occipital leads, with eyes open, and are associated with saccadic eye movements when looking at geometric patterns.

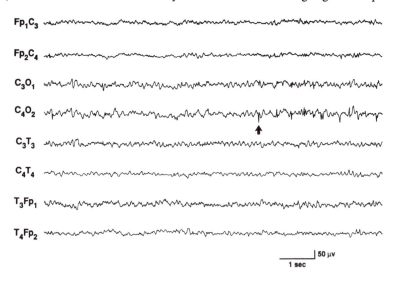

Lambda waves (arrow) in the occipital leads in an individual looking at a geometric design.

    3. Positive occipital sharp transients of sleep = positive sharp waves that appear in the occipital leads during NREM sleep.

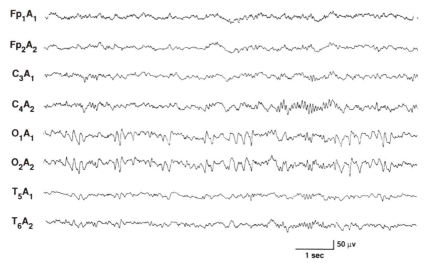

Positive occipital sharp transients of sleep.

34. What are the typical clinical characteristics of a patient whose EEG shows bursts of generalized 2-Hz spike and slow-wave activity?

They have varying degrees of developmental and mental retardation. These patients experience multiple types of seizures, most commonly atonic, tonic, atypical absence, and generalized tonic-clonic. Partial seizures may also occur. These seizures are generally refractory to anticonvulsant therapy, and such patients will often be treated with polytherapy. This constellation of clinical and EEG features is often referred to as the Lennox-Gastaut syndrome, or slow spike/slow wave syndrome.

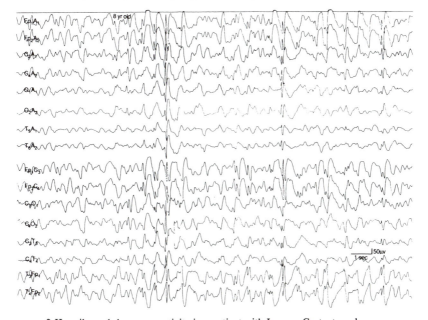

2-Hz spike and slow-wave activity in a patient with Lennox-Gastaut syndrome.

35. What are the usual effects of NREM and REM sleep on interictal generalized or focal epileptiform discharges?

In general, NREM sleep greatly enhances the frequency of interictal generalized spike and wave or focal spike activity, particularly the first NREM sleep episode of nocturnal sleep. On the other hand, REM sleep is usually associated with a marked attenuation or total abolishment of epileptiform activity.

36. What types of EEG changes may be seen postictally?

Immediately after a generalized tonic-clonic seizure, there is marked depression of background activity in all regions, followed by an increase in the voltage and frequency of the background activity, and a gradual return to the baseline state. Focal slowing may also occur postictally in a patient who has experienced a generalized tonic-clonic seizure. Following a partial seizure, the EEG frequently shows regional or hemispheric depression of the background activity over the ipsilateral hemisphere and/or focal slow-wave activity over the ipsilateral hemisphere. The duration that the postictal changes will persist in the EEG is highly variable. In general, the longer the duration of the seizure, the longer the postictal changes persist. This is particularly true in children, who may show diffuse and/ or focal postictal changes for days following a prolonged seizure or an episode of status epilepticus.

37. What four EEG patterns with an epileptiform morphology are classified as patterns of uncertain diagnostic significance?

1. The 14- and 6-Hz positive bursts (14 and 6 per second positive spikes)

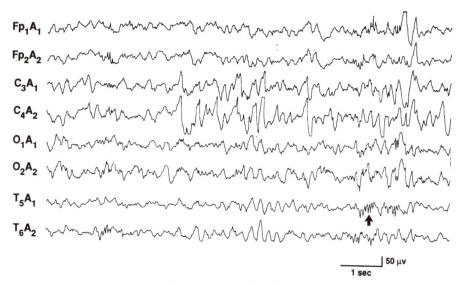

14 and 6 per second positive spike pattern.

2. The rhythmic temporal theta bursts of drowsiness (psychomotor variant pattern)

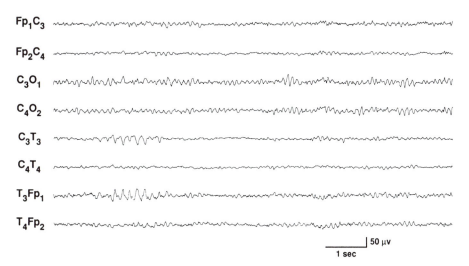

Psychomotor variant pattern.

3. The 6-Hz spike and wave pattern (phantom spike and wave pattern)

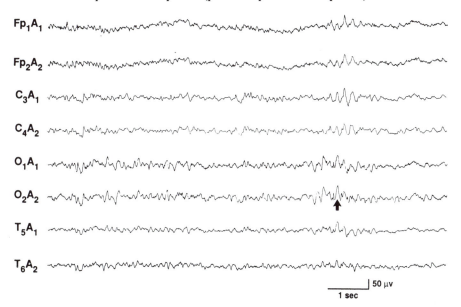

Phantom spike and wave pattern.

4. The small, sharp spike pattern (benign epileptiform transients of sleep)

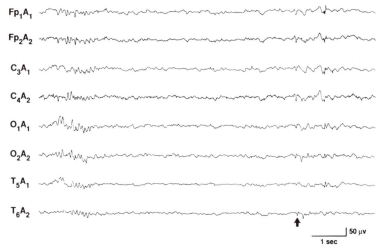

Small sharp spike pattern.

The 14 and 6 per second positive burst pattern is a pattern of childhood and adolescence, whereas the remaining three patterns are usually seen in adulthood.

38. What is the significance of a suppression-burst pattern? Which conditions may produce this pattern?

The suppression-burst pattern consists of brief paroxysms of activity occurring between periods of little or no discernable electrical activity. The activity during the bursts may consist of alpha, theta, or delta frequencies and/or sharp waves. The suppression-burst pattern indicates the presence of a severe diffuse disturbance in brain function. It may be seen in a variety of conditions, including anoxic insult, drug overdose, and severe head injury.

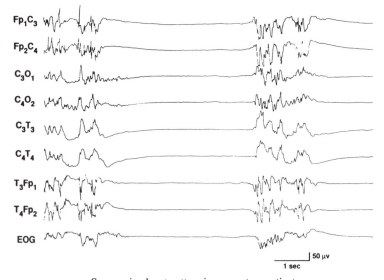

Suppression burst pattern in a comatose patient.

39. What are some of the patterns that may be seen following an anoxic insult?
Depending on the degree of the anoxic insult and the timing from the insult to the EEG, a variety of patterns may be seen. With mild insults, the EEG may be normal or show only slight diffuse slowing. As the severity of the insult increases, so does the degree of slowing of the background rhythms. In addition, periodic diphasic and triphasic sharp waves, superimposed upon a slow-background, alpha coma pattern, and suppression-burst patterns may all occur in the postanoxic state.

40. What are the three brainstem coma patterns? Which pattern generally has the best prognosis?
Alpha coma, spindle coma, and theta coma. Of these, spindle coma usually carries the best prognosis.

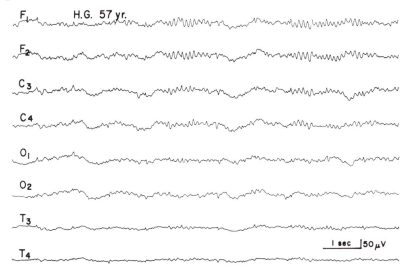

Alpha coma pattern in a comatose patient following a brainstem infarction. Note alpha frequency activity in frontal deviations.

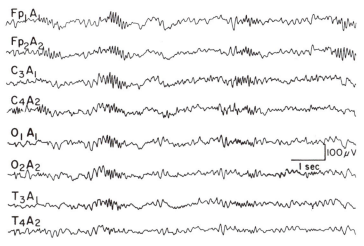

Spindle coma pattern in a comatose patient following a midbrain contusion.

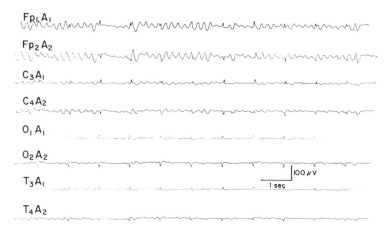

Theta coma pattern in a comatose patient following a cardiorespiratory arrest. Periodic low-voltage sharp waves represent EKG artifact.

41. What are the major criteria for recording a case of suspected brain death?

- A minimum of 8 scalp electrodes and earlobe reference electrodes should be used.
- The inter-electrode impedances should be under 10,000 ohms, but over 100 ohms.
- The inter-electrode distances should be at least 10 cm.
- The sensitivity should be changed from 7 mv/mm to 2 mv/mm during most of the recording with inclusion of appropriate calibrations.
- A time constant of 0.3–0.4 seconds should be used during part of the recording.
- The integrity of the entire recording system should be tested.
- Monitoring techniques (e.g., EKG, ambient noise, respiratory, etc.) should be used as needed to identify other physiologic signals and artifacts as not being of brain origin.
- The EEG should be tested for reactivity by intense stimulation such as pain and loud sound.
- The EEG should be recorded for at least 30 minutes.
- The recording should be made only by qualified technologists.
- A repeat EEG should be performed if there is any doubt about electrocerebral silence.
- Telephone transmission of an EEG should not be used for determination of electrocerebral silence.

42. What are the two conditions that may produce temporary, reversible, electrocerebral inactivity?

The two conditions that may result in reversible electrocerebral inactivity are overdoses with CNS depressants and hypothermia.

BIBLIOGRAPHY

1. Daly DO, Pedley TA (eds): Current Practice of Clinical Electroencephalography, 2nd ed. New York, Raven Press, 1990.
2. Fisch B (ed): Spehlman's EEG Primer, 2nd ed. Amsterdam, New York, Elsevier, 1991.
3. Niedermeyer E, Lopes da Silva F (eds): Electroencephalography, 2nd ed. Baltimore–Munich, Urban & Schwarzenberg, 1987.

26. ELECTROMYOGRAPHY

James M. Killian, M.D.

1. What is an electromyogram (EMG)? How is it recorded?

An electromyogram is an electrical recording of resting and voluntary muscle activity. It is transmitted from a needle electrode via a pre-amplifier and amplifier to a loudspeaker and oscilloscopic or digital visual display.

2. What are the clinical indications for ordering an EMG?

An EMG is usually ordered to determine the localization and severity of neurogenic disorders, and to differentiate them from myogenic disorders.

3. What are the characteristics of normal single motor unit potentials?

Normal muscle potentials appear as waveforms with a duration from 5 to 15 ms, with 2–4 phases, and from 0.5 to 3 mv in amplitude (depending on the size of the unit and type of recording needle electrodes).

4. What are polyphasic units? When are they seen on EMG?

These are voluntary motor units with more than four phases. They are seen in both myogenic and neurogenic disorders.

5. What are the characteristics of abnormal single motor unit potentials?

Abnormal motor unit potentials are classified as either neurogenic or myogenic. Neurogenic motor units appear of longer duration and higher amplitude than normal potentials and are usually polyphasic. Myopathic potentials are just the opposite, with shorter durations and smaller amplitudes than normal potentials. They are also usually polyphasic.

6. What are the EMG characteristics of fasciculation potentials?

A fasciculation is an involuntary firing of a single motor neuron and all its innervated muscle fibers. This is displayed by EMG as a single motor unit and visible in the patient as a brief irregular undulation of muscle.

7. What are the EMG characteristics of fibrillation potentials?

Fibrillations are involuntary contractions of single muscle fibers and cannot be seen through the skin. Electrically, they appear as regular short small action potentials that sound like static or cooking bacon. Fibrillations are always abnormal and indicate loss of innervation of a single muscle fiber from a variety of causes.

8. What is the importance of insertional activity?

Insertional activity is the discharge of single muscle fibers during insertion of an EMG needle, and does not indicate abnormality. The discharges appear similar to fibrillations on the EMG. Increased insertional activity may indicate irritable muscle fibers, such as from denervation.

9. What are positive sharp waves?

Positive sharp waves have the same pathologic implication as fibrillation potentials (i.e., denervation) and appear on the EMG as a downward wave formation after needle irritation of a group of denervated muscle fibers.

10. What electrical activity can be measured from the endplate?
High-frequency, short-action potentials can be seen when the EMG needle is close to or in the motor endplate, and is called endplate activity. This activity is not pathologic, but may be confused with fibrillation potentials.

11. What is the appearance of myotonia on an EMG?
Myotonia refers to a delayed relaxation of muscle. Two types of myotonia are seen: true and pseudo. The former occurs in myotonia dystrophica and myotonia congenita, and is represented by muscle action potentials that vary in amplitude and frequency and are heard on the loud speaker as "dive bombers." Pseudo-myotonia has a stable frequency resembling an airplane in steady flight, with abrupt endings. Pseudo-myotonia occurs in both muscle and nerve disorders, including polymyositis, glycogen storage diseases, hyperkalemic periodic paralysis, root disease, and anterior horn cell disorders.

12. What are the characteristics of muscle activity recorded in a myopathy?
The motor unit potentials are smaller and shorter because of a reduction in the size of the muscle fibers, without any change in the firing rate. There will still be the full pattern of discharging motor units seen on the EMG screen.

13. What are the characteristics of muscle activity recorded from a denervated muscle?
Fibrillations and positive sharp waves are seen in resting muscles 7–14 days after the onset of axonal denervation. When partially denervated muscle is voluntarily contracted, clinical weakness from axonal loss is seen on EMG as a reduction in motor unit firing patterns.

14. How long after a nerve is transected does it take for electrical changes to develop?
After transection of a nerve, there is immediate loss of voluntary activity, and therefore no electrical motor units are seen with attempted contraction. Spontaneous abnormal EMG activity from the muscle takes 7–10 days to develop, and is maximum at approximately 14 days.

15. How do the recruitment patterns differ in normal muscles, myopathies, and neuropathies?
The patterns of motor activity are no different between normal muscles and those with myopathic abnormalities. Neuropathies, however, show a dropout of motor units, which reduces the recruitment pattern according to the severity of the neurogenic pathology.

16. What are the clinical indications for ordering nerve conduction velocities?
Nerve conduction velocities are ordered to anatomically localize abnormalities of the peripheral motor and sensory systems and to assess the degree and severity of axonal or demyelinative nerve pathology.

17. What is the normal nerve conduction velocity?
This varies among nerves, but is usually in the range of 50–55 meters per second in the arm and 42–47 meters per second in the leg.

18. What is the amplitude of a normal motor action potential?
The amplitude varies with the muscle that is stimulated, but in the hand would be above 6 mv and in the foot above 1 mv in amplitude.

19. What is the amplitude of a normal sensory nerve action potential?
The amplitude varies depending on the size and accessibility of distal nerves, and ranges from 10 to 100 μv, approximately 1/20th the size of the motor action potential.

20. What is the H-reflex? How is it useful clinically?
The H-reflex is the electrical counterpart of the ankle jerk, and gives clinical information on any pathology in the S1 afferent-efferent reflex arc. The H may be prolonged or absent in neuropathies, S1 radiculopathies, or sciatic mononeuropathies.

21. What is the F-wave? How is it useful clinically?
The F-wave is a delayed motor potential following the normal motor action potential (M-wave), and represents the antidromic response seen when a motor nerve is powerfully stimulated. An F-wave may be obtained on any peripheral motor nerve, and gives information about conductibility across proximal nerve segments, since the stimulation will travel proximally and then return down the nerve to contract the muscle.

22. After nerve transection, what happens to nerve conduction in the distal segment?
Nerve conduction in the distal segment is retained for 3 days after proximal transection of the nerve. Wallerian degeneration rapidly interferes with nerve conduction, and at between 3 and 5 days all conductibility is lost.

23. What are the earliest changes on the EMG after acute nerve transection or injury?
Nerve conduction in the distal segment is more valuable than muscle analysis with the EMG, as the loss of conduction becomes evident at 3–5 days, whereas spontaneous EMG changes do not develop for 7–10 days.

24. What will repetitive nerve stimulation show in a patient with myasthenia gravis?
Approximately 65–85% of patients with myasthenia gravis show a decremental motor response of 10% or greater to slow repetitive stimulation of a motor nerve at 2–3 Hz. The highest yield is in the spinal accessory nerve, with measurement of the trapezius muscle action potential, but distal motor nerves and even the facial nerve can also be used.

25. What will repetitive nerve stimulation show in a patient with Lambert-Eaton myasthenic syndrome (LEMS)?
Repetitive stimulation in LEMS shows low amplitude muscle action potentials that double or triple in size following exercise (post-exercise facilitation), due to increasing release of acetylcholine at the motor nerve terminal. However, there may also be superimposed decremental responses similar to myasthenia gravis.

26. What is the role of single-fiber EMG?
Single-fiber EMG measures the delay in transmission between terminal nerve fibers and their muscle fibers (jitter). A delay beyond normal, known as prolonged jitter, indicates an abnormality in neuromuscular transmission at the motor endplate. Special needles and recording apparatus are necessary for this procedure, and it is used mainly in the diagnosis of early cases of myasthenia gravis, where it has a sensitivity of 90–95%. However, it is a nonspecific measurement and may be abnormal in motor neuron disease, neurogenic disorders, and some myopathies.

27. How can the EMG and nerve conduction studies help differentiate a demyelinating peripheral neuropathy from an axonal peripheral neuropathy?
Demyelinating neuropathies show moderate to severe slowing of motor conduction, with temporal dispersion of the muscle action potential, normal distal amplitudes, reduced proximal amplitudes, and delayed distal latencies. Axonal neuropathies show a milder slowing in conduction velocity, with generally low muscle action potential amplitudes at all sites of stimulation. The EMG shows denervation abnormalities early in axonal neuropathies and only later in demyelinating neuropathies, when axons begin to degenerate.

28. What does the EMG show in polymyositis?
The typical triad of myopathic motor units, fibrillations, and pseudo-myotonia are the classic EMG findings in polymyositis.

29. What does the EMG show in amyotrophic lateral sclerosis?
The EMG shows widespread proximal and distal denervation with fasciculations and giant units in at least two extremities, plus either denervation in the tongue or in thoracic paraspinous muscles.

30. What does the EMG show in the Guillain-Barré syndrome? How can this be useful prognostically?
In early Guillain-Barré syndrome, the EMG simply shows reduction in motor unit firing patterns, depending upon the degree of paralysis. After 14–21 days, spontaneous denervation activity (fibrillations and positive sharp waves) indicate wallerian degeneration (axonal loss). The EMG is useful prognostically because greater axonal loss generally implies longer recovery time. Conduction velocities show marked slowing in motor conduction, compatible with demyelination, beginning 3–5 days after onset.

31. How can the EMG be useful in brachial plexus lesions?
The main value of the EMG is in delineating the presence and degree of denervation in the appropriate arm muscles, and thus localizing damage in the roots, trunks, cords, or distal branches of the brachial plexus. When the plexopathy is diffuse, motor and sensory conduction studies in the arm will be severely abnormal.

32. What is the role of EMG and nerve conduction studies in evaluating a patient with a suspected radiculopathy from cervical or lumbar disc disease?
EMG can confirm the root distribution of muscle weakness noted on clinical examination and also give information about muscles that were not well examined because of pain or lack of full cooperation.

33. What is the carpal tunnel syndrome (CTS)?
CTS consists of nocturnal hand paresthesias caused by compression of the median nerve at the wrist from thickening of the flexor retinaculum, possibly in conjunction with congenital narrowing of the carpal tunnel, or, rarely, in association with other conditions that cause thickening of the median nerve.

34. What is the best test for an electrical diagnosis of CTS?
Sensory nerve action potential latencies of the median nerve will be delayed twice as often as motor latencies. The most sensitive of the sensory latencies is the palmar latency. CTS is diagnosed electrically by a delay in sensory conduction latencies from the index finger or mid-palmar area to the wrist. Needle EMG is of limited value, indicating denervation in the thenar muscles in more advanced cases.

35. What are other conditions associated with median nerve entrapment at the wrist?
The differential diagnosis of CTS includes (1) pregnancy, secondary to fluid retention, (2) hypothyroidism, (3) diabetes, (4) amyloid, and (5) Charcot-Marie-Tooth type I.

36. What is the therapy for CTS?
Wrist splints at night can be helpful for mild to moderate cases that show mainly sensory abnormalities on nerve conduction studies. More severe or persistent cases require surgical sectioning of the transverse carpal ligament (flexor retinaculum), which should be decompressed to the distal margin of the ligament in the upper palmar region.

37. What are the commonest causes of ulnar nerve entrapment at the elbow?
External pressure over the nerve in its shallow groove, flexion dislocation of the nerve over the medial epicondyle, and compression of the nerve as it enters the aponeurosis of the flexor carpi ulnaris (cubital tunnel syndrome) all can cause ulnar nerve lesions at the elbow. Arthritis from an old fracture (tardy ulnar palsy) and rheumatoid arthritis are less common causes.

38. What is the role of EMG and nerve conduction studies in diagnosing ulnar nerve entrapment at the elbow?
Motor and sensory conduction studies can confirm ulnar nerve entrapment at the elbow in 60–80% of cases, with the EMG indicating the distribution and degree of denervation in the ulnar-innervated hand and forearm muscles.

39. What is the best conduction test for diagnosis of ulnar nerve entrapment at the elbow?
Both motor and sensory conduction are helpful in this diagnosis. The motor conduction across the elbow segment may show the earliest motor delay. The amplitude and velocity of ulnar sensory conduction may be affected more than motor slowing. In early cases, studies may be normal.

40. What is the best therapy for ulnar nerve entrapment at the elbow?
Therapy varies according to the underlying mechanism of entrapment. Elbow protectors are helpful in mild to moderate pressure lesions, but surgery is indicated for more persistent or severe entrapments. Surgery may involve sectioning of the flexor digitorum aponeurosis in cubital tunnel syndromes, or medial epicondylectomy in flexion nerve dislocations and tardy ulnar palsies. Rarely, translocation of the nerve to the forearm may be necessary.

41. How can you differentiate a lesion in the C8 root from a plexus or ulnar nerve lesion?
  1. With a lesion in the C8 root, the EMG shows denervation in the following muscles: (a) extensor carpi ulnaris (radial), (b) abductor pollicis brevis (median), (c) first dorsal interosseous, abductor digiti quinti, flexor carpi ulnaris (ulnar), and (d) C8 paraspinous muscles. Motor and sensory conductions are normal in the ulnar and median nerves.
  2. With a lesion in the plexus (lower trunk or medial cord), there will be denervation in all of the above muscles with the exception of normal C8 paraspinous muscles. Conduction studies will be abnormal in the sensory ulnar and medial antebrachial cutaneous forearm nerves. Motor conduction is normal or minimally slow.
  3. Ulnar nerve lesions will have a normal EMG in the radial and median-innervated C8 muscles, but denervation in the ulnar-innervated muscles of the forearm and hand. There will also be abnormal motor and sensory ulnar conduction studies, with normal medial antebrachial cutaneous forearm nerve action potential.

42. What is the key muscle in differentiating a radial nerve palsy from a C7 radiculopathy?
Flexor carpi radialis, which is a C7–8 muscle innervated by the median nerve.

43. How can you differentiate a radial nerve palsy from a brachial plexus posterior cord lesion?
Abnormalities in the deltoid muscle indicate a lesion in the posterior cord of the brachial plexus.

44. How can you differentiate a suprascapular nerve lesion from a C5–6 radiculopathy?
Preservation of the deltoid, biceps, and rhomboid muscles, with abnormalities in the supraspinatus and infraspinatus muscles, indicate a suprascapular nerve lesion.

45. How can you differentiate a long thoracic nerve palsy from a C5-6 radiculopathy?
A long thoracic nerve palsy will cause winging of the scapula from weakness of the serratus anterior muscle, with normal C5-6 shoulder and arm muscles (deltoid, biceps, etc.). The serratus anterior muscle is not routinely studied by EMG.

46. How can you differentiate a peroneal nerve palsy from an L4-5 radiculopathy?
The invertors of the foot (posterior tibial muscle) are abnormal in L4-5 radiculopathies.

47. How can you differentiate a femoral nerve lesion from an L3 radiculopathy?
Abnormalities in the hip adductors and the quadriceps muscles are present in L3 radiculopathies.

48. What is the value of motor conduction velocities in Bell's palsy?
Facial nerve conduction studies 3-5 days after the onset of Bell's palsy can indicate prognosis: for example, complete loss of conductibility indicates wallerian degeneration, whereas normal latencies and amplitudes at 5 days indicate an excellent prognosis for recovery.

ADDITIONAL READING

1. Hammer K: Nerve Conduction Studies. Springfield, IL, Charles C Thomas, 1982.
2. Kimura J: Electrodiagnosis in Diseases of Nerve and Muscle: Principles and Practice. Philadelphia, F.A. Davis, 1989.
3. Sethi R, Thompson L: The Electromyographer's Handbook. Boston, Little, Brown & Co., 1989.

27. NEURORADIOLOGY

Loren A. Rolak, M.D.

Care has been taken to include in this book representative examples of the most common radiographs and images that appear on examinations and boards. These have been located in their appropriate place in the text, but they are specially indexed here to facilitate a neuroradiology review. The radiographs in this book, representing the major areas of neuroradiology, are cross-referenced below by chapter and page number.

28. NEUROLOGY TRIVIA

Questions You Will Often Be Asked By Attendings, But Which Are
Not Important For Understanding Science Or Taking Care Of
Patients, And You Should Not Have To Answer Them

Loren A. Rolak, M.D.

1. Who performed the first spinal tap?

Probably Dr. E. Wynter, in 1891, to drain cerebrospinal fluid from children with
tuberculous meningitis. Dr. H. Quinke that same year developed the instruments and
technique still used today.

Gorelick PB, Zych D: James Leonard Corning and the early history of spinal puncture.
Neurology 37:672–674, 1987.

2. Who suffered the first spinal tap headache?

The first post spinal tap headache was reported by Dr. August Bier in 1899, who described
it as a consequence of a spinal tap performed on himself by his laboratory assistant in the
course of studies on spinal anesthesia. The fate of the assistant is unknown.

3. How do you pronounce the last name of Dr. Georges Guillain, the French neurologist who helped describe the Guillain-Barré syndrome?

According to Dr. Joseph Rogoff, writing in the *Journal of the American Medical
Association*, "The mispronunciation of Dr. George Guillain's name by English-speaking
physicians has bothered me for many years. Even the medical dictionaries (e.g.,
Dorland's) give the pronunciation as "ge-yan," which is incorrect. I was Dr. Guillain's
extern in 1939, and I never heard him called anything but "ghee-lain " (with the final 'ain'
nasalized). If Guillain wanted his name pronounced thus, why should we insist on
changing it?"

4. What is the smallest amount of light the human eye can detect?

The human eye has 125 million rods, each one containing 1000 folds in its photoreceptor
membrane, with each fold containing 1 million molecules of photoceptor. This extraordinary
light-sensing array can detect one single photon, which is 10^{-11} watts. (Wow!)

5. What does the word "myelin" mean?

Myelin is the Greek word for "marrow" and comes from the belief that the white matter was
the marrow of the brain, much like the central portion of the bone is the marrow of the
bone.

6. What is Baltic myoclonus?

It is another name for Unverricht-Lundborg disease. Does that help? (It is a type of progressive myoclonic epilepsy.)

7. Why are the zigzag, scintillating, shimmering lights that often precede classic migraine headaches referred to as fortification spectra?

They are called fortification spectra because of their resemblance to the star-shaped, zigzag
fortifications constructed in Europe during the Renaissance to protect cities and military
compounds.

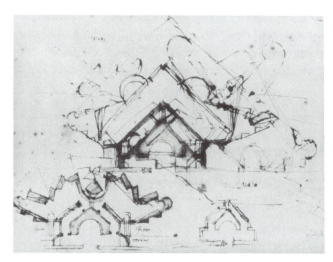

A drawing by Michelangelo for a proposed fortification, showing the triangular, zigzag defensive plan.

8. A lesion that transects the lateral half of the spinal cord will produce a Brown-Sequard syndrome of weakness and loss of proprioception ipsilaterally, with contralateral numbness. Who was Brown, and who was Sequard?
This is a trick question. Brown-Sequard was only one person, Charles Edward Brown-Sequard. His father was an American sailor, and his mother was of French descent, from the island of Mauritius. He took the unusual course of combining his mother's and his father's last names. He became one of the preeminent neurologists of the 19th century, holding professorships, at various times, in America, England, and France.

9. What happened to Charles Edward Brown-Sequard when he ate chocolate?
He developed gustatory perspiration and broke out in a sweat.
    Gooddy W: Charles Edward Brown-Sequard. In Rose FC, Bynum WF (eds): Historical Aspects of the Neurosciences. New York, Raven Press, 1985, pp 371–378.

10. Jules Dejerine was a brilliant pupil of the great French neurologist Charcot, and ultimately succeeded him at the Salpetriere. He described Dejerine's syndrome (medial medullary infarction) and collaborated with other colleagues of Charcot's to describe the syndromes of Dejerine-Landouzy (muscular atrophy), Dejerine-Roussy (thalamic pain), Dejerine-Thomas (cerebellar-brainstem atrophy), and Dejerine-Sottas (neuropathy and tremor). But who was the Klumpke of Dejerine-Klumpke (lower brachial plexopathy)?
Sorry, wrong Dejerine. When Augusta Klumpke married Jules Dejerine, she hyphenated her last name, in a fashion now popular with modern women. An accomplished physician herself, the syndrome of brachial plexus injury is named after her, not her husband. Like Brown-Sequard (sort of), Dejerine-Klumpke is one person.

11. A meningioma arising from the olfactory groove can extend to compress the optic nerve, producing anosmia, optic atrophy, and unilateral papilledema, a constellation of findings known as the Foster Kennedy syndrome. Who was Foster, and who was Kennedy?
This is another trick question. Dr. Foster (first name) Kennedy (last name) was a prominent American neurologist in the first part of this century, at one time president of the American Neurological Association. This use of first names is rare, but it gets even more confusing—the famous eponymic Marcus Gunn pupil comes from the *middle* name of the Scottish

physician Robert Marcus Gunn. Exactly how names are applied to diseases is one of medicine's great unsolved mysteries.

12. Who first used the word "neurology"?
The word first appears in Pordage's English translation of Thomas Willis's book *Cerebri Anatome* in 1664. Incidentally, Willis assembled a collaborative research team composed of the greatest minds of his time: Christopher Wren, Robert Hooke, Robert Boyle, Isaac Newton, and William Harvey. In a sense, these men formed the first "Circle of Willis."

13. What was the first description of a neurologic disease?
The first description of a neurologic disease appears in the Smith papyrus, which is the oldest known medical text. This ancient papyrus, translated by Edward Smith, consists of a number of "case reports" of different diseases, presented and discussed by an unknown Egyptian author, written about 3300 B.C. One of the cases is a person with a traumatic head injury, which is the earliest known description of a neurologic problem.

14. Neurology, more than most other specialties, abounds with eponyms and mellifluous phrases that roll off the tongue. For example, what is the torcular herophili?
It is the confluence of the straight, lateral, and sagittal sinuses, where much of the venous drainage occurs in the brain. A torcula is a cistern or well, sometimes used to collect the liquor from a wine press, and Herophilus (335–280 B.C.) was the ancient Greek anatomist who described this region of the brain.

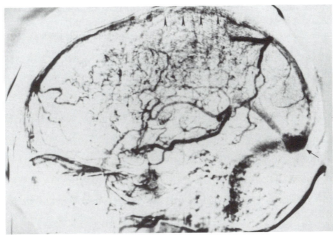

Venous phase of a cerebral angiogram, showing the venous drainage into the torcular herophili (arrow at the right of photo). This patient also has a thrombosis of his superior sagittal sinus (small arrowheads).

15. Refsum's disease is an inherited peripheral neuropathy with ataxia and accompanying retinitis pigmentosa, characterized by accumulation of phytanic acid. What is phytanic acid?
Phytanic acid is 3,7,11,15-tetramethyl-hexadecanoic acid.

16. If you place a human skull on the ground and begin piling weight on top of it, how much weight can you add before it cracks?
If the weight is applied slowly, the human skull can support 3 tons. (Wow!)

17. What does the word "carotid" mean?
It is derived from a Greek word meaning "to put to sleep," because pressure on the carotid arteries can cause loss of consciousness (as any fan of the World Wrestling Federation is aware).

18. What did Aristotle say was the function of the brain?
To cool the heart.

19. In 1909, Korbinian Brodmann divided the human cerebral cortex into 47 cytoarchitecturally distinct regions and gave each one a "Brodmann's number." What is found in Brodmann's areas 13-16?
Nothing. For some reason, Brodmann left out numbers 13-16, which do not appear anywhere on his cortical maps. The reason for the omission has never been discovered (see figures on facing page).

20. Who first described transient ischemic attacks (TIAs) and noted that they were warning signs of a future stroke?
Hippocrates first described TIAs, noting "unaccustomed attacks of numbness and anesthesia are signs of impending apoplexy."

21. What are the five diagnoses neurologists most dread telling a patient (according to a recent survey of practicing clinical neurologists)?
The most distressing diagnoses to tell a patient, in order, are:
1. Amyotrophic lateral sclerosis   4. Multiple sclerosis
2. Malignant brain tumor   5. Epilepsy
3. Traumatic paraplegia

22. What are the four drugs most commonly prescribed by neurologists in America?
1. Acetaminophen   3. Phenytoin (Dilantin)
2. Aspirin   4. Amitriptyline (Elavil, Endep)

23. How many pounds of aspirin are consumed each year in the United States?
Americans ingest 30 million pounds of aspirin per year.

24. Why did Rene Descartes choose the pineal gland as the seat of the soul?
He believed it was the only unpaired structure in the brain and occupied the brain's exact center.

25. What was Gilles de la Tourette's first name?
George.

26. Who did Gilles de la Tourette believe was the greatest neurologist of the century?
Himself. He died of general paresis, at age 47, in a state of grandiose megalomania.

Guilly P: Gilles de la Tourette. In Rose FC, Bynum WF (eds): Historical Aspects of the Neurosciences. New York, Raven Press, 1985, pp 397-413.

27. What percentage of all visits to a doctor are visits to a neurologist?
One percent of all doctor visits are to a neurologist, which is reasonable because 1% of all doctors in America are neurologists.

28. Who described the first reflex, and what was it?
In 1662, Rene Descartes described the blink reflex, where a blow aimed at the eyes causes a person to blink. The word "reflex" derives from the sight of an approaching object causing a "reflection" in the brain.

29. Why are cerebral infarctions called strokes?
According to the Oxford English Dictionary, a sudden, inexplicable cerebrovascular accident was first likened to a "stroke of God's hand" in 1599. The relationship of a cerebral

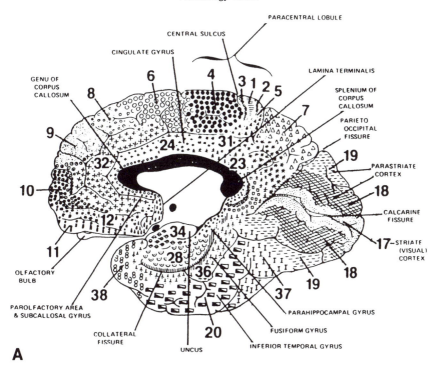

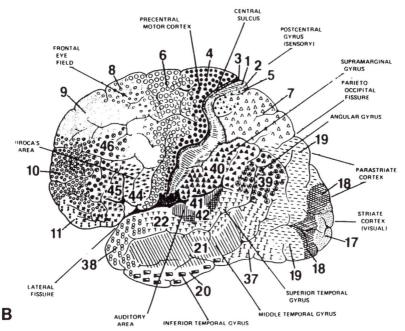

Diagram of Brodmann's areas of the brain—note the absence of numbers 13–16. (Reprinted with permission from Garoutte B: Functional Neuroanatomy, 2nd ed. Greenshore, CA, Life Press, 1990.)

infarction to an act of God exists in other cultures as well: the Greek verb "plesso" means to "stroke, hit, or beat," and the derivative "plegia" gives us our term hemiplegia.

Dirckx JH: Stroke. Stroke 17:559, 1986.

30. The Babinski sign is produced by stroking the lateral aspect of the foot with a noxious stimulus and observing whether the great toe dorsiflexes. What did Babinski call the Babinski sign?

There is no more pompous figure in medicine than the posturing attending physician on rounds expounding pedantically on the supposed oxymoron of a "negative Babinski sign" and extolling the "extensor plantar reflex." In fact, in his original papers, Babinski referred to his sign as "the phenomenon of the toes," but on rounds with his pupils he always insisted it be called "the great toe sign."

By the way, Babinski referred to the failure of the platysma to contract on the side of a hemiparesis as the "Babinski sign."

Babinski J: Sur le reflexe cutane plantaire dans certaines affections organiques du system nerveux central. C R Soc Biol (Paris) 48:207–208, 1896.

Babinski J: Du phenomene des orteils et de sa valeur semiologique. La Semaine Medicale 18:321–322, 1898.

31. There are many, minor, generally useless variations of the Babinski sign, most of them with eponymic names bestowed by egotistical neurologists (Chaddock, Oppenheim, etc.). But sometimes pyramidal tract lesions cause hyperactive plantar flexion of the toes, a movement opposite to the Babinski sign. How many variations of this reflex can you name?

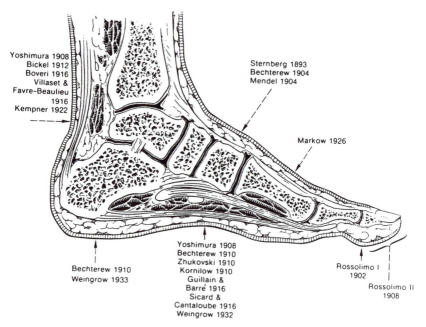

Yoshimura 1908
Bickel 1912
Boveri 1916
Villaset &
Favre-Beaulieu
1916
Kempner 1922

Sternberg 1893
Bechterew 1904
Mendel 1904

Markow 1926

Bechterew 1910
Weingrow 1933

Yoshimura 1908
Bechterew 1910
Zhukovski 1910
Kornilow 1910
Guillain &
Barré 1916
Sicard &
Cantaloube 1916
Weingrow 1932

Rossolimo I
1902

Rossolimo II
1908

Some of the variations of the Rossolimo sign of toe flexion ("grasp reflex of the foot") with pyramidal tract disease. (Reprinted with permission from DeJong RN: The Neurologic Examination, 4th ed. Hagerstown, MD, Harper & Row, 1979, p 462.)

32. What are crocodile tears?

After damage to the facial nerve, such as from Bell's palsy, regenerating fibers may become misdirected such that impulses to mouth and lip muscles instead stimulate the lacrimal gland. As a result, chewing food will cause the patient to weep. The expression comes from old African folklore that crocodiles felt compassion and remorse for their prey, and wept with sorrow whenever they ate.

33. The first successful treatment for epilepsy was bromides. Why was an obstetrician the first person to recommend their use?
It was believed in the mid-19th century that excessive sexual activity, especially masturbation, contributed greatly to epilepsy. Because bromides were known to cause impotence, Sir Charles Locock, personal obstetrician to Queen Victoria, proposed in 1857 that their suppression of sexual function (and menstruation) would result in suppression of seizure activity. He was right, for the wrong reason.
     Scott DR: The discovery of anti-epileptic drugs. J Hist Neurosci 1:111–118, 1992.

34. Ondine's curse refers to a neurologic lesion, usually in the medulla or high cervical cord, that destroys the pathways for automatic, rhythmic breathing, thus forcing the patient to breath voluntarily. Who was Ondine, and what was his curse?
Nobody, and nothing. Ondine is simply the French word for mermaid, and refers to the (unnamed) mermaid in the French version of Hans Christian Andersen's fairy tale, "The Little Mermaid." In this story, based on old Germanic legends, mermaids can assume human form, but only as part of a pact or bargain (not a curse) that requires them to return to the ocean if their human lover is unfaithful to them. The mangled approbation of Ondine's curse, referring to a neurologic deficit that interrupts automatic breathing, is derived from the 1939 play "Ondine" by the French author Jean Giraudeux, in which he embellished the story by having the mermaid's hapless knight punished for his infidelity by the cessation of all his automatic functions (not just breathing). The Ondine (mermaid) loved (not cursed) her human prince, and was always faithful. No Ondine, no curse, no one stops breathing.
     Giraudeux J: Ondine. New York, Random House, 1954.

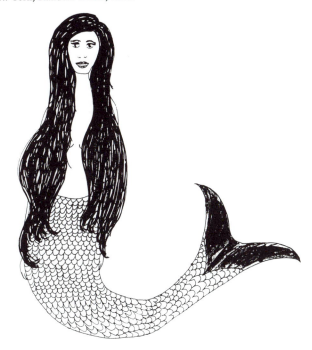

35. What are Finnish snowballs?
These are osmophilic, globular, intracellular inclusions seen with electron microscopy in patients with neuronal ceroid lipofuscinosis. They really don't look anything like Finnish snowballs.

36. What is the softest sound that can be detected by the human ear?
The decibel scale is set at 0 for the softest audible sound, which represents vibratory energy striking the eardrum at an intensity of 0.0002 dynes per square centimeter, which is a range of vibration scarcely larger than the width of several atoms.

37. What is the lowest form of life that sleeps?
Some insects sleep. The reason why animals sleep—its evolutionary or survival advantage—is unknown. There are many theories to account for the existence of sleep, but none of them really makes much sense.

38. Most humans have a clearly dominant hand (usually the right one). What is the lowest form of life that shows such a preference or dominance? Why are most people right-handed?
Birds, which have neuronal populations in the left hemisphere that regulate their song production, are the lowest phylum with a convincing laterality or dominance. The reason for dominance—its evolutionary or survival advantage—is unknown. There are many theories to account for the existence of dominance, but none of them really makes much sense.

39. What is the smallest concentration of a substance that can be smelled by the human nose?
The more than 10 million specialized neuroepithelial cells that make up the olfactory sensory receptors can detect some substances, such as musks, in concentrations of 10^{-12} moles, which is scarcely more than a few molecules.

40. What are the most common movements seen in dead people?
The Lazarus sign is a quick flexion of both arms up over the chest, beneath the chin, observed in brain-dead patients. It may represent spontaneous firing of hypoxic cervical spinal cord neurons.

Ropper AH: Unusual spontaneous movements in brain-dead patients. Neurology 34:1089–1092, 1984.

NEUROLOGIC BIOGRAPHIES

41. This shy, serious university mathematics professor had an alter ego. Using a pseudonym derived from a latinization of his own name, he wrote a series of playful "nonsense" books and poems, which, although ostensibly for children, were derived from chess games, mathematical logic, probability theory, and political satire. A neurologic syndrome of altered body image and time perception has been named after one of the characters in his books who suffered from similar bizarre distortions. **Who was this author, and what was his neurologic disease?**

Charles Lutwidge Dodgson, under the pseudonym of Lewis Carroll, achieved immortality with works such as *Alice's Adventures in Wonderland* and *Through the Looking Glass*. In the first book, Alice, trying to follow a white rabbit through an underground hallway and into an enchanted garden, must change sizes to accommodate various obstacles. She does this by drinking bottles marked "Drink Me," eating cakes marked "Eat Me," and swallowing magic mushrooms. Distortions of body size, which can be produced by lesions affecting the nondominant posterior parietal lobe, have been termed the Alice in Wonderland syndrome, and are virtually pathognomonic for migraine headaches. Like many Victorians, Lewis Carroll kept a diary, and from this we know he suffered from classic migraine headaches, which he described as "bilious headaches," preceded by visual disturbances and fortification spectra. Although he never described body distortions accompanying his migraines, some experts speculate that he drew upon personal experiences for these scenes in his book, and that "Alice trod the paths of a wonderland well known to her creator."

Rolak LA: Literary neurologic syndromes: The Alice in Wonderland syndrome. Arch Neurol 46:353, 1992.

42. The Tony-award-winning Broadway musical "The Mystery of Edwin Drood" (later shortened to just "Drood") tells of a love triangle and a mysterious murder. The play uses a gimmick of asking the audience to choose who they believe the murderer is, and then substituting the appropriate ending based upon the vote. **What is the neurologic reason why the playwrights had to use this trick?**

Charles Dickens, arguably the greatest novelist of all time, was writing his book, *The Mystery of Edwin Drood*, when he suffered a massive left hemisphere stroke and slumped forward on his desk, the pen sliding across the paper as he collapsed unconscious. He died shortly afterwards, only 58 years old. Because he had never revealed his intended solution to the murder, audiences must now guess the identity of the villain.

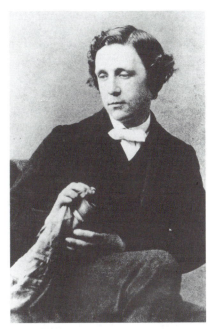

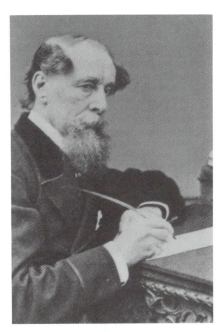

Lewis Carroll, a pioneer in early photography, took this photograph of himself polishing a camera lens.

Charles Dickens

43. This author, a minor French nobleman, was a brilliant observer of human foibles, and was gifted with a phenomenal memory. He made his reputation almost entirely through his short stories, which tell isolated, small, but revealing anecdotes about human behavior. Many of his stories have an ironic twist, and the overall tone is often sardonic and misanthropic. One of his stories, "The Horla," is believed by many critics to be an autobiographical description of his own neurologic sufferings. **Who was this writer, and what was his neurologic disease?**

Guy de Maupassant is considered one of the greatest short story writers of all time. Some of his stories, such as "The Queen's Necklace," are among the most famous ever written. Unfortunately, he contracted syphilis at an early age and subsequently developed neurosyphilis and general paresis. Demented and delusional, he had to be instutionalized. "The Horla," an intense psychological thriller, tells of a man's mounting terror as he becomes increasingly obsessed with the conviction that his mind has been invaded by an evil demon. It is a gifted writer's description of his own paranoid delusions and progressing insanity. Guy de Maupassant finally died, in status epilepticus, at age 45.

44. This Russian writer, the son of a minor land owner, saw his father killed in a peasant uprising and was himself later arrested and threatened with execution. His harsh life left him a friendless, embittered man through most of his adult years. His bleak books, considered among the first great Russian novels, frequently included characters with the same neurologic problem from which he himself suffered. **Who was this writer and what was his neurologic problem?**

Fyodor Dostoyevksy established his talent with such works as *The Brothers Karamazov, The Idiot,* and *Crime and Punishment.* He had his first epileptic seizure at age 7, and suffered from complex partial seizures most of the remainder of his life. Interestingly, his aura was one of ecstasy and extreme joy. He once wrote about his aura, "During a few moments I feel such a happiness that it is impossible to realize at other times, and other people cannot imagine it. I feel a complete harmony within myself and in the world, and this feeling is so strong and so sweet that for a few seconds of this enjoyment one would readily exchange ten years of one's life—perhaps even one's whole life."

Alajouanine T: Dostoiewski's epilepsy. Brain 86:209–218, 1963.

45. This French writer produced a number of notable works, but his reputation rests primarily on one supreme masterpiece, a single book that he spent much of his life writing, revising page by page, and even word by word, counting the number of syllables in each line. He was unpopular with many of his contemporaries, some of whom felt his great acclaim was due to sheer plodding work rather than talent, and some of whom were jealous of his extraordinarily beautiful mistress. His enemies even circulated the rumor that his neurologic problem was hysterical. Nevertheless, he remained generous and good humored, and when his masterpiece was condemned as being immoral and he was placed on trial for indecency, many of the leading artistic figures of his age rallied to his defense. **Who was this writer, and what was his neurologic disease?**

Gustave Flaubert's reputation rests upon his novel *Madame Bovary,* which tells the story of a restless woman unfulfilled by her marriage to a provincial country doctor. The great French writer Emile Zola defended Flaubert and his use of realism during the trial against his book, at which Flaubert was acquitted. Beginning at age 22, Flaubert suffered from seizures, which had the unusual manifestation of visual phenomena. He described "a hundred thousand images jumping up and down together, like illuminated rockets during a firework display." Candles, flames, and Japanese lanterns danced before his eyes during his seizures. Modern authorities speculate that these seizures with visual symptoms arose from occipital lobe damage suffered when Flaubert fell backward off of his horse as a young man. His death was also neurologic—he suffered an intracerebral hemorrhage, reportedly while making love to his young servant.

Gastaut H, Gastaut Y, Broughton R: Gustave Flaubert's illness: A case report in evidence against the erroneous notion of psychogenic epilepsy. Epilepsia 25:622–637, 1984.

46. This musician, a gifted "child prodigy" at the piano, achieved even more success as a composer than as a performer. He was at the height of his fame when he suffered an apparent-ly trivial head injury, but afterward experienced a decline in abilities. He noted speech difficulties, memory loss, and an inability to express any of his musical ideas in writing or performance. Indeed, he wrote essentially no further compositions. A very bitter and public feud arose among the many physicians called in at various times to treat this famous patient, culminating when one of the doctors "kidnapped" the composer when his primary physician was on Christmas vacation. Surreptitious exploratory neurosurgery was performed, which the patient did not survive. **Who was this composer, and what was his neurologic disease?**

Maurice Ravel (1875–1937) was injured in Paris when a taxi cab carrying him from the theater to his hotel collided with another cab on October 10, 1932. He suffered facial injuries and the loss of two teeth, but jokingly dismissed the trauma as minor. It was some months later that he began experiencing his mental decline and frustrating inability to compose. His neurologist, Theophile Alajouanine, believed that Ravel was suffering from a degenerative progressive aphasia, which today we would probably diagnose as Alzheimer's disease. Many of Ravel's friends were convinced that this decline was caused by the automobile accident, possibly by enlarging subdural hematomas or hydrocephalus. They persuaded the famous neurosurgeon, Clovis Vincent, to operate on him; the surgery revealed only a shrunken, atrophic brain. Ravel did not survive the operation.

47. This American composer began playing the piano and performing at age 12, and, using the media of American popular culture—Broadway musicals and Hollywood motion pictures—became one of the wealthiest and best-loved American musicians. He was a critical success as well, winning a Pulitzer Prize for his music, and later composing America's first true opera. Wealthy and respected, with a huge Hollywood estate and a series of beautiful lovers, he nevertheless remarked at one point, "I am 38 years old, wealthy and famous, but I am still deeply unhappy." Indeed, his neurologic problem was long diagnosed as psychiatric in nature, and not recognized as organic until two days before it finally killed him. **Who was this composer, and what was his neurologic disease?**

George Gershwin won a Pulitzer Prize in 1932 for "Of Thee I Sing," and completed his opera "Porgy and Bess" in 1935. On February 11, 1937, while conducting his "Piano Concerto In F Major" with the Los Angeles Philharmonic Orchestra, he experienced a repulsive and nauseating smell of burnt rubber, followed by a 10–20-second alteration of consciousness. Although he remained upright, he stopped conducting for several bars while staring into space, a lapse that was quite noticeable to the audience. He had increasing headaches and mental apathy, diagnosed as "hysteria" or "neurosis" until he collapsed on July 9, 1937, and was rushed to the hospital, comatose with a left hemiparesis. He was operated on for removal of a cystic right temporal lobe glioblastoma multiforme, but died without regaining consciousness on July 11, 1937, at age 38.

Ljunggren B: Great Men with Sick Brains. Park Ridge, IL, American Association of Neurological Surgeons, 1990, pp 91–100.

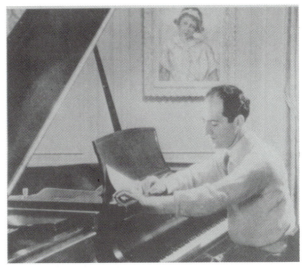

George Gershwin

48. This wealthy, refined, witty, kind, and generous composer was the antithesis of the romantic conception of the impoverished artist suffering in his garret while pouring out his heart into his music. Instead, this privileged musician, whose very name means "happy," came from a respected and talented family, and his own music is generally bright and vivacious. His contributions were unfortunately cut short by his sudden and early death from a neurologic problem—the same one that killed his grandmother, father, and sister (herself a child musical prodigy). **Who was this composer, and what was his neurologic problem?**

Felix Mendelsohn, the grandson of distinguished philosopher Moses Mendelsohn, and the son of wealthy banker Abraham Mendelsohn, demonstrated considerable musical talent as a child, as did his sister, Fanny. On May 14, 1847, Fanny suddenly became pale and nauseated, her upper extremities numbed and paralyzed, and she mumbled incoherently. She slipped quickly into unconsciousness and was pronounced dead of an intracranial hemorrhage, the same condition felt responsible for the deaths of her father and grandmother. On November 1 and 2, 1847, Felix suffered a similar hemorrhage, with severe headaches, a stuttering paralysis, unconsciousness, and death.

O'Shea J: Was Mozart Poisoned? Medical Investigations into the Lives of the Great Composers. New York, St. Martin's Press, 1990, pp 118–123.

49. These brothers, during 14 years of entertaining with the circus, achieved such fame that they literally became a household word. When they retired, they married sisters on adjoining farms and raised large families. Legendary for their closeness, when one of them died of a neurologic disease, the other died just hours later. **Who were these famous brothers, and what was their neurologic problem?**

Chang and Eng, Siamese twins, were joined at the thorax, with a common liver and diaphragm. Early on the morning of January 17, 1874, Chang suffered a fatal stroke (he had had a minor cerebral thrombosis in 1870). Eng, terrified and panic-stricken, was inextricably joined to his now dead brother. A physician was summoned to attempt a separation, but before he could arrive, Eng also died. Both brothers were autopsied, and it was felt Eng had collapsed from massive sympathetic stimulation, with neurogenic pulmonary edema and cardiac arrhythmias—he had literally died of fright.

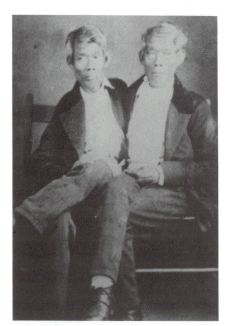

The Siamese twins Chang *(left)* and Eng *(right)*

50. In 1951, Dr. Richard Asher published a paper in the *Lancet* entitled "Munchausen's Syndrome," describing patients who simulate physical illness for the sole purpose of obtaining medical treatment, with no other recognizable motive. Asher chose this name in honor of a famous teller of dramatic and untruthful folklore, Baron von Munchausen. **What was von Munchausen's neurologic problem?**

There was a real Munchausen, namely Hieronymus Karl Friedrich Freiherr von Munchausen (1720–1797). He was a minor nobleman and country gentleman with a large estate near Hannover, Germany, who was locally famous for his hospitality and clever storytelling. Several of his good-natured tales were plagiarized by a notorious rascal, Rudolf Eric Raspe, who published them anonymously in the 1785 monograph *Baron Munchausen's Narrative of His Marvelous Travels and Campaigns in Russia.* Ironically, the real Baron von Munchausen became an embittered and irascible old man as he unsuccessfully pursued a series of lawsuits and other actions to stop the plagiarism and protect his name. Approaching ruination, at age 74, he tried to console himself by marrying an 18-year-old girl, Bernhardine Von Brunn, who, however, was said to have her eye on the remainder of his estate. Three years later, in 1797, he died of a massive left hemisphere stroke.

51. What congenital neurologic problem almost cost James Buchanan the presidency?
James Buchanan, the 15th President of the United States, served just before Lincoln from 1856 to 1860. He had a habitual head tilt forward and to the left, which was probably caused by a congenital right superior oblique palsy (cranial nerve IV). This well-known head tilt was the focus for a rumor circulated by Buchanan's opponents in the presidential election. In 1819, at age 28, Buchanan (who was the only bachelor president America has ever had) was engaged to marry Annie Coleman of New York, when she broke off the wedding at the last minute because of gossip about Buchanan's philandering. Shortly afterward, she committed suicide. Although this unfortunate incident was true, Buchanan's adversaries fabricated a sequel stating that Buchanan's head tilt was the result of his own attempted suicide by hanging in an effort to escape the vengeance of his fiancé's brother. The abortive hanging attempt was supposed to have twisted Buchanan's neck for life. Buchanan overcame this early example of "negative campaigning" to win the election.

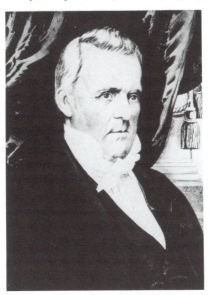

President James Buchanan

52. This 39-year-old, right-handed white male civil servant described his neurologic problems in his own words: "I first had a chill in the evening which lasted practically all night. On the following morning, the muscles of the right knee appeared weak and by afternoon, I was unable to support my weight on my right leg. That evening, the left knee began to weaken also, and by the following morning I was unable to stand up. This was accompanied by a continuing temperature of about 102° and I felt thoroughly achy all over. By the end of the third day, practically all muscles from the chest down were involved. Above the chest, the only symptom was a weakening of the two large thumb muscles, making it impossible to write. There was no special pain along the spine and no rigidity up the neck. For the following two weeks, I had to be catheterized and there was a slight, though not severe, difficulty in controlling the bowels. The fever lasted for only six or seven days, but all the muscles from the hips down were extremely sensitive to the touch and I had to have my knees supported by pillows. This condition of extreme discomfort lasted about three weeks." **What is your diagnosis?**

This is Mr. Franklin Delano Roosevelt's own description of the onset of his polio on August 10, 1921. His physician initially diagnosed, "A clot of blood from a sudden congestion has settled in the lower spinal cord temporarily removing the power to move though not to feel." Only subsequently was the correct diagnosis of polio established. Unfortunately, Roosevelt never regained any use of his lower extremities whatsoever, and remained with complete flaccid paralysis for the rest of his life. Interestingly, his disability was a well-kept secret, guarded by a press that considered it undignified to mention, and a tenor of the times that forbad such personal scrutiny. Photos of Roosevelt were always composed to conceal the disability (though a discerning eye can guess at the weakness and atrophy in the photo below, taken on his yacht in 1933, shortly after his first election to the presidency), and the general public never learned of his paralysis.

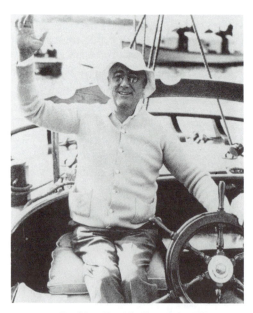

President Franklin Roosevelt, 1933

53. The former president of an Ivy League University, this man was one of America's most intellectual presidents, and also one of the most liberal and socially-minded. He was not any more reliable, however, because he ran for office with the slogan, "He kept us out of war," and then plunged the country into one four months after his inauguration. One of his most visionary and potentially greatest achievements was never realized, however, because he developed a serious neurologic problem while in office. **Who was this president, and what was his neurologic disease?**

Woodrow Wilson, America's 28th President, was a passivist who did not wish to become embroiled in World War I, but felt compelled to do so by April of 1918. He suffered a variety of ailments throughout his life, including probably an intraocular hemorrhage, writer's cramp, viral encephalitis, and, on September 1, 1919, he suffered a right hemisphere stroke with resultant left hemiparesis and considerable mental clouding. His wife sequestered him in the White House, refusing all visitors and access, and the nature of his ailment was never revealed to the public or to most members of the government. Although his mental capacities were obviously impaired, he never relinquished command, and thus the nation was essentially without a president for the final 20 months of his administration. Some historians speculate that he could have persuaded Congress and the public to endorse his proposal for a League of Nations had he not become ill.

A photographer snapped this photograph of a haggard, demented President Wilson in one of the rare moments when he was outside of the White House, propped against the right side of his automobile, with hat and clothing strategically draped to conceal his left hemiparesis.

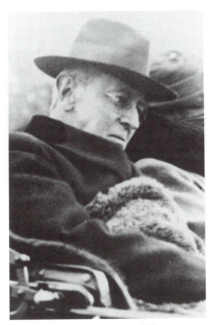

President Woodrow Wilson

54. This man was the smallest U.S. President, standing scarcely over 5 feet tall and weighing little more than 100 pounds, with a "discouraging feebleness of the constitution" much of his life. He was nevertheless a brilliant thinker who reshaped political philosophy and was one of the most intellectual presidents. His wife was renowned for her charm and grace, and became one of the most famous First Ladies. He had to overcome the stigma of a lack of military service, however, which was due to a neurologic condition. **Who was this President, and what was his problem?**

James Madison, the 5th President of the United States, helped Thomas Jefferson write the Declaration of Independence. He had many hypochondriacal and hysterical symptoms as a young man, many of which disappeared as he grew older. However, among the most prominent was "a constitutional liability to sudden attacks of the nature of epilepsy," which were known by his friends to be bizarre spells he suffered in response to stress. When he tried to enlist for military service in the Revolutionary War, he was rejected because of his "epileptoid hysteria" and told to go home, study less, and increase his exercise outdoors. These spells disappeared in his 30's, and indeed he enjoyed good health and vigorous leadership as President.

55. The patient is a 35-year-old female who gradually developed fatigue and dizziness, and began complaining of stiffness and pain in her legs, especially the calves. She developed a fine tremor involving the entire body, but most prominent in the limbs, and more so in the arms than in the legs. The tremor was present at rest and resembled a trembling or shivering movement. These symptoms progressed over a period of a day or two, at which time she complained of a fairly steady epigastric pain with nausea and then persistent vomiting. By the third day, the fatigue had progressed to lethargy, and she became bedridden. It was noted that her pupils were slightly large and sluggish, and she had developed protracted hiccups. Her general physical examination showed her temperature to be slightly subnormal, and her pulse irregular. She had constipation and decreased urine output, and her tongue was large and red. The conjunctivae were also infected. Her gastrointestinal distress continued and she had very diminished bowel sounds. On the fifth day of her illness her lethargy progressed to stupor and she became unarousable. She died on the seventh day. The patient lived on a farm, and the middle-aged man and wife on an adjacent farm had died of identical symptoms one week prior to the onset of the patient's illness. Another neighbor who lived half a mile away died several days later. This patient had directly nursed and cared for both of those families. **Can you identify this patient and her illness?**

The patient is Nancy Hanks Lincoln, the mother of Abraham Lincoln, who died at age 35 on October 15, 1818, when her son was 9 years old. Apart from the fact that she was born out of wedlock, the illegitimate daughter of Lucy Hanks of Elizabethtown, Kentucky, very little is known about Lincoln's mother. There are not even any reliable physical descriptions of what she looked like.

Nancy Lincoln died of a disease known as the "trembles" or "staggers," named for its primary symptom of tremor. The first references to this disease appeared in colonial days, but the cause was unknown and variously attributed to infections, noxious gases, or poisonings. Outbreaks of the illness occurred frequently as settlers migrated westward, causing "an appalling loss of human life." It was not until 1927 that the cause was finally found to be a toxic substance in the leaves of the white snakeroot plant, a flower that grows native in the Midwest, reaching a height of 2 to 3 feet, with sharp-toothed leaves and white or purple bell-shaped flowers. It grew only in dense woods, and so when land was sufficiently cleared for pastures and farming, the plant disappeared. Outbreaks of the disease were caused by settlers moving into an area that had not been cleared sufficiently to provide adequate grazing land for their cattle. The cows would forage in the woods, eat the snakeroot, and the toxin would accumulate and concentrate in their milk. When ingested by humans, this milk would produce the disease. Indeed, the other name for the disease was "milk sickness."

The toxin was named "trematol" because of the tremors which were the primary symptom of the disease. Trematol is an aromatic alcohol, with a pleasant odor, and a chemical structure of $C_{16}H_{22}O_3$. Ingestion of this compound causes ketosis and elevated acetone levels, but the exact nature of its action in tissues, especially the nervous system, was never determined. Autopsies performed on patients who had died of milk sickness never showed any gross changes in the brain. With the continued westward migration and clearing of land, the natural habitat of the white snakeroot diminished. Although the plant has not become extinct, the last recorded case of milk sickness was in 1938.

INDEX

Entries in **boldface** type indicate complete chapters.